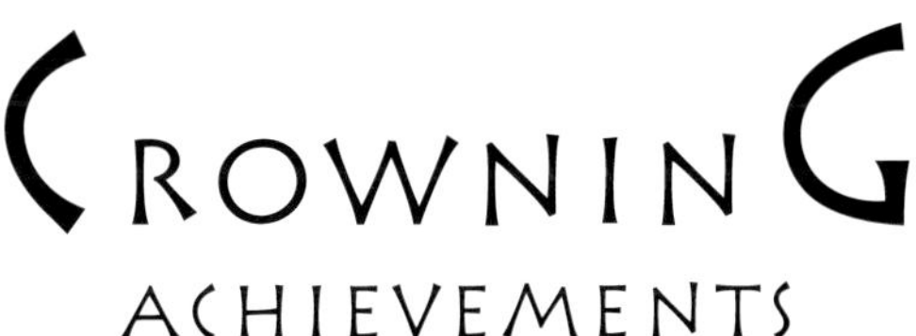
CROWNING
ACHIEVEMENTS

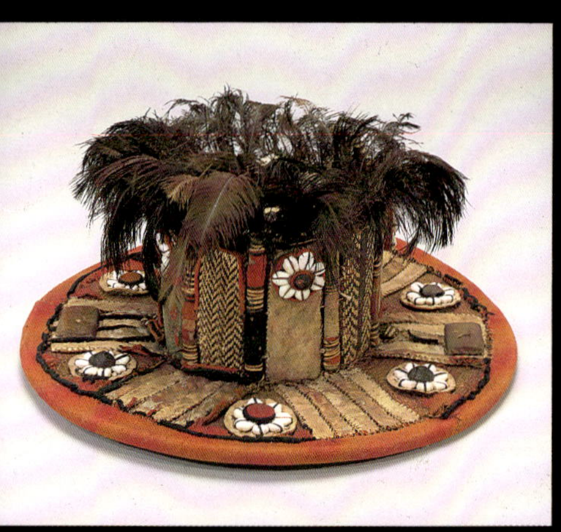

TO ROY SIEBER
TOP HAT

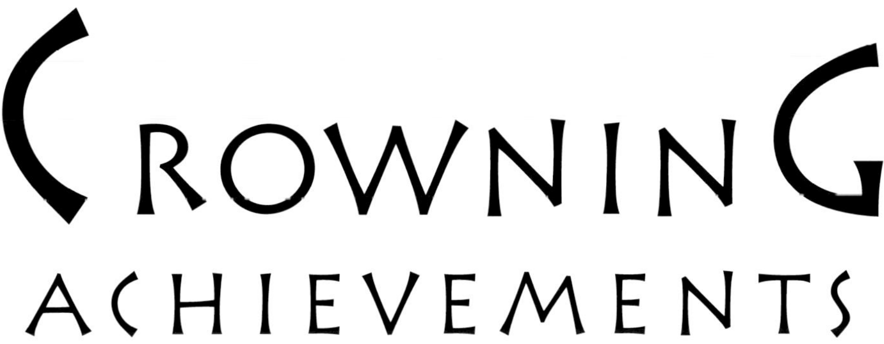


## African Arts of Dressing the Head

Mary Jo Arnoldi and Christine Mullen Kreamer

with contributions by

Michael Oládèjo Afoláyan and Betty Wass
Elisabeth L. Cameron
Patricia Darish and David A. Binkley

Fowler Museum of Cultural History
University of California, Los Angeles

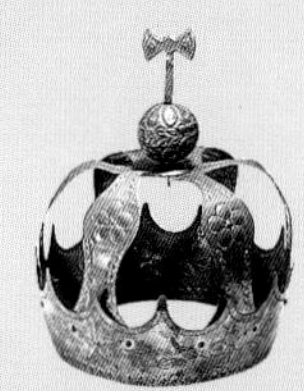

**Front cover:** Hat. Nkutcu, Zaire (see page 85).
Background: Chief's hat *(mpu)*. Kongo, Republic of Congo and Zaire (see page 42).
**Page 2**: Man's hat. Gola, Liberia. Photograph by Diane L. Nordeck (see pg. 30).
**Page 4**: Xangô crown. Salvador da Bahia, Brazil (see pg.178).
**Page 5**: Dancer's hat. Mossi, Burkina Faso (see pg. 22).



Fowler Museum of Cultural History
University of California, Los Angeles
405 Hilgard Avenue
Los Angeles, California, USA 90095-1549

Printed on acid-free paper and bound in Hong Kong by Pearl River Printing Company, Ltd.

Library of Congress CIP Information Data on file.

ISBN 0-930741-42-0 (hard cover)
ISBN 0-930741-43-9 (soft cover)

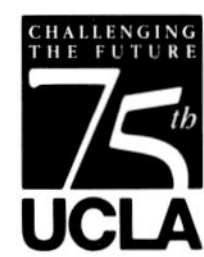


This catalogue and associated exhibition were supported by funding from the following:

THE AHMANSON FOUNDATION

THE NATIONAL ENDOWMENT FOR THE HUMANITIES CHALLENGE GRANT

THE TIMES MIRROR FOUNDATION

MANUS, THE SUPPORT GROUP OF THE UCLA FOWLER MUSEUM OF CULTURAL HISTORY

## LENDERS TO THE EXHIBITION

MARY JO ARNOLDI AND CRAIG A. SUBLER
DAVID A. BINKLEY AND PATRICIA DARISH
MORT DIMONDSTEIN
LITINA EGUNGUN
JOANNE B. EICHER
ROBERT ALAN FRIEDMAN
JEROME L. JOSS
OWEN F. MOORE
NATIONAL MUSEUM OF AFRICAN ART
NATIONAL MUSEUM OF NATURAL HISTORY
NEUTROGENA CORPORATION
TOM PATCHET
FRANCES TABBUSH
THREE ANONYMOUS LENDERS

# CONTENTS

# PREFACE

In 1988 the Fowler Museum of Cultural History had the pleasure of lending eight African hats from its collections to an exhibition curated by Dr. Mary Jo Arnoldi at the University of Missouri, Kansas City. When an opening appeared in our exhibition schedule, Dr. Arnoldi, joined by Dr. Christine Mullen Kreamer, agreed to develop an exhibition around a selection from the Fowler Museum's collections and to organize and write a catalogue. We are extremely grateful to both of them for their extraordinary efforts on behalf of this project. They met unconscionable deadlines with original ideas, careful attention to detail, and considerable good humor. We are also greatly appreciative of the work of our contributors Elisabeth Cameron, Patricia Darish and David Binkley, and Michael Oládèjo Afoláyan and Betty Wass. Emily Meyer and Pravina Shukla provided invaluable research assistance. The energy and conscientiousness of all assured the successful completion of this project.

The staff of the Eliot Elisofon Archives at the National Museum of African Art are true collaborators in this volume. Christraud Geary, Amy Staples, Anita Jenkins, and Audrey Johnson provided an enviable model of collegiality and professionalism in the hunt for elusive photographs.

The substantial collection of African headwear housed in the Fowler Museum was augmented by a number of key loans. We sincerely thank all the lenders listed at the beginning of this volume for sharing their wonderful pieces with the Los Angeles community. The exhibition has benefitted enormously from their participation.

For each of the Fowler Museum's exhibition and publication projects, it is the collective efforts of the Museum's staff (listed at back of this volume) that have ensured success. Still, I would like to single out the work of staff photographer Denis Nervig. Long hours both before and after the birth of his first child clearly merit a dramatic tip of the cap from all involved.

Irina Averkieff wore two different hats on this project: those of editor *and* publication designer. With the combined talents of juggler and magician, she repeatedly exchanged these hats with impressive speed and grace. Her remarkable efforts are greatly appreciated.

Director of Publications Danny Brauer provided project oversight and critical coordination with the printer, Pearl River Printing Company, Ltd., of Hong Kong. I would especially like to thank Alan Scott Jordan, Charles Lee, Paula Gasparello, and Jeanette Leehr of Pearl River for their substantial contributions to ensuring the timely publication of this book.

The exhibition was designed by David Mayo, with considerable imagination and appreciation of the subject matter. Each of his installations since our reopening in 1992 has had a remarkably distinctive look, providing a perfect complement to the materials being displayed.

Both the publication and exhibition were made possible by endowments funded by the National Endowment for the Humanities Challenge Grant, the Ahmanson Foundation, the Times Mirror Foundation, and the Jerome L. Joss Endowment Fund.

*Doran H. Ross*
*Deputy Director*

# ACKNOWLEDGMENTS

This exhibition and catalogue could never have been realized without the extraordinary enthusiasm, encouragement, and goodwill of many people. It has been our great pleasure working with the staff of the UCLA Fowler Museum of Cultural History. We would particularly like to thank Owen Moore, David Mayo, and Denis Nervig, who cheerfully worked with us solving the many thorny problems associated with objects, exhibit design, and object photography. We would also like to thank Elisabeth Cameron, David Binkley and Pat Darish, and Michael Oládèjo Afoláyan and Betty Wass whose essays have greatly enriched the catalogue.

Smithsonian colleagues also gave generously of their time. Susan Crawford and Natalie Firnhaber of the Anthropology Department, National Museum of Natural History, worked on the Smithsonian hats for this exhibition. Valerie Singer, Jeremy Prestoholdt, and Letty Bonnell assisted us with the library and archival research. Doc Dougherty of the Smithsonian Office of Printing and Photographic Services expedited the photography, and Diane L. Nordeck took the photographs of Smithsonian objects.

A very special thanks is due to Christraud Geary, Amy Staples, Anita Jenkins, and Audry Johnson of the Eliot Elisofon Archives at the National Museum of African Art. They cheerfully helped us locate, select, and process a large number of appropriate historical and contemporary context photographs. We would also like to thank Virginia-Lee Webb of the Metropolitan Museum of Art and Martha Labelle of the Photographic Archives, Peabody Museum of Archaeology and Ethnology, Harvard University, for their help finding several key historical photographs. We are grateful to Dr. Christine Siege, the Museum für Volkerkunde, Leipzig, and Dr. Gustaaf Verswijver, Musée Royal de l'Afrique Centrale, Tervuren for granting us permission to publish historical photographs from their collection.

Many colleagues generously shared with us their information and insights about African headwear. A number also provided us with important contemporary context photographs. We would like to thank Marla C. Berns, Kristyne Loughran Bini, David Binkley, Herbert M. Cole, Michael Conner, Christine Conte, Patricia Darish, William Dewey, Henry Drewal and Margaret Thompson Drewal, Joanne Eicher, Christraud Geary, Gordon D. Gibson, Walter Goldschmidt, Carolee Kennedy, James Payne, Philip Ravenhill, Allen Roberts, Doran H. Ross, and Betty Wass. Mark Auslander, Michael Atwood Mason, and Robert Leopold read parts of the manuscript and we appreciate their helpful advice and criticism.

We are greatly indebted to Irina Averkieff, the editor and designer of the catalogue, for her generosity and patience and her unwavering commitment to this project. Finally, this entire project would not have been possible without the tireless efforts of Doran H. Ross, the Deputy Director of the Fowler Museum. His curatorial and editorial expertise and his intellectual involvement were central, and his support of our efforts never faltered, even in the face of seemingly insurmountable deadlines.

*Mary Jo Arnoldi and Christine Mullen Kreamer*

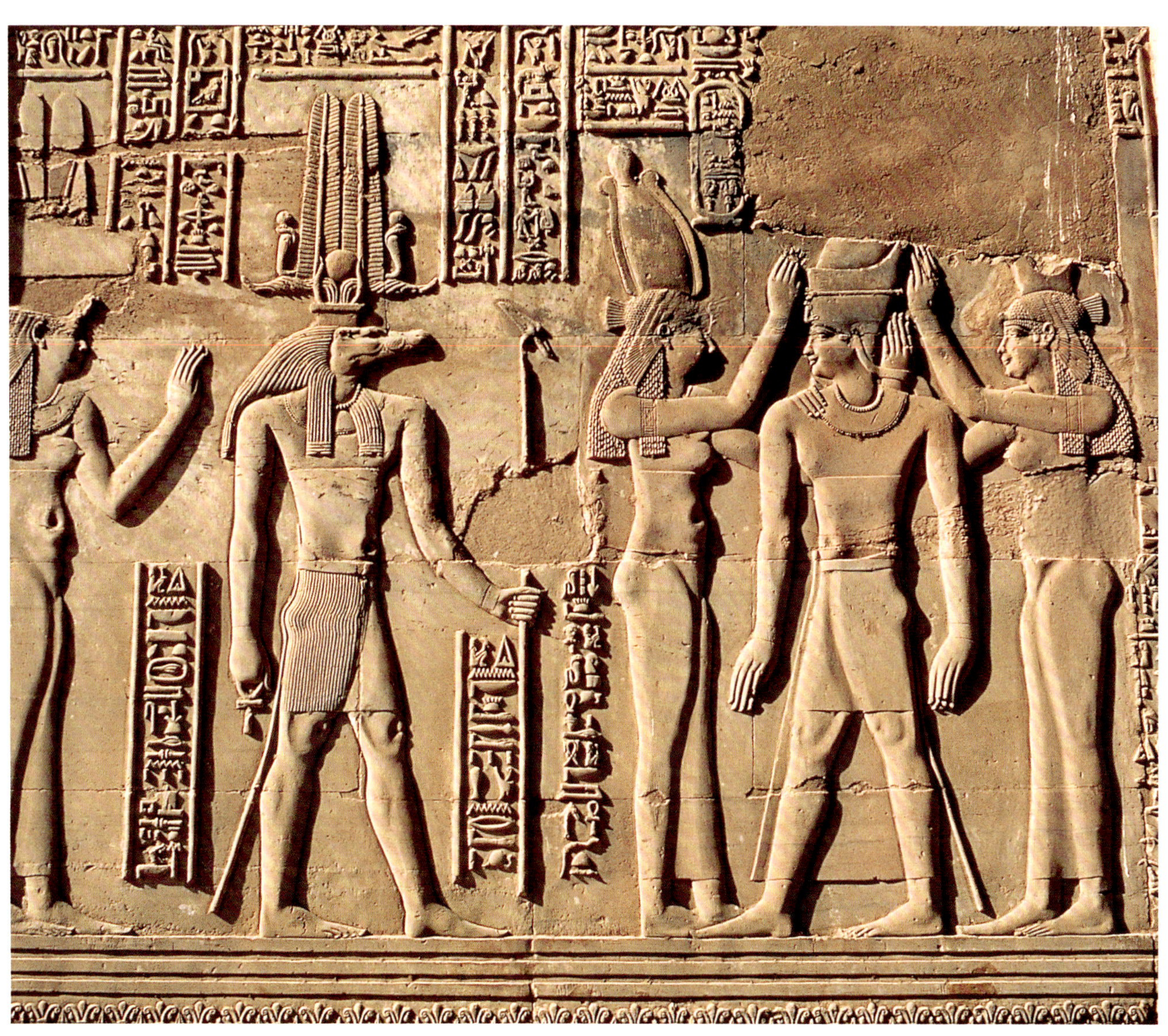

# 1 INTRODUCTION

## MARY JO ARNOLDI

African men and women throughout the continent and in the African diaspora adorn their heads in creative and distinctive ways. The head, high and center, is an ideal site for the aesthetic and symbolic elaboration of the body. In many African languages, as in English, the word "head" is used metaphorically. Some common meanings of *kun*, head, in the Bamana language spoken in Mali include leader, main, premier, highest, superior, chief, and source. Among the Karamojong of Uganda the word head, *ekasikout,* also means elder and signifies a person with great wisdom, experience, and moral influence (Pazzaglia 1982:96). There are similar meanings associated with the word "head" in many other African languages and these associations shape the ways people conceptualize and use headwear.

The many hats, caps, diadems, crowns, and hair styles that African men and women wear throughout the continent and elsewhere are important features of daily and ceremonial display.[1] From ancient Egypt to the present, Africans have regularly invested this "headwork" and its permanent or ephemeral products with heightened value. Certain headdresses can recall founding myths or historical episodes. Hats and hair styles can celebrate the achievements of individuals or glorify an office. Some forms and materials may be important symbolically, others may speak to pragmatic solutions to the problems of physical comfort. When imported forms or materials are incorporated into headwear they provide historical information about important trading networks that have linked African societies to one another and Africa to the Middle East, Asia, and Europe for thousands of years (Fig. 1.1).

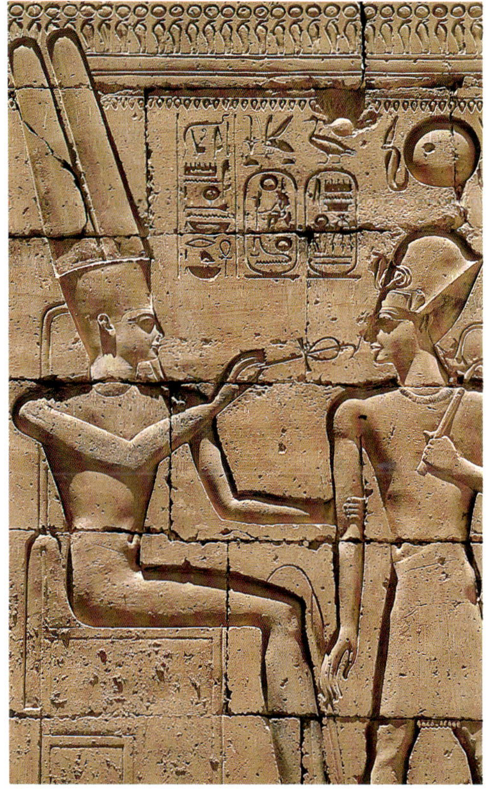

**Figure 1.1**, above. Hieroglyphic detail. Kom Ombo, Egypt. Photograph by Gerard Champlong, 1984.

**Opposite**. Temple of Karnak. Luxor, Egypt. Photograph by Giuliano Colliva, 1991.

Recent attention to social practices and the nature of power have clarified our understanding of how social relationships are produced and reproduced in ritual and in everyday practices (Arens and Karp 1989, Bourdieu 1977, Giddens 1990, Hardin 1993, Jackson and Karp 1990, Ortner 1984). These insights have also affected our understanding of the active role that objects, like hats, can play in people's everyday and ceremonial lives. Headgear and hair styles can no longer be viewed simply as passive reflections of culture. They not only mean something, but through the mediation of human action, they can do something as well. Hats and hair styles, as well as other material objects, need to be understood as one of the technologies that people use to construct social identities and to produce, reproduce, and transform their relationships and situations through time.[2]

Despite the centrality of headgear in the material repertoire of many African societies, there have been, until recently, only sporadic descriptions of headwear and clothing in travelers' accounts and in ethnographies. Daniel Biebuyck noted that most references to African headwear and dress offer only a "piecemeal, casual and superficial treatment" of these important objects (Biebuyck and Van den Abbeele 1984:17). More systematic studies of African headgear and dress as an art form, cultural artifact, material symbol, economic good, and as fashion are being undertaken and the results of this research will make significant contributions to our understanding of the multiple dimensions of African dress, but much work remains to be done.[3]

## THE HEAD AND BODY IN THE AFRICAN IMAGINATION

Throughout Africa, as elsewhere in the world, people devote a great deal of thought and attention to the human body. Our bodies are not only natural, but cultural entities. As Bryan Turner stated so succinctly, "There is an obvious and prominent fact about human beings; they have bodies and they are bodies. More lucidly, human beings are embodied, just as they are enselved" (1984:1). Our bodies mediate all our reflection and action, and it is through both the lived experience of our bodies and our awareness of our culturally objectified body, that we come to know ourselves and to know others. We project ourselves upon and into the world through our bodies. Bodily adornment, attitudes, demeanor, and gestures say precise things about the society in which a person lives, the constraints and expectations a society puts upon its members, and the degree to which individuals are or are not integrated into their society. The presentation of self through the presentation of the body in everyday and ritual contexts can profoundly shape a person's relationships to others.[4] Many of the culturally specific bodily practices we learn that enable us to project ourselves into our environment become habits that we reproduce with little reflection, even though at some somatic level, these practices must still "feel right." Other practices are more often subject to conscious and repeated reflection and modification. Headgear and hair styles seem to fall more often within this latter category of practices.

While there is a universal concern in human society with elaborating the body, this elaboration is achieved differently throughout the world. Terence Turner notes that

> The surface of the body, as the common frontier of society, the social self, and the psycho-biological individual, becomes the symbolic stage upon which the drama of socialization is enacted and bodily adornment . . . becomes the language through which it is expressed (1980:112).

Processes of socialization are not natural, but cultural, and replete with expectations and contradictions. Every society must deal with the basic tension between the individual and the collective, and much of the philosophy, and ceremonial and ritual life of any society is directed towards defining personhood throughout the life course and coming to terms with the competition between individual and collective interests and actions.

Most cultures use the physical body as a metaphor for the social body, the larger community. Illness, whether physical or mental, is often interpreted as a powerful metaphor for conflict within the community. In Jean Comaroff's study of Zionism as a form of Tshidi resistance to the hegemony of the South African state she notes that:

> Not surprisingly, the metaphors of social contradiction deployed by these cults are often rooted in the notion of the body at war with itself, or with its immediate social and material context and desired transformations focus upon "healing" as a mode of repairing the tormented body, and through it, the oppressive social order, itself (1985:9).

Among the Ndembu of Zaire, as in many societies, an individual's illness is often interpreted as a sign of sickness in the social body (V. Turner 1967:359–360). In twentieth century America, cancer persists as a pervasive and powerful metaphor for individual and societal vulnerability and decay (Sontag 1977).

Bodily metaphors are as widespread in Africa as elsewhere, and these metaphors extend and shape people's understanding of their environment and their material experience. For example, images of the body and bodily processes are central metaphors for the house and the built environment among the Tamberma in the Republic of Benin and the Kaguru in Tanzania (Blier 1987:118–139; Beidelman 1972, 1993). Among certain Igbo groups in Nigeria the entrance of a titled man's house was formerly distinguished by a carved door flanked by several carved wooden panels. The doorway was called the "mouth" and the central motifs on the carved panels were described as the "eyes" (Cole and Aniakor 1984:65). In those African societies that practice smelting and ironworking, the body, and more specifically the female body, operates as the central metaphor for the smelting furnace. Bodily processes, specifically gestation and birth, are principle metaphors for the smelting process and are associated with pottery technology in Africa (Herbert 1993). Anthropomorphic ceramic vessels, most reserved for ritual contexts, have been widely documented across the continent. Among various ethnic groups living in the Upper Benue valley in Nigeria, anthropomorphic vessels are used to localize ancestral and other spirits in order to mediate the relationships of these forces with the living (Berns 1986; Fig. 1.2).

In the thought and moral imagination of many African and African diaspora societies, the head, itself, is a potent image that plays a central role in how the person is conceptualized. Among the Yoruba of Nigeria, for example, the head (*ori*) is the seat of personal destiny. The physical head, visible to the world, surrounds the "inner head," and the physical head becomes the focus of many important rituals. Some rituals addressed to the head center on the person of the king as the embodiment of the destiny of his people. Individuals, too, perform regular rites to their inner head at

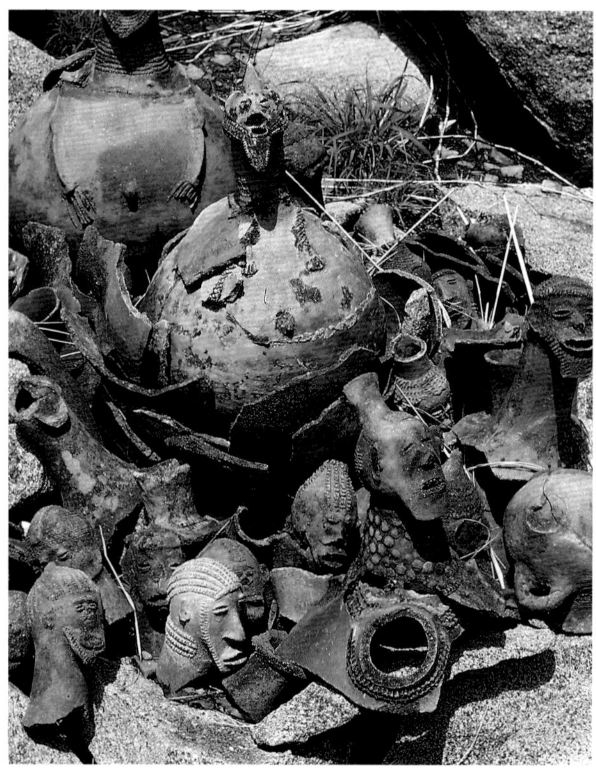

**Figure 1.2.** Shrine with ceramic ancestral pots called *wiiso*. Yungur, Nigeria. Photograph by Marla C. Berns, May 1981.

personal altars of the head (Abimbola 1973:77–85). Robert Farris Thompson (1993:146–7) reports that in 1982–83 when the singer Sunny Ade experienced a serious illness, he composed the now popular song, *"Jà fún mi,"* as a supplication to his "inner head."

In many other African societies the head is also given special emphasis. Among the Kaguru of Tanzania, the top of the head should be respected and one should avoid touching others in this spot. The head connects persons to birth and ultimately to the land of the dead (Beidelman 1993:64). The head, and specifically the forehead, is the locus for the spirit, *teme,* that controls a person's behavior among the Kalabari Ijo of southeastern Nigeria (Barley 1988:16). For the Tabwa of Zaire, the center of the forehead is regarded as the seat of wisdom, of prophecy, and of dreams (Roberts 1990:42).

Many African societies regard the head as the seat of intelligence, while strong emotions are lodged elsewhere in the body. For example, among the Bamana of Mali intelligence and reflection are located in the head, while character and passion are located in the liver. An individual's lifelong moral struggle is to bring the two into balance (Cissé 1973:147, 156–7). In a similar way, among the Iteso of Kenya, the head and heart embody two different capacities of the individual. Knowledge, perception, and skill are located in the head, while the heart is the site of the stronger emotions. Qualities associated with the head are cumulative and can grow over time, thus enabling people to manage themselves and their affairs. Mental illness and drunkenness, for example, are described as illnesses of the heart because they entail an individual's loss of control over the head. When someone becomes possessed by spirits, people say that "the spirits are sitting on the head," and the possessed person must struggle through a ritual process to regain control of the head (Karp 1990:86).

Our attention is directed towards the head as a site for special regard and elaboration in many African sculptures created at quite different times and places. Throughout the archaeological record there are numerous figurative objects that emphasize the head. The celebrated terra-cottas and bronzes from Nok, Igbo-Ukwu, Ife, and Benin in Nigeria are well-known sculptures where the head is given a particular emphasis in both its proportional relationship to the body and the amount of decoration lavished upon it (Fig. 1.3). Somewhat lesser-known sculptures including the terra-cotta figures from the Komo culture of northern Ghana, the Sao culture in Chad, the Nomoli stone figures from Sierra Leone, the ceramic heads from South Africa, and the Akan and Anyi terra-cotta heads, also stress the head over the rest of the body, and hair styles, facial scarification, and headgear are carefully rendered (Fig. 1.4). There are also many historical and contemporary African objects where the head is exaggerated including the Kuba *ndop* king figures (which date from ca. 1750

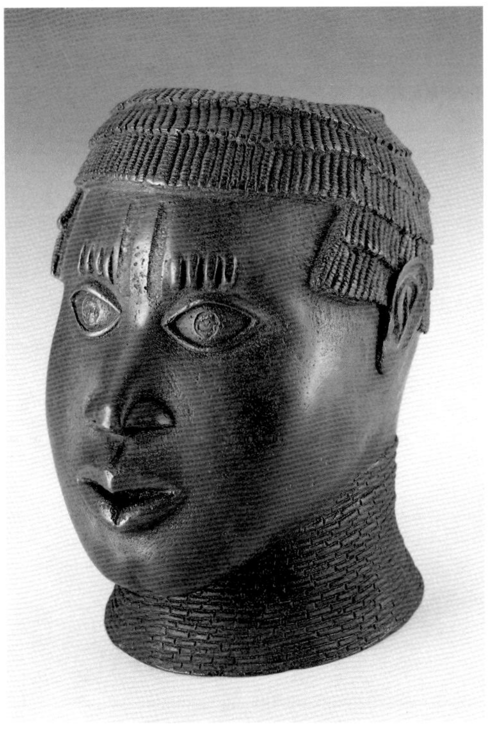

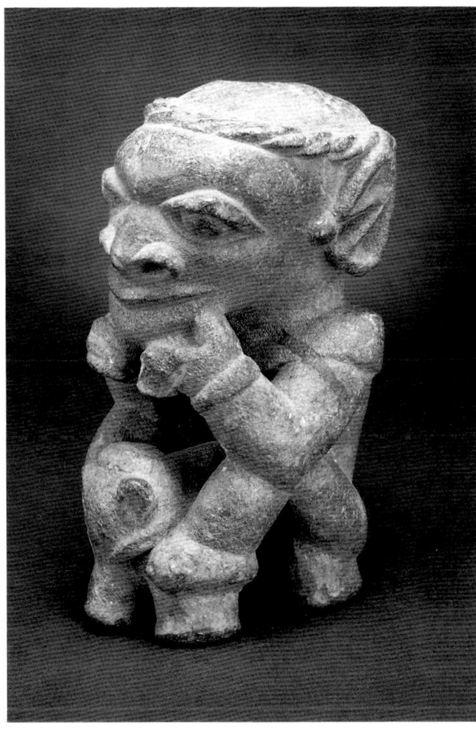

**Figure 1.3**, far left. Male head. Late fifteenth–early sixteenth century. Edo, Benin Kingdom, Nigeria. Copper alloy, iron. H. 22.2 cm. Purchased with funds provided by the Smithsonian Collections Acquisition Program, 82-5-2. Photograph by Franko Khoury. National Museum of African Art. These heads express the Bini belief that a person's fate depends upon thinking, judgment, and will power and on the senses of hearing, sight, and speech associated with the head.

**Figure 1.4**, left. Figure. Nomoli style, Sierra Leone and Guinea. Steatite. H. 19 cm. Photograph by Jeffery Ploskonka. National Museum of African Art. The proportion of the head to the body is 1:4.

**Figure 1.5**, below. Reliquary figure. Kota, Gabon. Wood, brass, copper ? H. 54.0 cm. FMCH X65.3802. Gift of the Wellcome Trust.

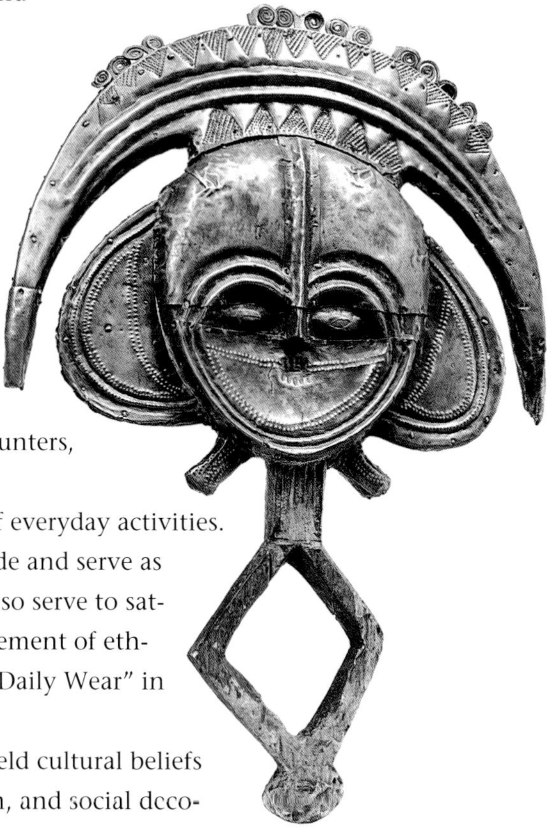

onwards), Luba figures from Zaire, Kota reliquary figures from Gabon (Fig. 1.5), and most Yoruba figurative art .

## DRESSING THE HEAD AS CULTURAL AND SOCIAL ACTION

In a more direct way, people regularly use headwear and hair styles to transform their heads and by extension their whole bodies into cultural entities. African headwear and the arts of dressing the head demand serious attention, not only as compelling artistic forms, but as significant cultural indices. Headdresses and hair styles can denote membership in certain religious and initiation societies, mark and celebrate changes in a person's life cycle, identify key participants at rituals and festivals, or they can designate such specialists as warriors, diviners, hunters, and musicians.

Hats, caps, and headties are also worn by men and women in the course of everyday activities. These hats and caps are practical and functional and are designed to provide shade and serve as effective rain gear. Besides protecting the wearer from the elements, they often also serve to satisfy the community's notion of decorum and modesty and can function as a statement of ethnic affiliation in a multiethnic environment (see "Practical Beauty: Headgear for Daily Wear" in this volume).

People use hats and hair styles to express and explore shared and deeply held cultural beliefs and values towards ethnicity, gender, life stages, status and authority, occupation, and social deco-

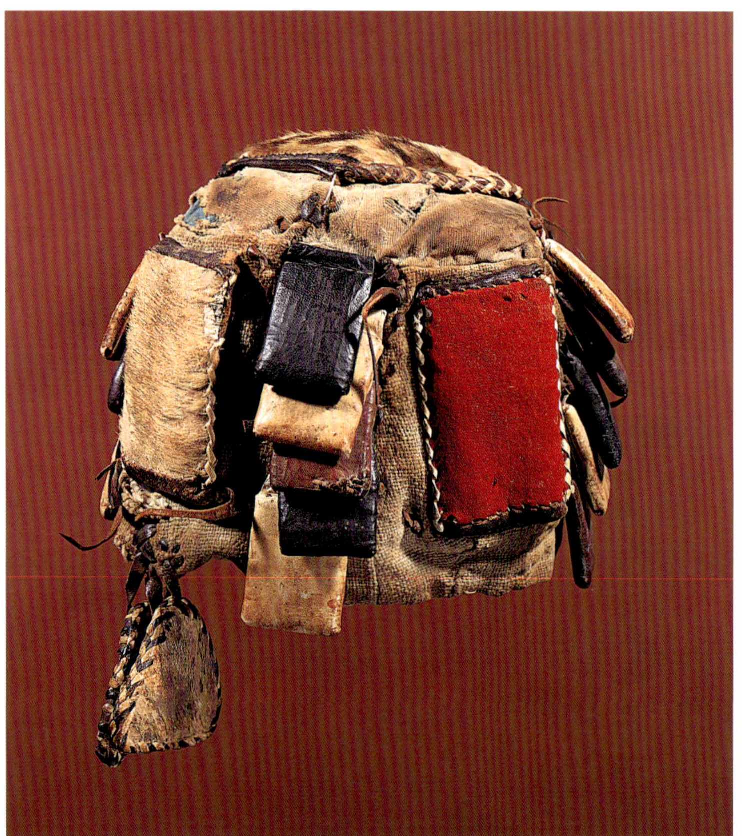

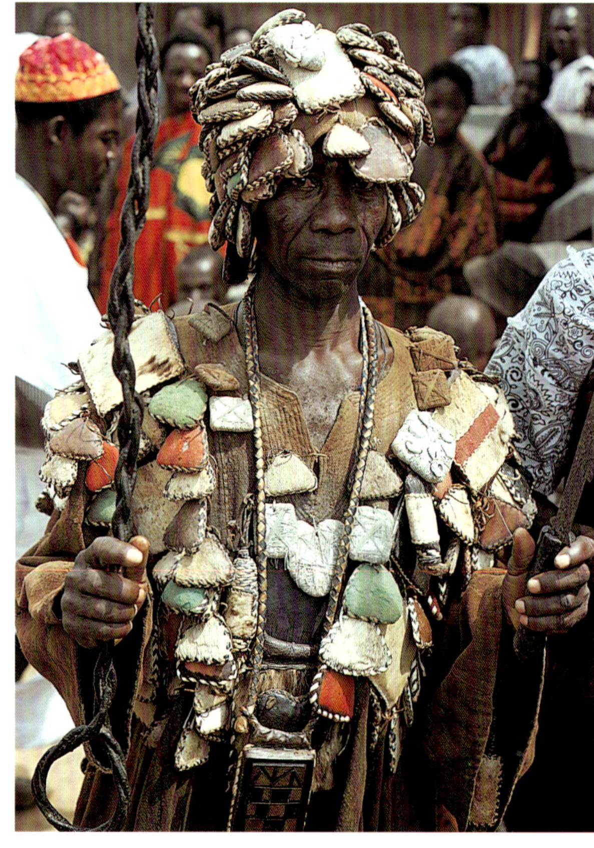

**Figure 1.6**, above. War hat. Akan, Ghana. Burlap, leather, cotton, felt, fur. H. 22.0 cm. FMCH X70.128. Museum purchase. Northern Ghanaian or Akan hats like this are typically worn with a similarly adorned war shirt. The leather-covered Islamic amulets contain passages from the Koran and are designed to provide spiritual protection for the wearer.

**Figure 1.7**, above right. Fante warrior chief *(asafohene)* wearing amulet-laden war shirt and hat during annual path-clearing festival *(Akwambo)* at the coastal town of Legu. Photograph by Doran H. Ross, 1976.

rum. Headwear and hair styles can also express personal aesthetic preferences and ideas about fashion and modernity. A single hat or hair style, when worn alone or as part of a larger costume ensemble, can be a multivocal symbol with layers of associations and meanings. A hat can communicate the wearer's personal aesthetic or it can convey mood. Hats and hair styles can also signal the wearer's endorsement or commitment to a particular role, status, or course of action. As a material "language," hats and hair styles can be put on, and taken off, manipulated, and invested with an aggregate of meanings depending on how and in what contexts they are put into play.

Tuareg adult men wear turbans and face veils everyday. When throughout the day, a Tuareg man adjusts and readjusts his turban and face veil, sometimes pulling it tighter and higher on his face, sometimes loosening it, he is articulating and responding to the shifting mood and behavioral expectations of his various social engagements. These shifting behaviors project him into his social world and actualize the deeply held Tuareg cultural values of respect and reserve that contribute to his own self-definition and serve as the basis for how others define, judge, and relate to him. When a man travels abroad either for schooling or business, he often chooses not to wear the face veil, although he may wear the turban on formal occasions. While abandoning the veil may indeed be a statement of his modernity, in these foreign settings a Tuareg man may feel no need to wear the veil precisely because his daily activities no longer involve interactions with either Tuareg elders or his affines. However, when he returns to his community, he usually resumes wearing the veil (see "Wrapping the Head" in this volume).

Other types of headgear are reserved for occupational specialists, such as hunters and warriors. This type of headgear generally combines practical serviceability with apotropaic functions. Amulets are attached to these hats and are intended to counter the dangerous powers associated with these highly charged occupations. The warrior's tunic and headgear assert that he is a man of action who attracts dangerous forces and who has accumulated the means to manage these forces (Figs. 1.6, 1.7).

Shared notions of social propriety, beauty, and solemnity dictate a variety of acceptable modes of decorating the head and the body. Special hair styles and headwear often figure prominently in rituals for major life passages such as birth, coming of age, marriage, and funerals. The Ndebele beaded back train *(nyoga)* along with other elements in a bride's costume, focus attention on the social transformation a woman undergoes during the marriage rites. When a bride dons her ensemble she announces her intention to move from one social state to another. This ritual not only transforms the bride, but her new identity as a married woman profoundly alters and shapes her future relationships with others and in turn theirs with her within her community (Fig. 1.8).

Throughout the Cameroon Grassfields, headgear and other forms of dress convert material wealth into symbolic capital within a political economy of prestige

**Figure 1.9**, below, left. Man's prestige cap *(ashetu)*. Bamun Kingdom, Cameroon. Cotton, wood pith, natural dyes. H. 20.0 cm. Neutrogena Corporation.

**Figure 1.10**, below. Two Bamun men attending the dedication of a drum house in the square in front of the palace at Foumban, Cameroon. One man wears an imported red fez to which feathers have been attached. The other man wears a local prestige cap with reinforced wood burl extensions resembling an elaborate hair style. Photograph by Christraud M. Geary, 1971. Eliot Elisofon Photographic Archives. National Museum of African Art.

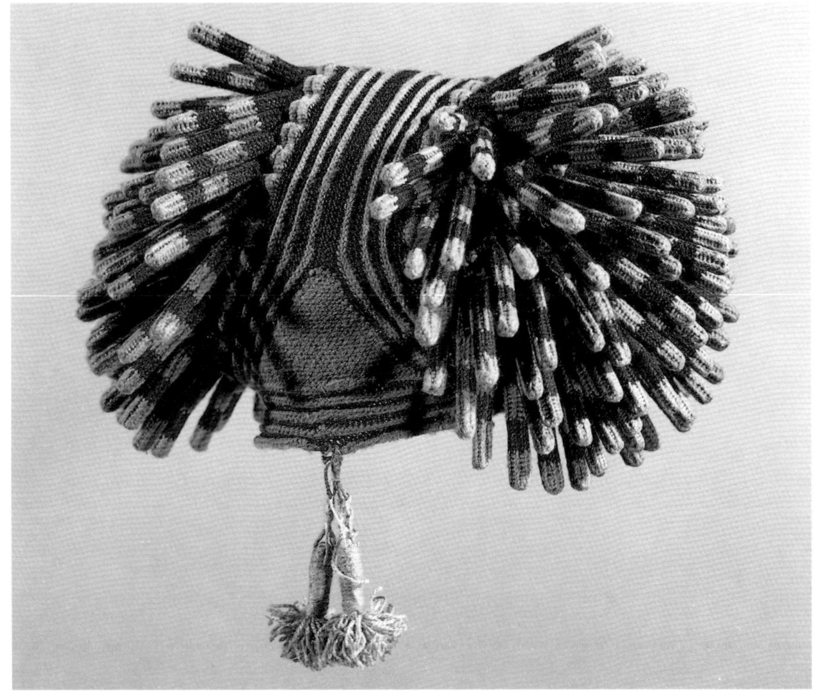

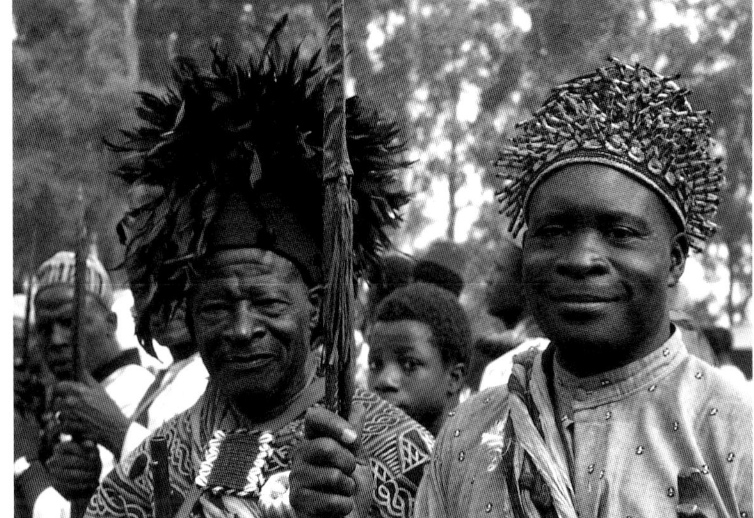

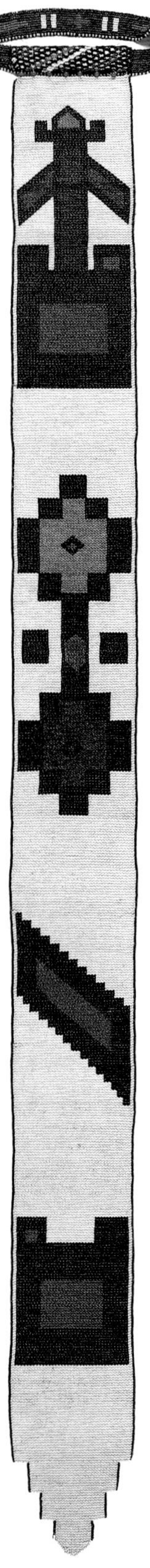

**Figure 1.8.** Bride's train *(nyoga).* Ndebele, South Africa. Twine, beads. H. 190 cm. FMCH X86.3190. Museum purchase, Manus Fund. This train is worn attached to the back of the head and trails to the ground. White beads are predominant in bridal headwear. The colorful geometric beaded designs in this veil identify it as a more recent style.

(Engard 1989). On formal occasions, when a Grassfields man wears the distinctive burled cotton cap *(ashetu),* his hat asserts his ethnic identity, alludes to Grassfields history and cultural values, and serves to underscore his social status and his sphere of influence within the community (Figs. 1.9, 9.10).

The violation or inversions of normative modes often occur at times of social disruption. Among the Tuareg, for example, when a woman undergoes curing rituals for spirit possession, she puts on a man's turban and face veil and performs the "head dance" *(asul)* in time to drumming and choral singing. The head dance, performed while in trance, is said to be directed by the occupying spirit. During the head dance the woman enacts behaviors that vacillate between the reserved and the flamboyant, expressing basic contradictions in Tuareg social life. Assuming the man's turban and face veil, protects the women's inner self in this period of crisis and transition (Rasmussen 1994:88–89, Rasmussen 1991a:109).

In many societies there are special practices associated with the head during *rites de passage,* initiation into religious societies, and the installation of leaders. When Temne and Kuba boys and Okiek girls enter the period of seclusion, their heads are shaved to symbolize birth. Later, during the public ceremonies when they are presented to the community for the first time as adults, they don special cloth hats, fiber caps, or beaded diadems (Lamp 1978, Kratz 1988, 1994; see "Headdresses and Titleholding Among the Kuba" in this volume). Among the Yoruba, an initiate to an *òrìṣà* cult is prepared to receive the god by shaving, anointing, and painting his head with spiritually potent substances and symbolic colors (Drewel, Pemberton and Abiodun 1989:75; Fig. 1.11). Initiates into *Candomblé,* a Yoruba-derived religion practiced in Brazil, also undergo similar treatments to the head in order to receive the *òrìṣà.* The head is shaved and intersecting lines are painted on top of the head dividing it into four equal quadrants. Where the lines intersect a small incision is made and rubbed with medicines (M. Drewal 1977:43). Young adult men among the Tuareg wear their hair long and braided under their turbans. However, when they become elders, they crop their hair short as a sign of their changed status. Similarly, when Maasai and Samburu warriors finally marry, they cut their hair short to symbolize their redefinition as elders.

Rituals surrounding death and funerals are also occasions when the head is modified and normal grooming patterns are inverted. Among the Merina of Madagascar, for example, widows untress their hair and leave it ungroomed during the period of mourning (Mack 1986:71). Among the Samburu of Kenya a young man, who normally invests many hours in dressing his hair, shaves it off completely when a close relative or age-mate dies, to ward off misfortune (Cole 1979:91). At Akuropon funerals of important chiefs, the townspeople wrap their heads with leaves and some gather beehives from the forest and wear them on their heads. These practices are fundamental statements about the state of disorder within the community following the death of a chief. In the funeral rites, participants bring the natural and cultural spheres together and the untransformed natural materials that they wear draw attention to the power located in the natural realm (Gilbert 1989:76).

During the colonial period people used headwear as a symbol of resistance to colonial authority. In the 1930s, during the Pende revolt against the Belgian colonial authority, the Pende wig *(mukotte)* was invested with a new meaning, repopularized, and became a symbol for Pende resistance (Fig. 5.9; Hoet 1936 as cited in Biebuyck and Van den Abbeele 1984:70). Jomo Kenyatta, one of the leaders of the nationalist movement in Kenya, was photographed on numerous occasions between 1946 and 1964 wearing different types of clothing and headwear from a European fedora to a tall colobus monkey hat. His choice of the colobus monkey hat along with other items of chiefly regalia, drawn from the universe of local forms shared by many groups in Kenya, was certainly a conscious act. The colobus monkey hat and cape are associated with power, spirit mediumship, and chiefly authority. The symbolism of the headwear and cape were widely understood and were objects around which people could unite in a common struggle.

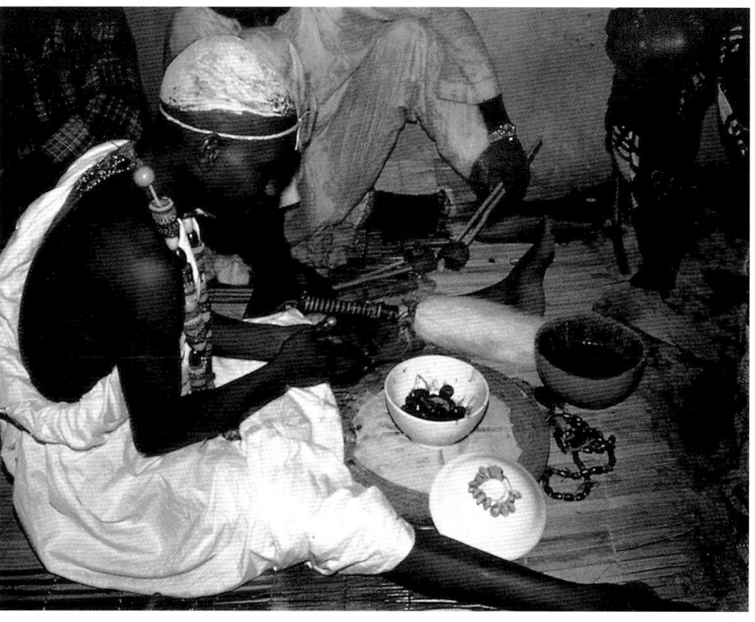

**Figure 1.11**, above. *Itefa* initiation, Imodi, Nigeria. Yoruba, Nigeria. Photograph by Henry John and Margaret Thompson Drewel, 1982. Slide no. YRB (A1992-028-02014). Eliot Elisofon Photographic Archives. National Museum of African Art.

During the *Itefa* ritual or the "establishment of self," diviners set out to interpret the nature of an initiates' "inner head." During one phase of the ritual, the initiate's head is shaved and painted with white chalk to symbolize rebirth. Each initiate learns the specific Ifa texts that will guide his or her new life. The white chalk makes a visual analogy between the newly defined personality and a shining star (M. Drewel 1992:63–65).

Many post-colonial politicians and leaders have consciously exploited particular forms of headwear and dress as symbols of the legitimacy of their power and authority. In Zaire, for example, President Mobutu regularly appeared in public wearing a leopard-skin cap as part of his presidential regalia (Fig. 1.12). While the form of the hat derives from a military cap, his choice of leopard skin was certainly calculated to exploit the symbolic association of the leopard with chiefly legitimacy and power that has a long history in many societies in this region. This hat style with its association with state authority and prestige was adopted by many local authorities. Eliot Elisofon photographed the Kuba king wearing this style hat and the distinctive suit worn by government functionaries in the 1970s. In the Kuba area, the "Mobutu" hat was overlaid with beadwork and designs from the local repertoire of prestige forms (Fig. 9.20).

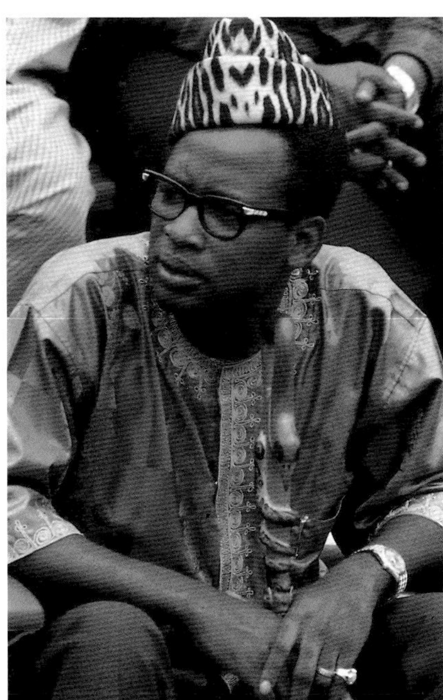

**Figure 1.12**, left. President Mobutu of Zaire at a parade of Corps Voluntier Republique in Kinshasa, Zaire. Photograph by Eliot Elisofon, 1967. Slide no. C ZAI 15.11 (2383). Eliot Elisofon Photographic Archives. National Museum of African Art. Mobutu's cap is probably derived from a French/Belgian military cap, "bonnet de police," that has been used since the Napoleanic Wars.

## THE DIVERSITY OF FORMS, MATERIALS, AND TECHNIQUES

African headwear and hair styles are fashioned in a variety of forms and materials that can enhance, alter, protect, reveal, and/or conceal the head. Societies like the Yoruba and the Kuba are geographically separated and have developed extremely different forms of leadership headwear Figs. 2.2, 9.4). In East Africa, however, forms such as the colobus monkey hat and the distinctive face ruffs worn by warriors were once distributed across a number of ethnic groups including the Maasai, Chagga, Kikuyu, and others (Fig. 1.13). These shared forms underscore the dynamic history of the region, which has also resulted in many shared attitudes and idioms among the various groups.

Materials are selected according to local criteria. Some may be chosen for their rarity or such qualities as sheen, color, or pliancy, or for their beauty (Figs. 2.17, 5.21). An incredible variety of local flora and fauna enters into the manufacture of headgear. Bark, cotton, palm fiber, animal manes, wool, hides and skins, as well as minerals such as clays, stones, and metal have been exploited in creative ways by various societies in the process of elaborating the head (see Figs. 2.7, 2.9, 5.1, 5.25). Many communities have also incorporated a rich variety of imported textiles, glass beads, and other materials into headdresses, and these elements bear witness to extensive historical and contemporary trading networks (see Figs. 2.1, 2.3, 2.7).

Techniques that African artists use for fabricating headwear are as varied as the materials they choose. Some artists make hats using basketry techniques like plaiting and twining (Figs. 4.4, 4.7, 4.8, 5.7). Others shape and sew cloth or leather and skin (Figs. 2.9, 5.19). Many people decorate their hats by painting, pyro-engraving, incising, dyeing, or appliqueing and embroidering the base materials (Figs. 2.11, 4.18).

Hats, caps, diadems, and headbands can be modest and formally

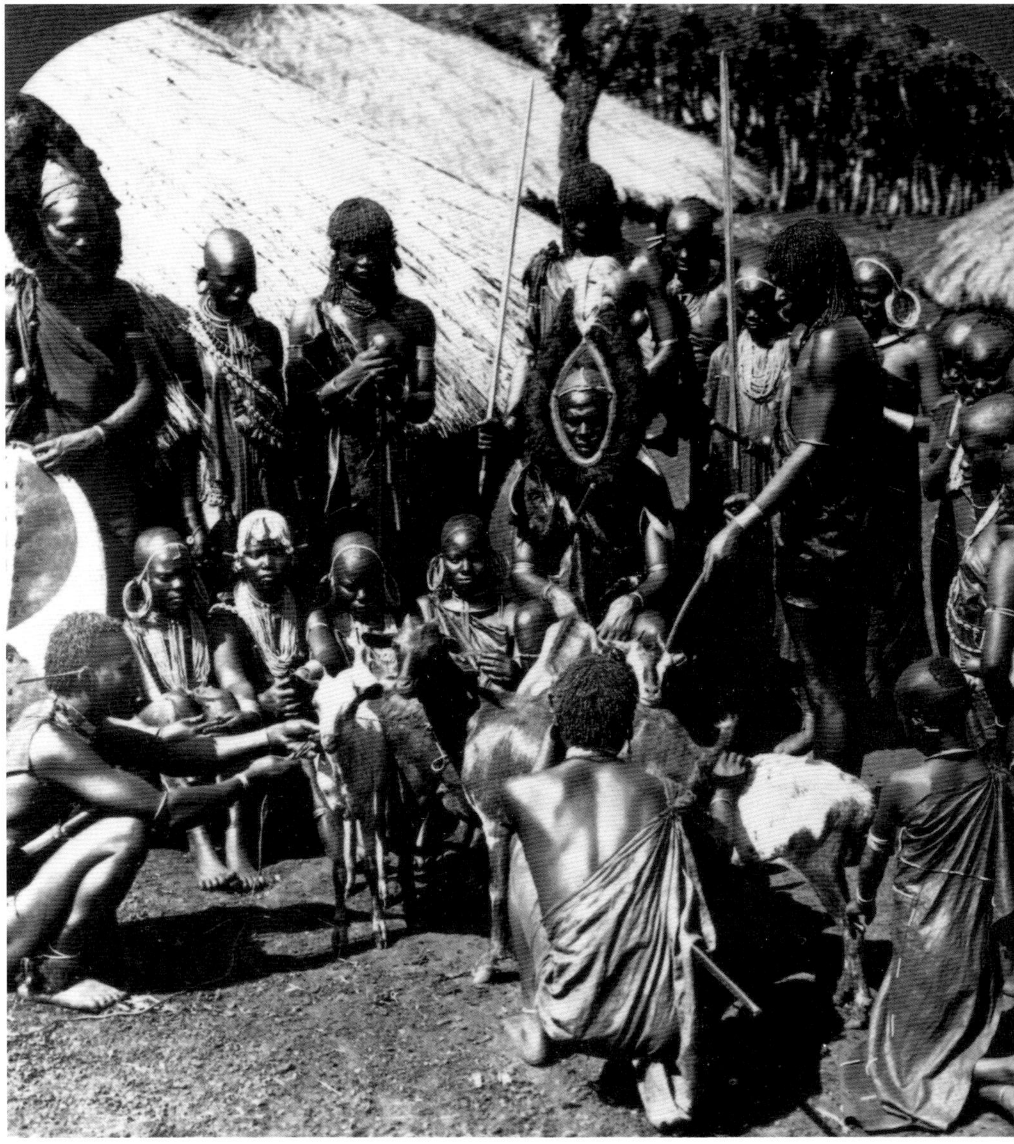

**Figure 1.13.** Stereograph of "A Kikuyu warrior buying a wife from her father, the King (payment in goats), East Africa." Kenya. Photographer unknown, ca. 1910. Underwood and Underwood, no. 10548. Stereograph Collection. Eliot Elisofon Photographic Archives. National Museum of African Art. The ostrich feather face ruffs designated the wearer as a member of the warrior age-grade. This style of headwear was once widely distributed throughout East Africa and worn by Kikuyu, Maasai, and Chagga warriors among others.

restrained, simply encircling the head and emphasizing its shape. Many of these types of hats are used for daily wear, for instance, Kuba men's hats (Fig. 4.6), Nigerian Muslims' knitted caps (Fig. 4.21), Himba unmarried girls' wigs (Fig. 4.13), Lega men's caps (Figs. 8.1), Goudour women's calabash hats (Fig. 4.2), !Kung ostrich-shell headbands (Fig. 4.1), and Bura calabash baby hats (Fig. 2.11; see "Practical Beauty: Headgear for Daily Wear" in this volume). Others of this type, like the Mossi leather-covered calabash hat (Fig. 1.14), are worn only on ceremonial and ritual occasions. This gourd is covered with appliqued and plaited leather designed to represent a face. Young men in dance troupes *(wiskwamba;* Roy 1979) wear this type of calabash hat when they perform at funerals of important elders to honor the deceased. There is an interesting visual play of the "head atop the head" in this Mossi example, where the dancer's own face becomes subordinated to the face on the hat .

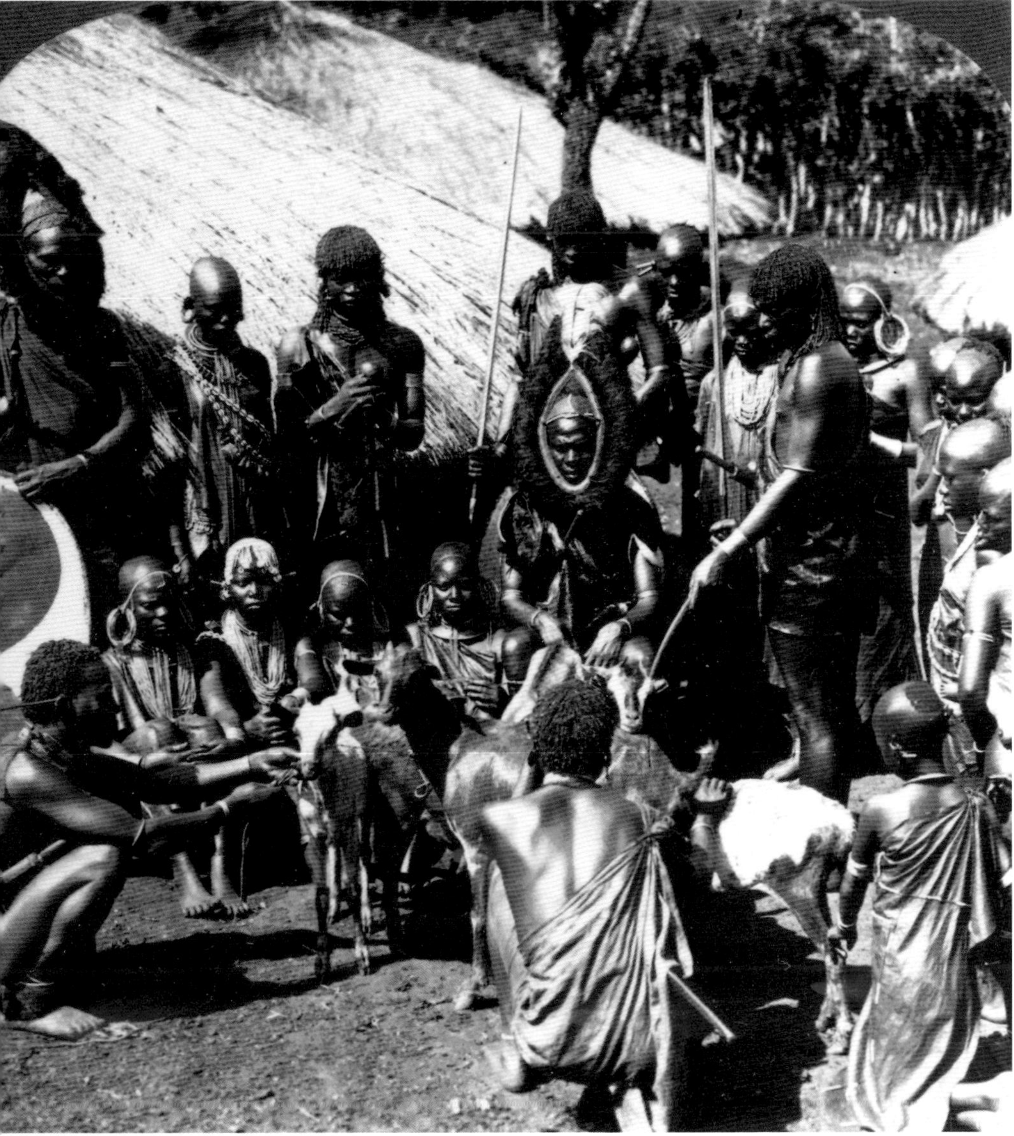

Many hats used on a day-to-day basis often receive the same care and attention from their owners as does more visually spectacular headwear reserved for ritual and ceremonial occasions. The proscriptions surrounding the use and care of the small Lega caps, for example, reveal them to be central forms in *bwami* regalia linked to the philosophy, knowledge, and tenets of the association (Fig. 8.1; see "Lega Hats" in this volume).

Several years ago when the Kuba king visited the Smithsonian, he and his official entourage wore European-style suits, but they also wore the small raffia caps that are central to notions of adult status and social propriety and are worn daily by Kuba men in Zaire. The care that some men take with their caps, the type of embellishment they choose, and their attention to personal grooming, go well beyond cultural concerns and are personal expressions of style and self-esteem (David Binkley, personal communication 1994).

Headgear and hair style forms can also be complex and voluminous, dramatically calling attention to the head, visually altering its shape, and extending it vertically and laterally. Many of these types of hats and hair styles are reserved for particular groups or offices and most are worn only for ceremonial or ritual occasions, although like the more modest forms, this is not unilaterally the case. Many of these hats including Yoruba Obas' crowns, Kongo chiefs' hats, emirs' turbans worn in northern Nigeria, and Yaka chiefs' hats are important symbols of leadership.

Yoruba kings are divine and their authority derives from a mythological/religious charter. When a beaded crown *(ade)* is placed on the king's head it unites the king's "inner head" with all past kings. With his face masked by a beaded veil, his humanity is concealed and his divinity revealed. The act of wearing the crown intensifies his performative powers and he assumes a heightened spirituality (Fig. 2.1; Drewal, Pemberton, and Abiodun 1989:75–76; Abiodun 1994).

Emirs in northern Nigeria derive their authority from a historical/religious charter that links them to Sheikh Usman dan Fodio, who through a *jihad,* founded the powerful early-nineteenth-century Sokoto Caliphate. While the contemporary Nigerian state invests these rulers with secular power, their political/religious authority derives from their direct descent from the ruling class within the Sokoto Caliphate. Their ample turbans fashioned from meters of prestige cloth and the "caliphate robes" they wear when appearing in public ceremonies are potent material reminders of the legitimacy of their authority (Fig. 6.2; see "Wrapping the Head" in this volume).

Among Kongo peoples, the authority of the ruler derives its potency from a mythical/religious charter. Chiefs' exceptional powers come from the ancestors of their matrilineal descent groups in whose name they rule. At their investitures, chiefs are anointed with many of the same medicines that are used by the *nganga*, diviners and healers, in constituting an *nkisi* power object. The regalia associated with chiefdom, including the tall caps and canes of office, legitimize the chief's authority and power to act as the intermediary between the living and the ancestors (Fig. 2.15; MacGaffey 1993:60, 95–96).

Northern Ghanaian musicians', hunters', and warriors' helmets with their sweeping horns (Figs. 1.15, 1.17), the tall complex Ekonda hat reserved for diviners and initiates (Fig. 2.17), the chain-mail helmets worn by nineteenth-century Sudanese warriors (Fig. 2.5), the Lega *bwami* association hat fashioned from a pangolin hide (Fig. 8.21), and the headgear of the *Asafo* military societies in Ghana (Fig. 5.19) are all dramatic forms of headgear that are reserved for particular groups within their respective societies. The hats, their forms, and the materials from which they are fashioned, embody important cultural, historical, and symbolic meanings (see "Spectacular Hats for Special Occasions" in this volume).

Yoruba women's headties, which are among the most sculptural forms of women's headdresses worn in Africa, are not restricted to specific ritual or ceremonial contexts, but are worn regularly when visiting friends, going to parties, or going to the market (Figs. 7.1, 7.7; see "Yoruba Headties" in this volume). Men's broad-brimmed, conical straw hats that seem to extend the head vertically and laterally are widely distributed throughout West Africa and are used as everyday wear. While these large straw hats clearly protect the wearer from the elements, the quality of the workmanship and decoration also satisfy a personal aesthetic (Fig. 4.8).

Many headwear forms have a long history: Ethiopian crowns, tall fiber Kongo hats, Yoruba conical crowns, and the Tuareg men's turbans and face veils — all of these have endured over centuries (Figs. 2.1, 2.7, 2.15, 6.5). Other examples like the chain-mail helmet from the Sudan and the Herero married women's leather horned headdress, are no longer being produced in the late twentieth century (Figs. 2.5, 2.9). Among the Herero, the older form of the leather cap began to be replaced by a cloth headwrap beginning in the late nineteenth century. Throughout the first half of the twentieth century, women who converted to Christianity generally adopted this cloth headwrap. This headwrap (known as the *otjikaiva)* however, retains an association with the older form. Horn elements constructed from cloth rather than leather were sewn onto the headwraps. Gordon Gibson notes that in the 1960s he did not see Herero women wearing the older leather horned hat, although some elder Himba women still wear them (personal communication 1994).

There are also a number of newer forms that have been inspired by older headgear. Others have been appropriated by one group from their neighbors, or they have been imported or inspired by hat forms from outside the continent. The Yaka chiefs' hats from Zaire are examples of the Yaka borrowing leadership regalia from their Pende neighbors, who previously borrowed it from the Lunda (Fig. 1.16). Zulu women's hats *(isicholo)* represent an interesting documented case of both the creation of a new hat form in the late nineteenth century and the changing patterns of its use over the twentieth century. Today, both the columnar and the flared styles of Zulu married women's hats (different regional variations developed in the early twentieth century) are considered to be an essential element of Zulu women's "traditional" dress. Both styles of hats were once worn as everyday headgear to indicate a woman's marital status, but now they are usually worn only on important ceremonial occasions. Carolee Kennedy (personal communication 1994) reported that many women wore these "traditional" hats during the agricultural fair and the wedding celebration for the Zulu king in 1977. These hats are also worn by the national dance troupe to project an image of "traditional" Zulu society. The hats themselves, which came into vogue in the late nineteenth century were inspired by and replaced a nineteenth-century married woman's hair style, which itself had evolved from a more modest eighteenth-century style (Fig. 3.3; Conner and Pelrine 1983; Kennedy 1978).

## LOCAL RESPONSE TO IMPORTED FORMS AND MATERIALS

For centuries Africans have been active in both long-distance trade within the continent and with the Middle East, Asia, and Europe. Many headdresses, in form or decoration, are creative expressions of this fluidity of goods and ideas. Many Islamic and European forms have been widely adopted or reproduced in local materials. In the nineteenth century during the Islamic reforms that swept West Africa, Islamic-style headwear was often adopted to proclaim the owner's adherence to the faith and often

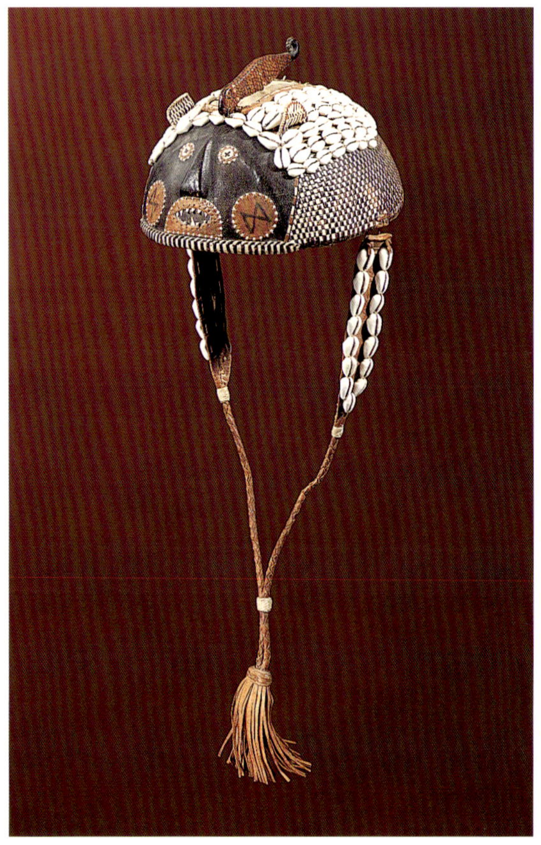

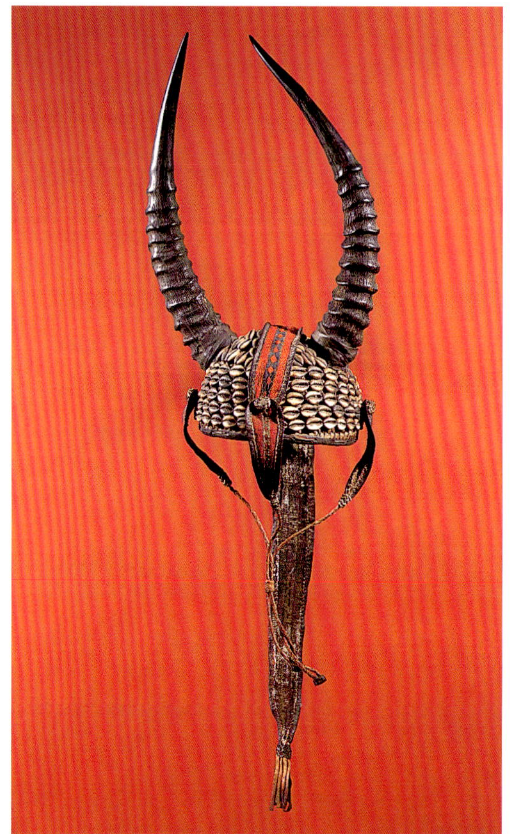

**Figure 1.14**, above left. Dancer's hat. Mossi, Burkina Faso. Gourd, leather, cowries. FMCH X64.93. This gourd hat, worn in funeral dances for elders, is covered with appliqued and painted leather representing an animal face (possibly a feline). Leather ears, a painted leather chameleon, and cowrie decorations are fastened to the base.

**Figure 1.15**, above right. Ceremonial helmet *(ipiedza)*. Konkomba, northern Ghana. Grass, cowrie shells, horsetail, leather, fiber, antelope horns, cloth, string. H. 106.0 cm. FMCH X74.1344. Gift of Katherine C. White. These helmets were used by many ethnic groups in northern Ghana and northern Togo, including the Moba, Tamberma, and Kabye.

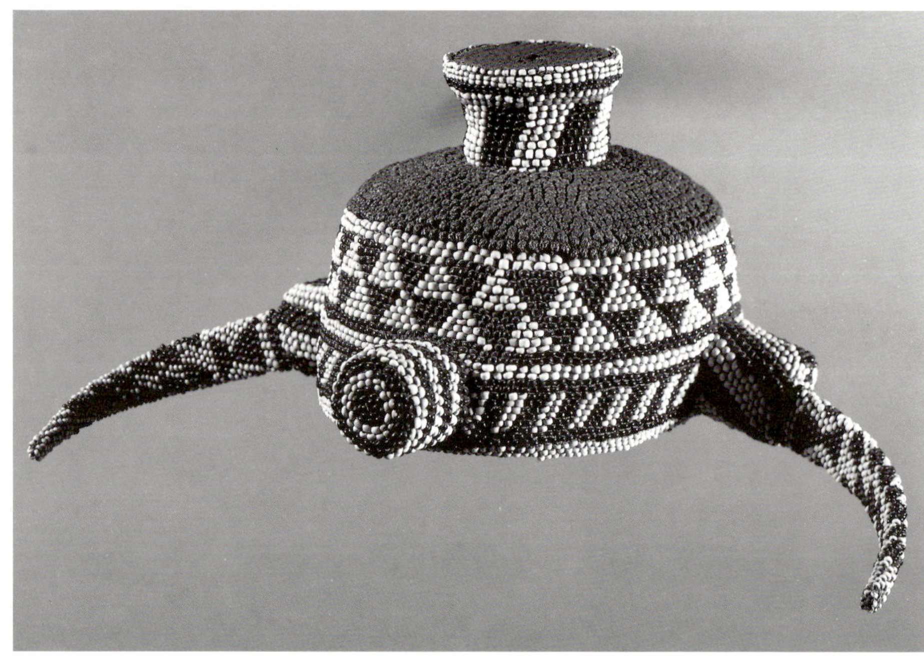

**Figure 1.16**, right. Chief's hat *(misango mayaka)*. Yaka, Zaire. Beads, fiber. H. 15.0 cm. FMCH X94.29.2. (See Figure 5.3). Museum purchase, Jerome L. Joss Endowment Fund.

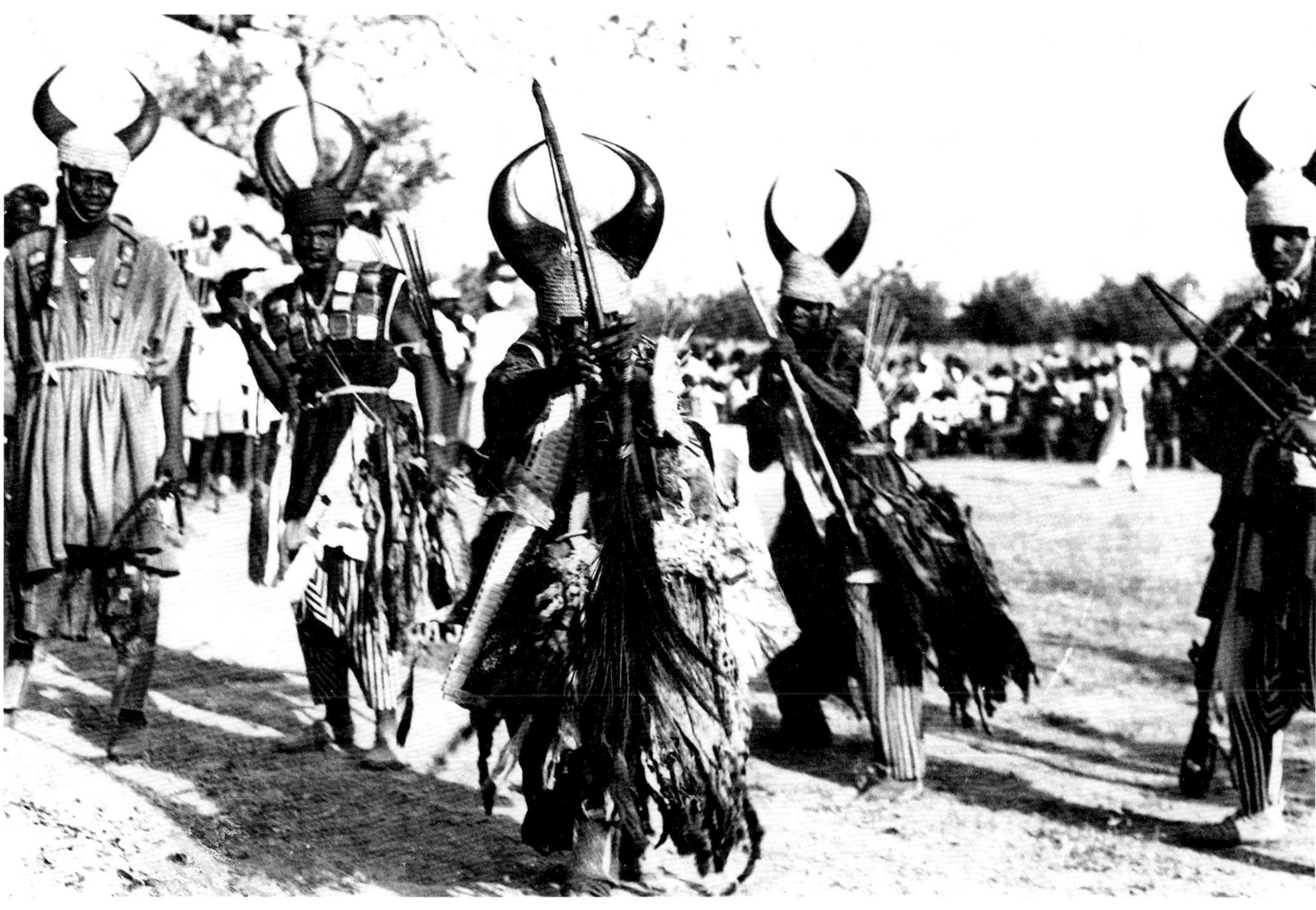

**Figure 1.17.** Horn and cowrie-adorned headdresses are worn among many peoples of northern Ghana and neighboring countries in festivals often associated with hunting and war. Photograph courtesy of Ghana Information Services, date unknown.

served to set him apart from his non-Moslem neighbors. The use of Islamic amulets and design motifs is widespread in Africa. While their adoption symbolically associates a person with the power of Islam, it does not oblige the individual to embrace the religion. Materials such as European brocades, velvets, and other textiles along with items like beads, buttons, glass mirrors, and brass tacks were imported from outside the continent and circulated through networks of intracontinental trade routes. Imported forms and materials are often combined with those manufactured or found locally, and the hat or headdress is invested with local value and symbolism that ultimately transcends any single element in its creation.

Some forms brought in from outside were domesticated through creative reworking of various elements to conform to local sensibilities and aesthetics. For example, the late-nineteenth-century top hat collected in Liberia demonstrates the creative reworking and elaboration of a Western top hat (Fig. 2.3). The hatmaker added a number of decorative objects to the hat that are associated locally with wealth and prestige or are invested with symbolic meaning. The cowrie shells, once a form of currency, speak to wealth and prestige. The ostrich feathers on the crown were probably imported from northern areas, and the red wool on the brim is a European import.

The top hat, itself, was introduced as elite ceremonial headwear into Liberian cities by the Americo-Liberian settlers, who brought the formal style of the top hat with them from America. Top hats soon were acquired and used as prestige headwear by high-ranking men and women in the Liberian countryside, or the hat form was reproduced in local materials and adapted for use as in the Gola example.

The Yoruba beaded crown in the shape of a barrister's wig is another example of the creative reworking of an imported form. The authority of the Yoruba Oba and that of British law are visually and symbolically brought together in this hat constructed entirely of white beads (Fig. 2.19). More recent examples of this process of adaptation and reinvention are the colorfully embroidered Hausa hats (Fig. 4.18). A small cylindrical white hat of the same type with white embroidery was already being worn in Hausaland in the nineteenth century, but Heathcote (1975:54) notes that ordinary men in rural areas during this period would have probably gone bareheaded. The inspiration for the colorful embroidered hats was most probably the hats brought back by pilgrims from Mecca; they gained popularity among the Hausa in the 1950s. The hats are generally worn by adult men as part of formal ensembles. Today, hats of this type are widespread throughout Nigeria and have been exported by traders to many parts of West Africa where they are purchased by Moslems and non-Moslems alike. In a recent video shot in Cameroon, the ruler of Fumban is shown conducting an annual ceremony wearing a "Hausa ensemble," which includes one of these colorful embroidered hats.[5] Embroidered "Hausa" hats have also recently become fashionable among young African-Americans in the United States as part of an Afrocentric fashion statement.

Hair styles and hats that are not associated with ritual contexts often undergo the most rapid transformations responding to the dynamics of fashion and taste. Today, both in Africa and in the worldwide African diaspora, popular hair styles for both men and women are featured in photographs in international and national magazines and many are promoted locally by barbers and hairdressers. For decades, African artists throughout West and Central Africa have created painted tableaux as advertisements for local hairdressers and barbers to promote the latest fashions. These tableaux along with photographic collages from magazines are put on display in the various shops. Many popular hair styles are given local names that relate them to contemporary events or highlight local notions of modernity.

The hats, caps, and crowns in this exhibit represent only a small sample of the headwear created and worn by Africans. These historical and contemporary forms stand as splendid artistic objects that enhance and beautify the body. Whether hats and hair styles are reserved for ceremonial and ritual purposes or are more generally popular, they communicate important messages about modes of life and the attitudes, values, and beliefs that shape the human experience.

The organization of the catalogue essays reproduces the conceptual framework of the exhibit. The central themes are explored in the opening section followed by a focus on twelve individual hats which are discussed in terms of their specific cultural histories, the technology of manufacture, the symbolism of designs, and their museum or collection histories. The next section examines hair and hair styles in Africa and is followed by two sections that highlight groups of hats from throughout the African continent organized into two categories: daily and formal headwear, and ceremonial and ritual hats. Turbans, headscarves, and headties in northern and southern Nigeria and in Niger are the subject of the next two essays. Notions of status and accumulation are addressed in essays on the Lega and Kuba which discuss the full range of headwear used in these two societies. The final essay examines transatlantic connections between Africa and the Americas both in the historical period and in the present.

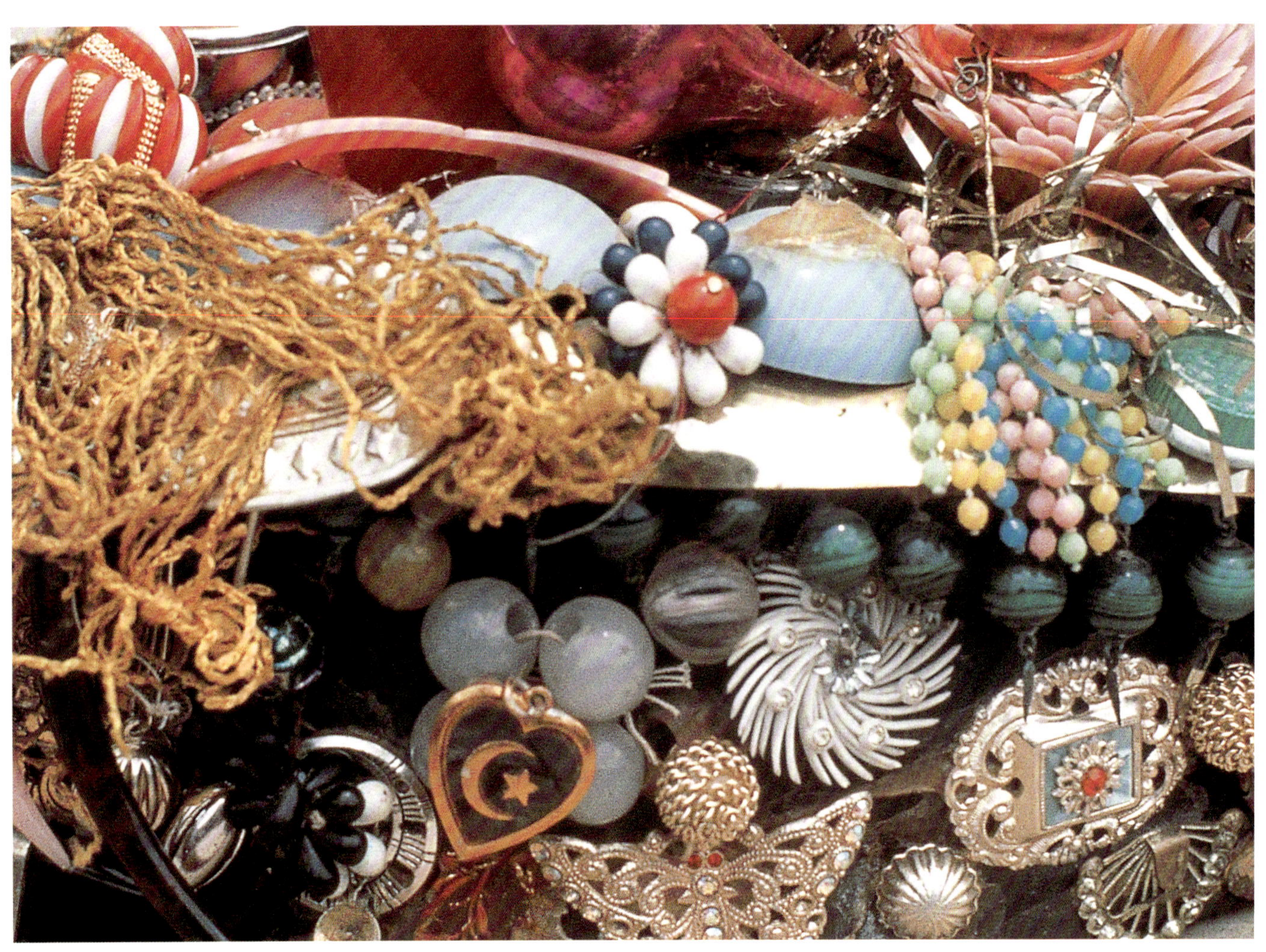

# 2 FOCUS ON TWELVE AFRICAN HATS

MARY JO ARNOLDI AND CHRISTINE MULLEN KREAMER

African headwear provides a window into the dynamic cultural history, social processes, symbolism, aesthetics, and technologies of societies throughout the continent and the African diaspora. In the exhibit, twelve individual hats are featured, each installed in its own free-standing case. Because hats not only mean something, but they do something, our visitors are asked to move around each hat in order to experience it from every angle, engaging with its form, examining its textures and materials, imagining how the hat is worn, how it encloses or extends the head into space, and how it feels on the head.

The dialogue with objects always raises many questions and we have tried to anticipate and answer some of them by organizing information into a series of four different labels. In the exhibit each label in the series is mounted on one of the four faces of the free-standing case. These labels include not only an explanatory text, but photographs of people wearing similar types of hats, and a map as a geographical orientation.

The first label (PEOPLE) addresses the questions of who made the hat and where they live in Africa. Label two (OBJECT) examines who wore the hat, how it was worn, for what occasions, and whether it is still being worn today. The third label (TECHNIQUE) speaks to how each hat was made and out of what materials, whether these materials were locally produced or imported, and what aesthetic or symbolic value these materials have to the owners. The final label (COLLECTION) looks at the life history of each hat and how it got to this American museum exhibition in the late twentieth century.

It is our hope that an active engagement between the museum, the object, and the audience will both answer questions and generate many more. Even though a catalogue can never replicate the visual and spatial dynamics of an exhibition, we have reproduced in schematic form, twelve individual case studies in order to approximate the experience.

**Opposite.** Detail of chief's hat *(ajibulu).* Kalabari Ijo, Nigeria. Collection of Joanne Eicher (see pg. 50).

## PEOPLE

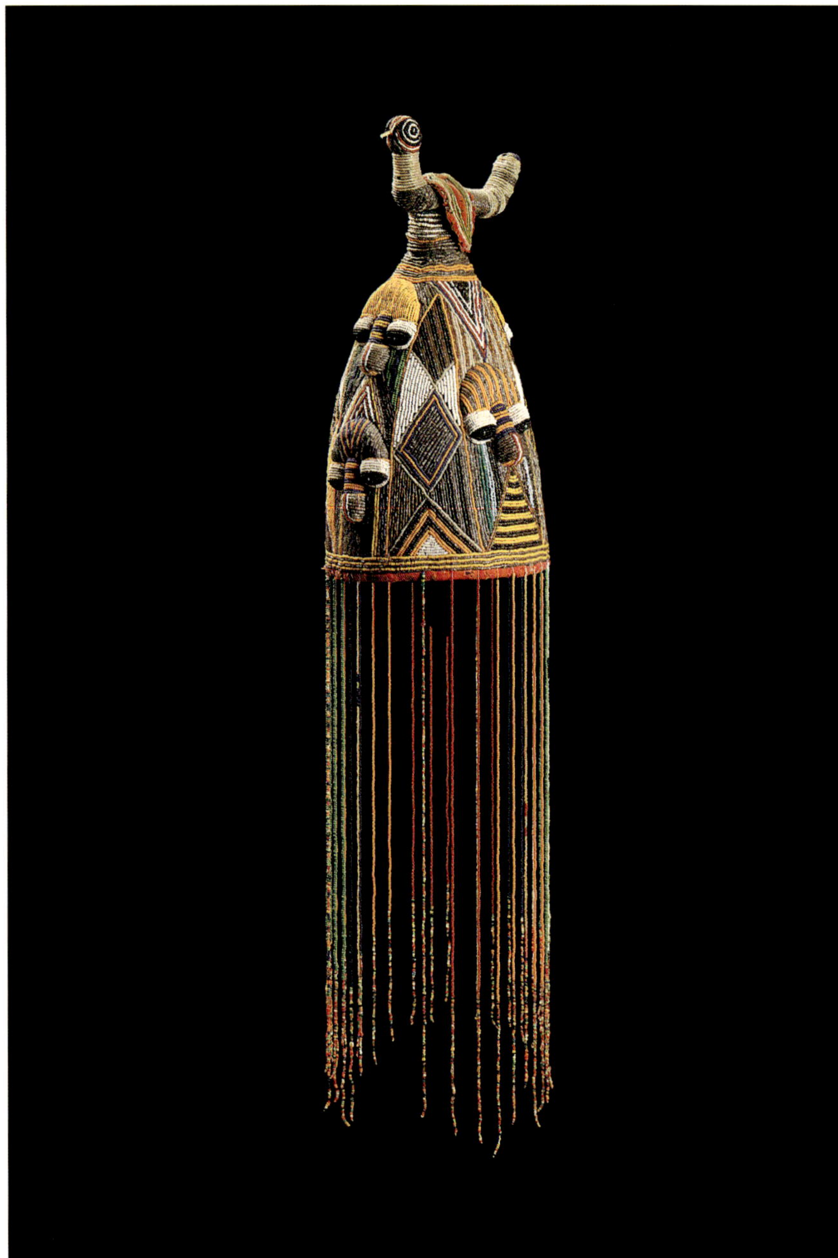

**Figure 2.1. King's crown *(ade)*. Yoruba, Nigeria. Fabric, glass beads, thread. H. 76.0 cm. Twentieth century. FMCH X86-1081.**

The Yoruba-speaking people live primarily in southwestern Nigeria and number over twenty million. They are one of the three largest ethnic groups in Nigeria today, and they have a long tradition of urban life. Historically, the Yoruba were divided into a number of independent kingdoms that were generally known by the name of their capital city.

The Yoruba creation myth provides a charter for Yoruba ritual and political organization. According to this myth the god Odua created mankind and gave the right of rulership to the first king of Ife, the Oni of Ife. Odua's other sons became the Obas of other Yoruba kingdoms. Because of changing historical circumstances including disputes over succession, the founding of new towns, and inter-kingdom warfare, there are hundreds of Obas, but in fact not all hold the same degree of authority, and only those who can trace descent from one of the sixteen sons of Odua can wear beaded crowns (Beier 1982:5, Smith 1976:128–129). At his installation, the Oba elect is ceremonially "killed" and symbolically "reborn" as a divine ruler. The Oba is generally referred to as *ekeji òrìṣà,* the brother of the gods.

### OBJECT

The crown *(ade)* is the most important of all the Oba's (king's) regalia, and Obas wear their beaded veiled crowns on all ceremonial and religious occasions. The king is the center of a complicated network of forces and the crown, imbued with medicines, gives the king the power to resist, direct, and control these forces. In its form and materials, the crown asserts Yoruba beliefs about the divine aspects of kingship and the wealth and authority these rulers hold in social, political, and religious realms.

A crowned Oba is the representative of the collective destiny of his people. Yoruba view the head *(orí)* as the locus of a vital force called *àse.* The head is symbolically linked to notions about destiny, individuality, intellect, and personal power. The crown's beaded veil *(iboju)* obscures the king's face, whose divine countenance is considered dangerous and powerful and must be shielded from public view (Thompson 1972:230). The crown, itself, can serve as a material substitute for the king. In such a case it would be publicly displayed on the throne and subjects would be expected to show it the same deference that they accord to the Oba.

### TECHNIQUE

The conical crown begins as a palm-rib wickerwork or cardboard frame. Starched unbleached muslin or stiffened cotton fabric is stretched over the form. Figures and designs in high relief shaped from pieces of cloth dipped in wet starch are attached to this basic form. Artists then string together beads of a single color to form a strand. Different colored strands are then tacked to the surface until the crown is completely covered.

Crownmakers work in the palace of the Oba. Prior to beginning their work they make a sacrifice to Ogun, the god of iron, honoring the needle they use, and to Olokun in remembrance of the fact that this *òrìṣà* (god) gave the first crown to the Yoruba (Beier 1982:34).

In every case, the important ritual crowns are surmounted by the image of a bird, who represents Okin, the royal bird. Many crowns also carry images of one or more faces. There are multiple interpretations of whom these faces represent. Some say they are merely decorative motifs; others claim they are representations of Oduduwa (Odua), the ancestor of all crowned Obas; and others interpret the face as a representation of Obalufon, the *òrìṣà* who invented beads (Beier 1982:24). In addition to the bird and faces, there are also a variety of natural and abstract designs that ornament the crowns. Beads of different colors are associated with particular gods, and since the Oba is a member of all *òrìṣà* cults, it is appropriate that his ritual crowns are made from all the colors associated with these gods.

### COLLECTION

This crown was acquired in the 1970s from an undentified dealer by Barbara Jean Jacoby, a lawyer and avid collector of African art. Ms. Jacoby received her Bachelor of Arts and law degrees from UCLA in 1951 and 1953. Upon her death in 1986, Ms. Jacoby's parents and her brother donated this crown and several other works of African art from her estate to the Fowler Museum in her memory.

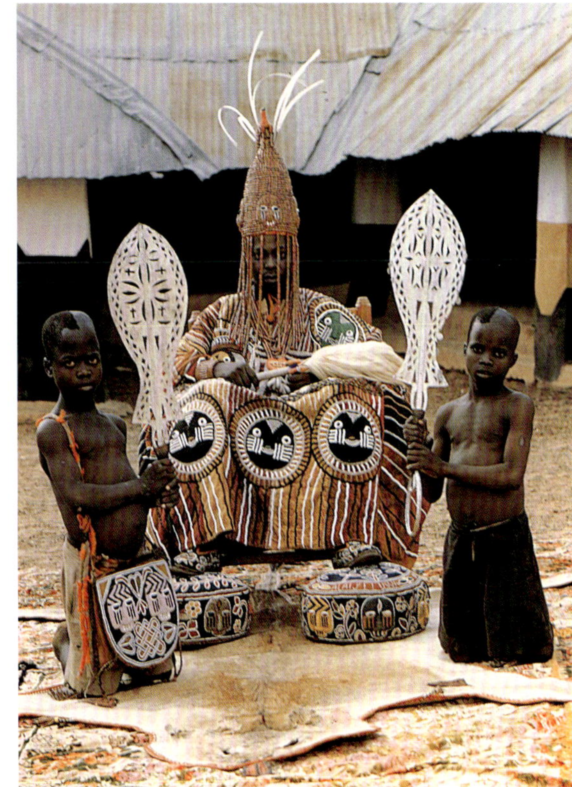

**Figure 2.2.** Oba Ademuwagun Adesida II, the Deji of Akure, on a throne in the courtyard of Akure palace, Nigeria. Photograph by Eliot Elisofon, 1959. Slide no. CYRB 12.4 (2077). Eliot Elisofon Archives. National Museum of African Art.

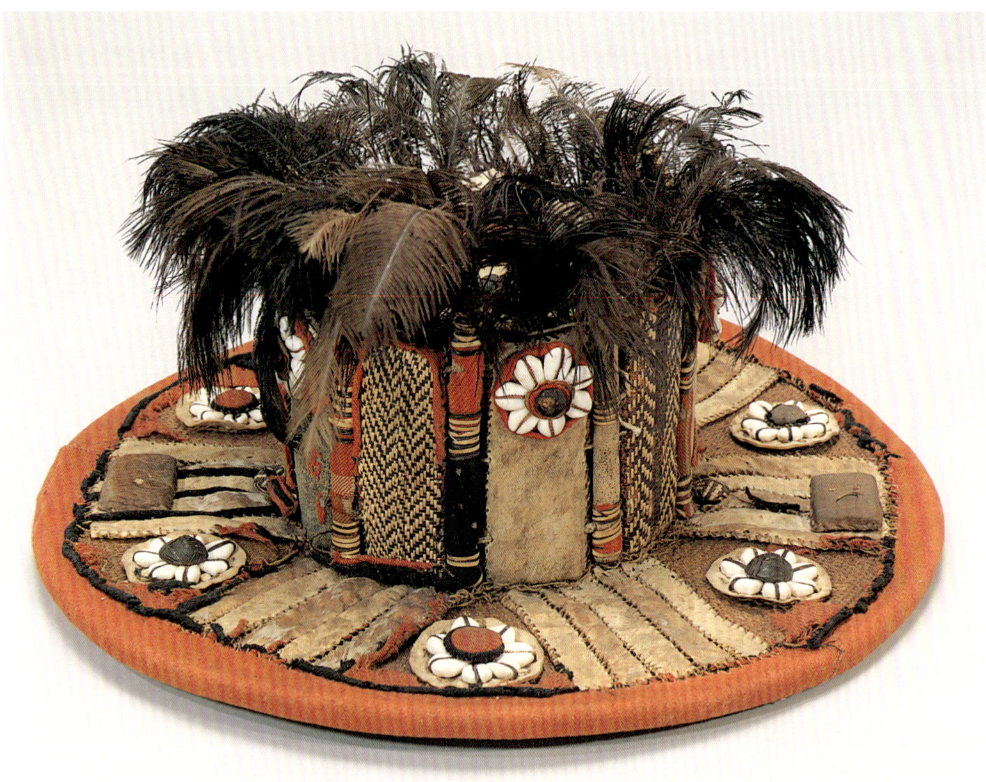

**Figure 2.3. Man's hat. Gola, northwestern Liberia. Fiber, cloth, cowries, feathers, leopard skin. H. 16.5 cm. Nineteenth century. Department of Anthropology, Smithsonian Institution NMNH E015,073. Photograph by Diane L. Nordeck.**

The Gola live in northwestern Liberia and are organized into many small chiefdoms. They are primarily agriculturists, with rice as the principal crop (d'Azevedo 1975:284–285). Today, the Gola regard themselves as a single ethnic group and share a common language and myth of origin. Prior to the nineteenth century, the region that now comprises present-day Liberia and Sierra Leone was ruled by a succession of federations under the control of powerful war chiefs. These federations were allied for long-distance trade and mutual protection, although many local communities were ethnically and culturally diverse and multilingual (d'Azevedo 1962:12–13).

In Gola society, the men's association *(Bon poro,* or *Poro)* and the women's association *(Sande),* are major avenues for the development of regional interrelationships. These organizations serve a number of critical social, political, and economic roles. One of their tasks is the maintenance of traditional institutions in the local community, but historically they were also important instruments of political and economic validation over the larger territories (d'Azevedo 1975:285).

## OBJECT

Adult men and women in Liberia wear head coverings in public as a matter of etiquette (Robert Leopold, personal communication 1994). On formal occasions, leaders might wear a hat like the one on display. The form and materials used on this hat suggest that it was worn by a prosperous Gola elder, for only the wealthiest individuals would have had access to imported wool, cowries, and ostrich feathers.

The oldest male and female members of high-ranking lineages (groups of families who trace their origins to the same ancestor) hold leadership positions in Gola communities and in the powerful men's *Bon poro* and women's *Sande* associations. Genealogical claims to important ancestors and to their great deeds are important factors in a person's self-esteem. A person of status knows his own worth because he knows his line of descent and its connections to the larger society (d'Azevedo 1962:16).

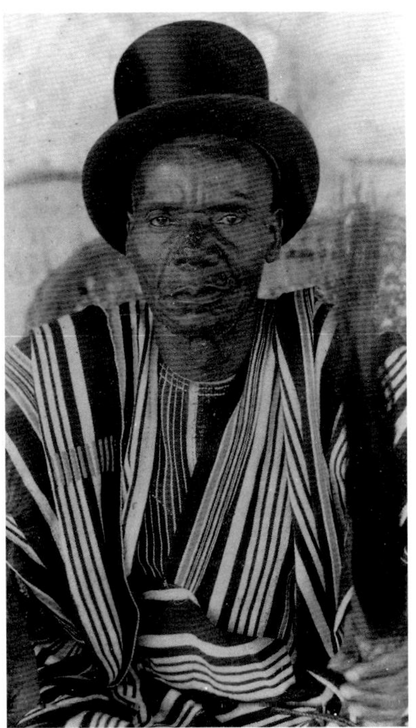

**Figure 2.4.** Chief Towai, Dan, wearing a top hat. Northeast Liberia, date unknown. Peabody Museum, Harvard University.

## TECHNIQUE

The hat base is a woven basketry form that is trimmed with imported red wool, leopard skin, and cowries, and embellished with ostrich feathers. The intricate cut leatherwork decorations are in a style that is similar to those still produced today by a professional caste of leatherworkers, who live and work not only in Liberia, but in also Guinea, Senegal, and Mali. In Gola society, only men who are members of the *Bon poro* association are entitled to wear the color red, and wearing leopard skin is an emblem of leadership. Cowries, once used as money throughout this region, symbolize wealth. Imported wool cloth and ostrich feathers, which are luxury materials, also symbolize wealth.

In 1822, the colony of Liberia was founded by African-Americans, who settled primarily on the coast. They called themselves Americo-Liberians. This new society was animated by nineteenth-century southern American Christian values. Americo-Liberian settlers reproduced many features of southern American culture, including the apparel; men wore top hats to all formal, public functions. The craftsman who made this hat appears to have been emulating the formal headwear of the urban Americo-Liberian gentlemen, while adding decorations that were meaningful to the Gola.

## COLLECTION

This hat was donated in 1874 by the Reverend Ralph Randolph Gurley of Baltimore, who was a prominent promoter of the new colony of Liberia and an agent for the American Colonization Society. In 1847, Liberia declared its independence from the American Colonization Society and became Africa's first independent Black republic. Americo-Liberians modeled their flag and constitution on the United States' and named their capital city, Monrovia, after President James Monroe. Gurley, along with Jehudi Ashmun, drafted the first provisional constitution. He visited Liberia in 1824 and again in 1849 after Liberia's independence. Throughout the nineteenth century, textiles and clothing, weapons, pottery, and tools from various ethnic groups in Liberia were regularly donated to the Smithsonian Institution by American missionaries, administrators, and military personnel, and merchants who had traveled or worked in Liberia.

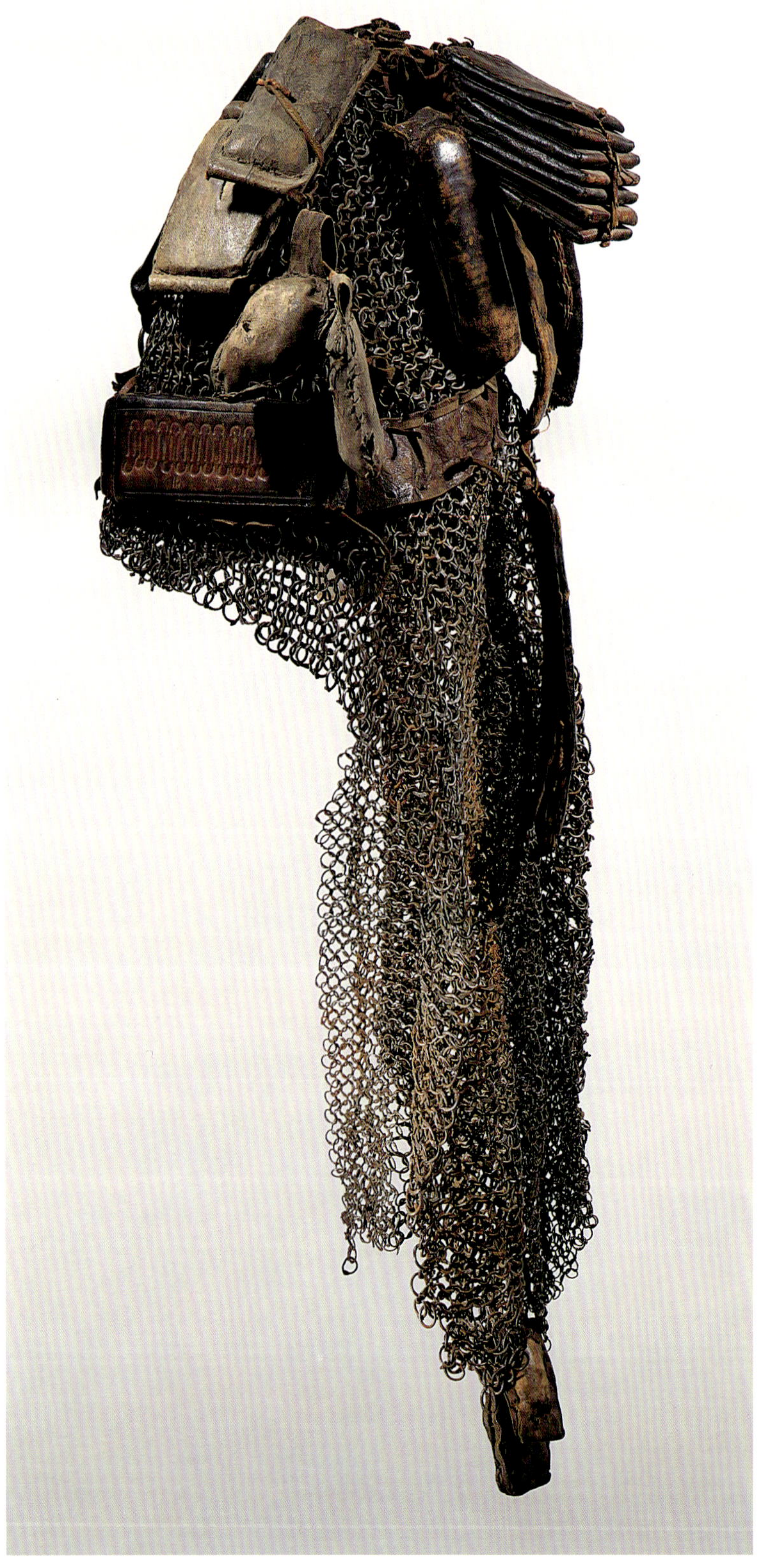

**Figure 2.5. Warrior's helmet. Sudan. Chain mail, leather, metal, string, cotton. H. 61.0 cm. Late nineteenth–early twentieth centuries. FMCH X65.8684**

Sudan has a population of between 15 and 20 million people and is culturally and ethnically diverse. In the northern areas most of the Arab peoples are identified on the basis of traditional genealogies with either the Juhayna or the Jaaliyyin-Danaqla. Non-Arab groups in this area include the Beja and the Nubians. Although Arabic is the official language of the country, over 115 other languages are spoken throughout the Sudan (Voll 1978:3–6).

During the Funj and Keira periods (between the sixteenth and nineteenth centuries), Islam was firmly established in the northern Sudan. In the early nineteenth century, the Turco-Egyptian forces of the Ottoman Empire conquered the northern and central areas, but by the late nineteenth century popular resentment towards these rulers had grown quite strong. Mohammad Ahmad al-Mahdi (1848–1885), a cleric, rose to prominence as a strong critic of the impiety of the Turco-Egyptian rulers. He mounted a *jihad* (holy war) against them in 1881 and ousted them by 1885 when the Mahdist forces took Khartoum and most of the northern Sudan. However, Anglo-Egyptian forces invaded the Sudan and eventually defeated the Madhist forces in 1898. In 1899 the British set up a new administration for the Sudan that lasted until its independence in 1956.

## OBJECT

For centuries, mounted warriors from north and central Sudan wore chain-mail armor to protect themselves during battle. Chain-mail headpieces protected the nape of the neck, while chain-mail tunics with sleeves and with side and back extensions well below the thigh, protected the body by deflecting blows from lances and swords. Chain-mail headpieces were worn with either a cloth turban or a metal helmet. In the nineteenth century, this armor was plentiful in the Sudan and every important chief *(melik)* was said to have had 200 to 300 chain-mail suits (Arkell 1956:83). Chain mail was worn by many of the Mahdist troops at the Battle of Omdurman in Sudan in 1898, and a number were brought back to England as battlefield trophies (Arkell 1956:83). Scholars have speculated that surplus armor from western Europe and from the Ottoman Empire and further east might well have found its way to Cairo merchants where it was exported into the Sudan (Spring 1993:36).

**Figure 2.6**, right. "Panzerreiter aus Dikoa" (rider in chain mail from Dikoa), Fulbe peoples, Northern Cameroon. Photographer unknown, ca. 1912. Kolonialkriegerdank, no. 1576. Courtesy of Museum für Volkerkunde, Leipzig, Germany. Protective chain-mail helmets and tunics were worn by the cavalry in the Sudan, northern Nigeria, and northern Cameroon.

## TECHNIQUE

Hamid Idris of Omdurman, interviewed in 1940 by A. J. Arkell, made armor for the Turco-Egyptian government and for the Mahdi in the last quarter of the nineteenth century. It was his opinion that armor made from individually riveted rings was imported from the "north" through Cairo (Arkell 1956:83). This headpiece has domed riveted rings and was probably imported from the Ottoman Empire or further east, rather than from western Europe where chain-mail armor had wedge-shaped rivets (Bivar 1964:83).

Both Omdurman and Sennar, the capital of the Funj kingdom south of Khartoum, were major centers for the production of chain-mail armor and tunics, and chain-mail tunics were made in Omdurman for ceremonial purposes as late as the 1940s (Arkell 1956:83). Local Sudanese craftsmen constructed their armor from butt-joined rings. According to Hamid Idris, it took about ten kilos of rings to make one tunic (Arkell 1956:83). The headpiece is built up by clipping together groups of rings. First, individual rings are linked together in groups of five, then an open ring is inserted into that grouping and closed. Then two groupings of five are clipped together by passing another open ring through a pair of closed rings from each group, and then the open ring is closed (Arkell 1956:84). The sewn leather packets attached to the headpiece are amulets, and on the Wellcome piece many of them probably contain passages from the Holy Koran. These amulets could be defensive or offensive charms and were used widely by warriors and others throughout Islamic Africa.

## COLLECTION

This helmet is part of a large collection of archaeological and ethnographic objects from Africa, India, Pakistan, Australia, the South Pacific, and Native America collected by Sir Henry Wellcome and donated to the University of California, Los Angeles in 1965. Wellcome (1853–1936) was born in the United States and went to England in 1880, where he founded the pharmaceutical firm of Burroughs-Wellcome. He later became a British citizen and was knighted in 1932. Wellcome directed archaeological excavations near Khartoum before World War I, but bought this piece at Sotheby's auction house in London.

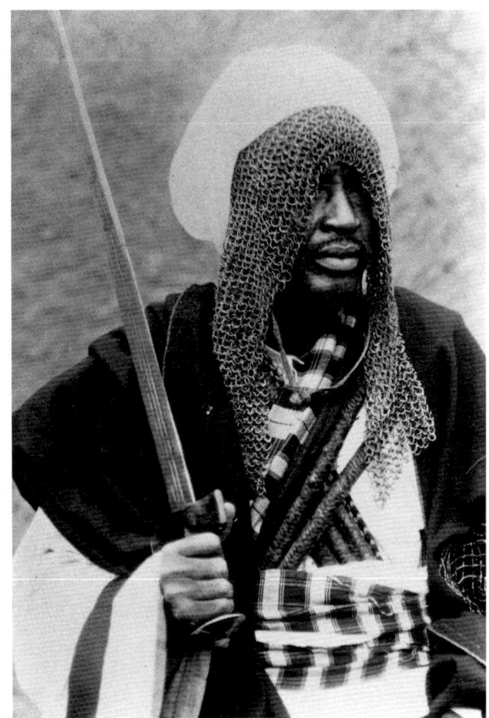

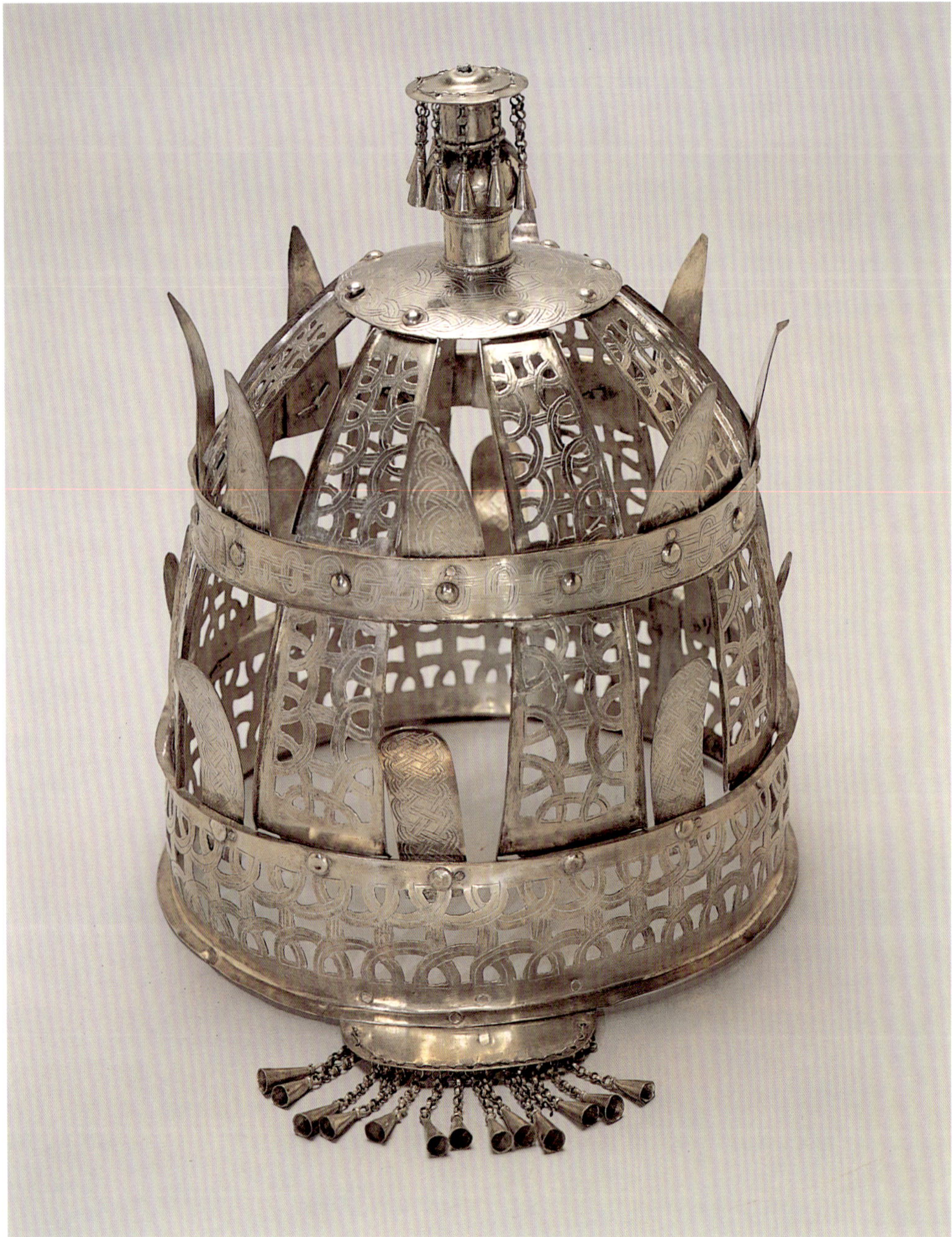

**Figure 2.7. Priest's crown *(aklil)*. Addis Ababa, Ethiopia. Silver. H. 27.0 cm. Late nineteenth–early twentieth century. Department of Anthropology, Smithsonian Institution NMNH E261,843. Photograph by Diane L. Nordeck.**

Ethiopia is one of the most ancient empires in Africa dating from the around 800 B.C. Christianity was introduced into the Aksumite Empire in the fourth century A.D. during the reign of the Emperor Ezana. Throughout the centuries, Christianity has provided a unifying force for the empire. In the seventh century, a series of struggles began between Moslems and Christians, and Aksum lost many of its ports on the Red Sea. During this period, the center of Ethiopian civilization shifted to the south in areas occupied by Amhara peoples, and the new Christian kingdom of Abyssinia arose. Throughout the next ten centuries, the Abyssinian kingdom's power waxed and waned. Following a period of decentralization, the emperors Theodore (1855–1867), John (1867–1889), and Menelik II (1889–1909) expanded their realms and increased control by reducing the power of the landed nobility and destroying the independence of regional dynasties. Menelik II reconquered the critical southern territories, as well as the northeastern and northwestern territories (Lewis 1965:20–44).

### OBJECT

Crowns *(aklil)* are part of the ecclesiastical vestments of the Ethiopian Christian Church and part of the Church treasury. Crowns are worn by priests and deacons during important religious festivals and at marriages (Buxton 1970:76). The first mention of crowns in Abyssinia dates from the seventeenth century, although crowns from Axum are known from a much earlier date (Buxton 1970:163–164). Today silver and brass crowns are generally worn over a colorful cloth turban. The Smithsonian's silver crown originally belonged to the Church of Saint George in Addis Ababa.

### TECHNIQUE

This crown is made of silver, which was scarce in Ethiopia until the end of the eighteenth century, when it began to be imported in large quantities in the form of Maria Theresa dollars. The Maria Theresa silver *thalar* (after which the American dollar was named) was common currency throughout Arabia and the horn of Africa after 1740 and was legal tender in Ethiopia until the mid-1940s (Buxton 1970:164).

Silversmiths melted *thalars* and beat the metal into sheets or used it for lost-wax casting. This crown consists of pierced metal bands: a brow band, a central band, and an apex plate that are secured to eight vertical, curving strips. A tubular structure is attached to the apex of the crown. Suspended from it by chains are ten little bells. A small oval plate juts out from the lower rim of the crown, which is fringed with bells and chains and resembles the visor of a cap. The designs engraved on the various bands consist of a series of self-involving loops which are found on other silver objects from this area.

### COLLECTION

Hoffman Philip (1872–1951) had a long and distinguished diplomatic career. In 1908–09, he served as the United States' minister resident to the Court of Emperor Menelik II and the consul-general to Abyssinia (present-day Ethiopia). In 1910, he loaned (donated in 1930) his collection to the Smithsonian which contained Ethiopian objects including coins, crosses, jewelry, religious paintings and scrolls, decorative shields and scabbards, and three hats. The three hats included the silver crown from the Church of St. George, a lion-mane headdress worn by high-ranking officers in the Abyssinian army, and an embroidered coiled basketry hat modeled after a brimmed European man's hat.

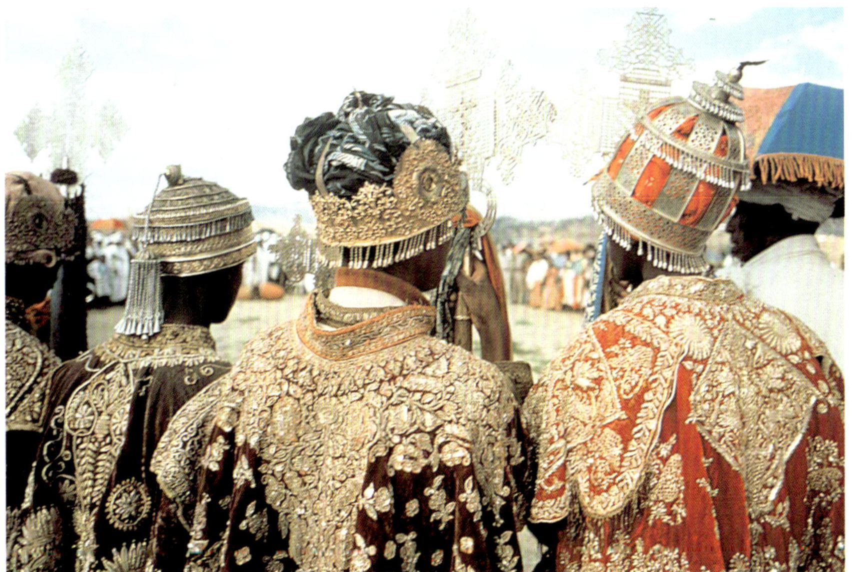

**Figure 2.8.** Timkat festival in Lalibela, Ethiopia. Photograph by James Payne, ca. 1975. Slide no. EP 58. Eliot Elisofon Photographic Archives. National Museum of African Art.

PEOPLE

**Figure 2.9. Women's headdress *(ekori)*. Herero, Botswana. Leather, iron beads. H. 48.0 cm. Twentieth century. Department of Anthropology, Smithsonian Institution NMNH E407,661a and E407,670b. Photograph by Diane L. Nordeck.**

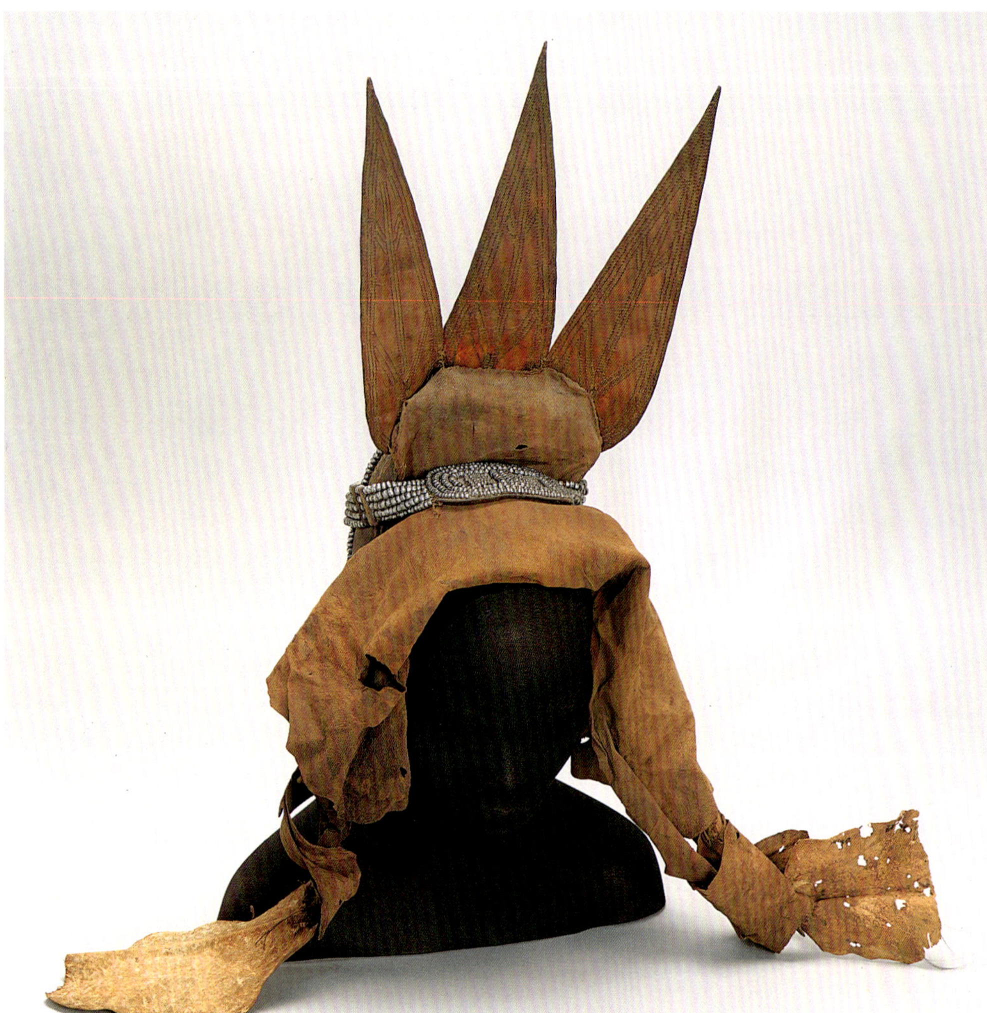

The Herero, a southwestern Bantu-speaking people, are divided into three geographically distinct groups called the Herero, the Mbanderu, and the Himba. Today the Herero subgroup lives primarily in Botswana. They share a common language, but historically they were not unified politically, nor did they share the same traditions of origin (Gibson 1956:111). Their primary occupation is cattle-herding, although they practice some agriculture. They formerly lived in dispersed settlements and practiced a form of nomadic pastoralism where younger men moved with the cattle to different grazing lands.

One or more household clusters formed the largest formal residential unit, the homestead *(onganda*; Gibson 1956:112). Each settlement is defended by an encircling thorn fence and dwellings are grouped in family compounds around a central open space that serves as the cattle corral. Members of the same homestead generally cooperate in political, economic, and ritual activities. The senior male member of a patrilineage is recognized as the ritual leader, and the symbols of his office are the sacred hearth, which occupies a prominent position in his homestead, his herd of sacred cows, and the milk vessels associated with the herd. Births, marriages, divorces, and deaths are announced to the ancestors at the sacred hearth (Gibson: 1956:123–125).

## OBJECT

This headdress *(ekori)* was worn on special occasions by Herero married women and this type dates from the nineteenth century or before. It is no longer worn by Herero women today. The metal bead decorations on the decorative band that is worn with the cap symbolize wealth. A variation of this style of leather headdress was also worn by Himba married women.

On most occasions, married women wore the leather veil rolled back off their faces. However, when a new bride was escorted to her husband's home, she unrolled the leather veil and covered her face. Several women would escort her, moving slowly, bent slightly forward from the waist and swaying back and forth imitating the gait of cattle. If she was widowed and chose to return to her natal home, she also arrived with the veil drawn down over her face. The form of the headdress, the materials, the decorative horns, and its use in rituals associated with marriage and widowhood seem a reminder of the ritual exchange of brideprice in cattle at marriage. While this exchange is minor in economic terms, it is important symbolically as a token of good faith on the part of the groom's family and a pledge of security for the wife (Gibson 1962:637).

Beginning in the late nineteenth century, Herero women, who became Christians, adopted a cloth headwrap. Like the old style leather headdress, the current cloth headwrap, known as the *otjikaiva,* also has two cloth projections, which the Herero refer to as horns.

## TECHNIQUE

The headdress consists of a curved leather cap *(ocipa)* to which three flat and peaked leather horns *(ozonya)* with ornamental stitching are sewn on top. A triangular soft skin veil is attached to the front of the cap, trailing downward to two decorative tails of sheepskin. An ornamental leather band *(ombeta)* with iron bead decoration is fastened around the cap. The cap itself is decorated with lines of stitching and rows of iron beads. The beads were made locally, not by the Herero, but by Ambo and Bergdama blacksmiths living among the Herero (Gibson 1962:621).

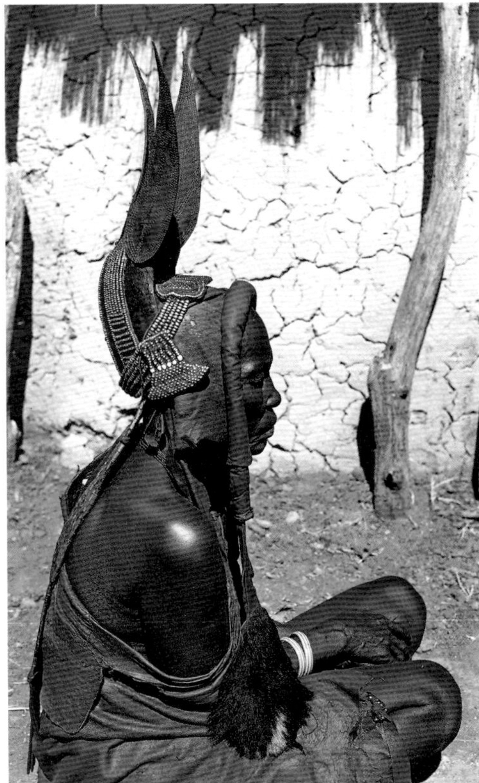

## COLLECTION

This headdress is part of a large collection of Herero and Himba material culture made by Dr. Gordon D. Gibson in Botswana in 1968. This collection includes items of dress as well as domestic objects. His field notes include local terms for the objects and information on their manufacture and use. During his field research, Dr. Gibson also took photographs and made several films about aspects of Herero and Himba life which are in the Human Studies Film Archive at the Smithsonian Institution. Dr. Gibson, an anthropologist, was the first curator of African ethnology at the National Museum of Natural History.

**Figure 2.10.** Herero woman, Mabanderu subgroup, Botswana. Photograph by G. D. Gibson, 1953.

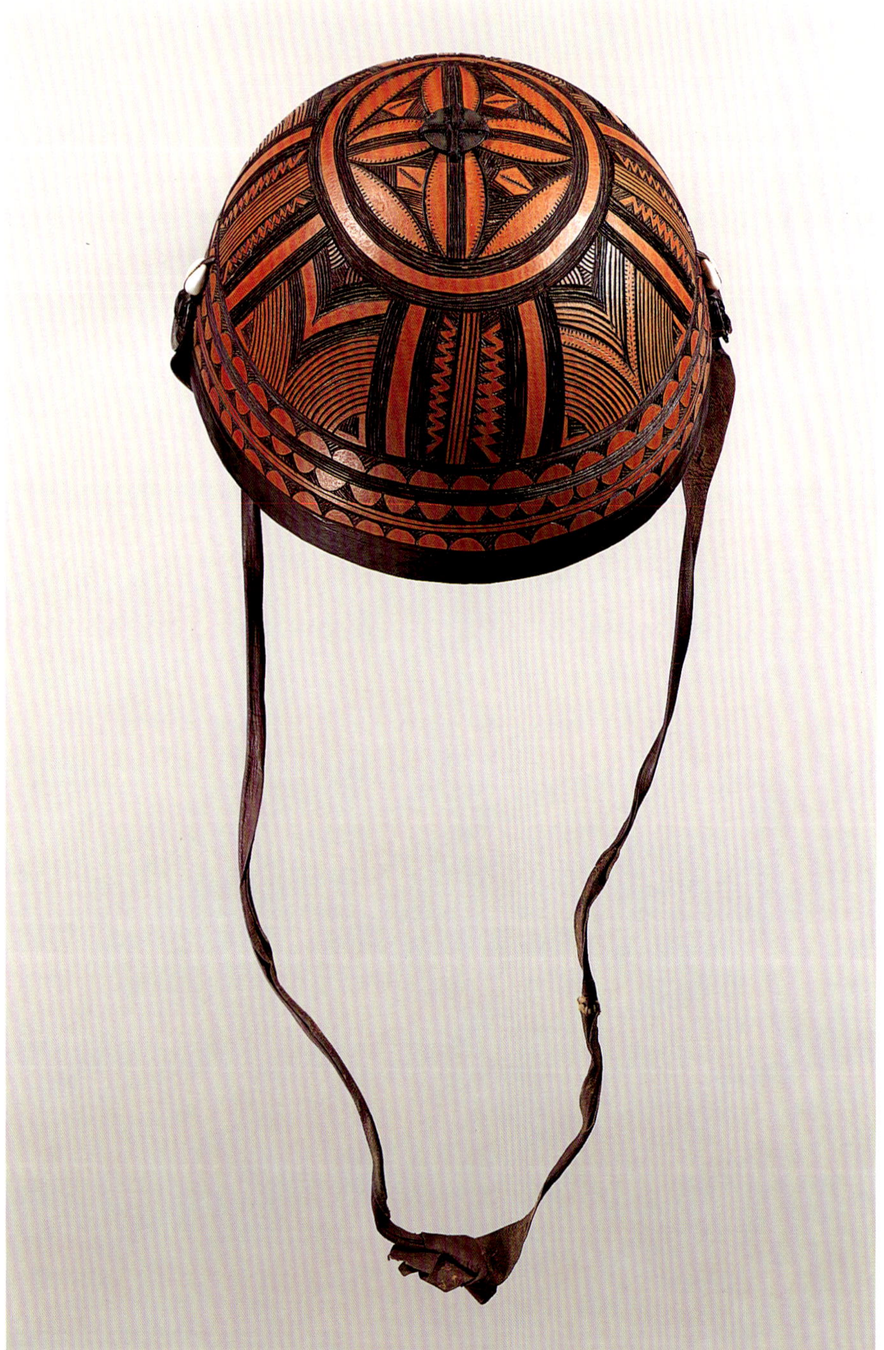

PEOPLE

**Figure 2.11. Baby's bonnet *(dambalem).* Bura, North East State, Nigeria. Gourd with cowries, Nigerian pennies, leather strap. Twentieth century. FMCH X83-760.**

The Bura people are one of a number of small ethnic groups that live in northeastern Nigeria. Their towns and settlements are located in the elevated grasslands of the Biu Plateau northeast of the confluence of Gongola and Hawal rivers.

The Bura speak a Chadic language and like many of their neighbors, the ancestors of the Bura migrated sometime in the remote past from the area around Lake Chad (Newman 1977, Sutton 1979). Until recently Bura villages remained culturally isolated and politically autonomous. Today, most Bura have adopted either Islam or Christianity.

## OBJECT

Decorated gourd sun hats *(dambalem)* are typically part of a baby's layette. For the first year or so of a child's life, the mother carries her baby on her back. The gourd hats, secured by a leather strap under the baby's chin, protect the child from the elements. However, these sun hats are more than merely functional. Bura women prefer traditional designs for objects of personal use like the baby hats. These designs communicate the ethnic identity of the mother and child. The care with which they are decorated clearly underscores their cultural value as objects of aesthetic display. These valued objects are regularly kept within families and passed down for use by its newest members (Rubin 1970:23, Berns 1985:40, Berns and Rubin Hudson 1986:56).

Decorated gourds communicate social, economic, and aesthetic values. Among many groups in the area, gourds are essential items of household equipment, and decorated bowls in a variety of sizes and shapes are made and owned by women (Berns 1985, Berns and Rubin Hudson 1986, Chappel 1977). Gourds play a central role in marriage rites and are an important symbol of a bride's transition to full marital status. Decorated gourds are an essential part of the groom's family's bridewealth payments; the bride's dowry, which is provided by her family, consists of a large collection of decorated gourds. This gourd capital, which she brings to her new home, symbolizes her economic status and her ability to set up her household (Berns 1985, Chappel 1977).

## TECHNIQUE

Gourd decoration is an ancient art in the area and probably began with the shift from a stone-based to an iron-based economy sometime after the fifth or sixth century A.D. (David 1976:237). Among the Bura, gourd decoration is a woman's art. The gourd is first prepared by soaking it until its contents rot. It is then cut open, the pulp is removed, and the shell is allowed to dry. At this stage it is ready for decoration.

Bura women pryo-engrave their gourds, which involves burning lines into the surface of the gourd with a hot metal blade. The women work with several forged iron tools. Leaf-shaped blades with long, straight shafts are embedded in circular wooden handles. The artist holds the tool in one hand and the gourd in the other. As she turns the gourd away from her body, the artist pulls the knife toward her, burning the design into the gourd's surface. Pyro-engraving allows the artist to produce long fluid lines. Bura designs are characterized by a dense overall decoration of the surface with little interplay between figure and ground. They are defined by a central circle framed by concentric circles or, in this example, by four vertical registers that are filled with symmetrical patterns. Some design names are based on organic referents, such as the cowrie design *(lakandam)* in the center circle of this baby sun hat. Other names describe particular techniques such as cross-hatching or curves (Rubin 1970:23). For decades Bura women have produced decorated gourds for the market and especially accomplished artists are known over a wide area.

## COLLECTION

This baby's sun hat was made by Patum, a Bura woman from the village of Zoana. It is part of a group of 214 decorated gourds that were donated to the Fowler Museum of Cultural History by Barbara Rubin Hudson. Rubin Hudson made this field collection between 1969–1971 in Northeastern Nigeria where she conducted research on decorated gourds among the Bura and neighboring groups. This collection was featured in the Fowler Museum's 1986 traveling exhibition *The Essential Gourd: Art and History in Northeastern Nigeria.*

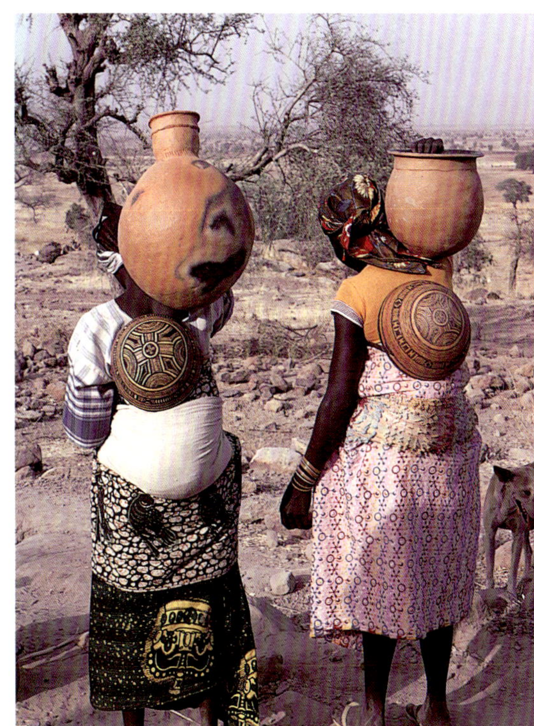

**Figure 2.12**. Waja women using gourd bonnets *(gakire)* to shield their babies from the sun when going to the well to fetch water. Talesse, Nigeria. Photograph by Marla Berns, 1982

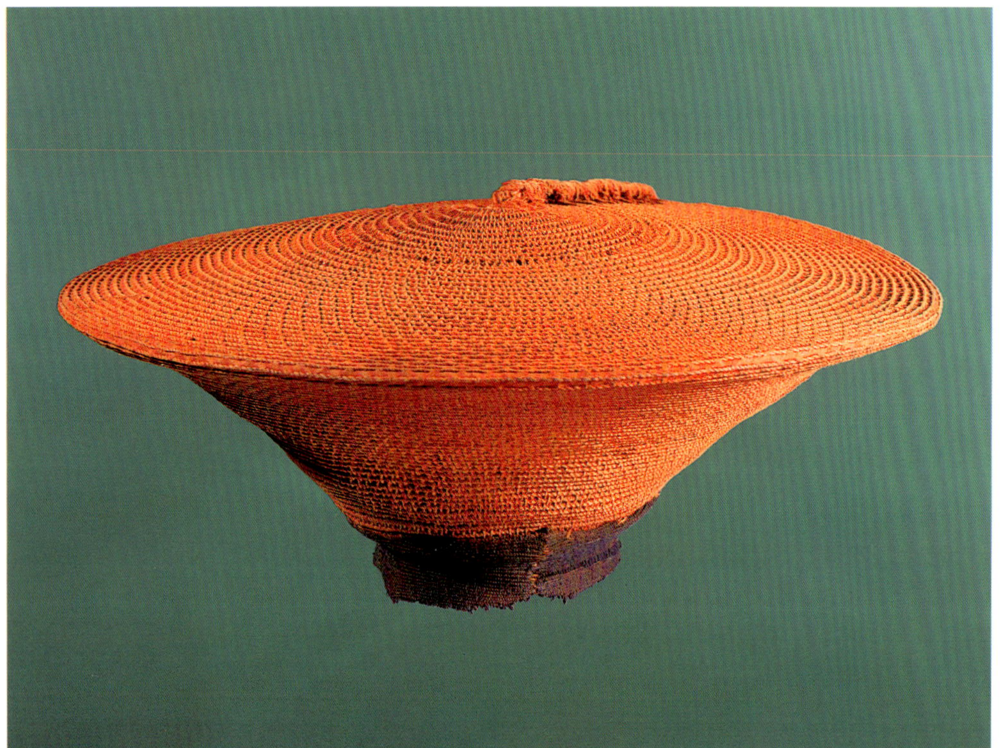

**Figure 2.13. Zulu woman's hat *(isicholo).* Misinga District, Natal province, South Africa. Grass/bast fiber, fat, ochre. H. 15.0 cm. Twentieth century. Neutrogena Corporation.**

The Zulu are Nguni-speaking peoples, many of whom still live in the Natal province in South Africa. In the early nineteenth century, the Zulu kingdom emerged as the central political authority in this area under the formidable leadership of Shaka ka Senzagakona. The Zulu expansionist period (1818–1828) coincided with the arrival of English settlers at Port Natal (1824). Throughout the nineteenth century, Zulu armies clashed with the English and the Dutch, who had pushed into the territory. Following years of confrontation, the Zulu army was defeated by British forces in 1879. Shortly thereafter, the Zulu kingdom was incorporated into the British Colony of Natal and the power of the Zulu kings was severely curtailed (Wilson and Thompson 1969).

In 1910, the provinces of South Africa were united and received independence within the British Empire. Blacks were systematically disenfranchised and in 1948 the Nationalist Party instituted the pernicious policy of "separate development" or apartheid. KwaZulu, a Zulu homeland, was created and though the Zulu retained a king, his power was more symbolic than real. In 1994, after decades of struggle, the system of apartheid was finally dismantled and Nelson Mandela was elected as the first president in post-apartheid South Africa.

## OBJECT

Zulu women's hats *(isicholo)* developed in the late nineteenth century and were based on a married woman's hair style also called *isicholo.* In the early nineteenth century, married women regularly shaved their heads leaving only a small tuft of hair on the crown which they smeared with a mixture of fat and ochre. During the latter half of the nineteenth century, women let this tuft grow several inches in length resembling a truncated cone (Fynn 1969:293–294). To give the hair cone its desired volume, grass or false hair was sometimes woven into the hair and the whole smeared with fat and ochre as before (Krige 1965 [1936]:372). Women also wore a woven fiber headband above the forehead as a sign of respect for adult men in their husband's family (Kennedy 1978:13). At the turn of the nineteenth century, this cone-shaped coiffure was replaced by a detachable woven hat. Today, most women wear Western fashions every day. However, in Msinga district, where the Zulu king resides, dress tends to be more conservative and *isicholo* hats are sometimes worn on a daily basis. Most Zulu women wear these hats only for special or ceremonial occasions (Kennedy 1978:15).

**Figure 2.14**, right. Zulu woman wearing a flared basketry hat at the agricultural fair in Mahlabatini, South Africa. Photograph by Carolee Kennedy, August 1977.

## TECHNIQUE

Several styles of women's hats have evolved from the cone-shaped coiffure. The most elaborate form is the wide flared hat with a woven headband attached to the base. This is the preferred style of married women in the area around Tugula Ferry (Kennedy 1978:15). A basketry foundation is overlaid with string dyed with a mixture of red ochre and fat, or with brightly colored commercial red yarn. Women regularly buy undecorated hats from shops and decorate them before wearing them. At the insistence of taxi drivers who complained that the dye on the hats left marks on the headliners of their cars, women responded by tying colorful imported scarves over the hats. This practice evolved quickly into a fashion statement and now women invest in new styles and colors of scarves as preferences change from year to year (Carolee Kennedy, personal communication 1994).

In other Zulu areas, women prefer a more columnar hat form. These hats are constructed using a basketry frame covered with nylon netting, string, or yarn which is covered with red ochre mixed with fat. Women often decorate these hats with beaded bands sewn on the top and center of the front of the hat. Both the older cone-shaped coiffure and the various styles of detachable woven hats are the material and symbolic equivalents of men's headrings, the *isicoco,* which are no longer worn. Like the women's coiffures and later the hats, the men's headrings were markers of a man's maturity and his marital status.

## COLLECTION

The Neutrogena Corporation purchased this hat from Mary Hunt Kahlenberg of Textile Arts Gallery, Santa Fe, New Mexico in 1989. The Neutrogena Collection is one of the largest corporate collections of art in the United States. It contains a broad range of expressive culture from a wide variety of countries and time periods and is especially recognized for its textile holdings from Japan, Indonesia, and Zaire. The objects in the collection were personally selected by its CEO and Chairman Lloyd Cotsen who is well-known for his leadership in support of educational and arts institutions. The collection is displayed at the company headquarters in Los Angeles in a truely unique work environment.

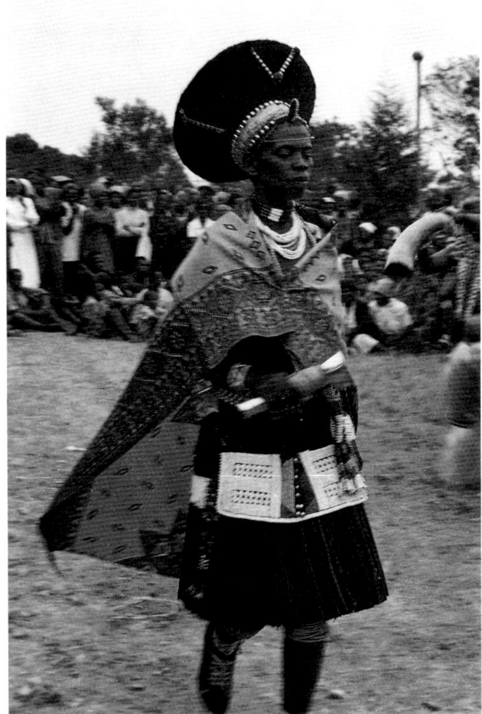

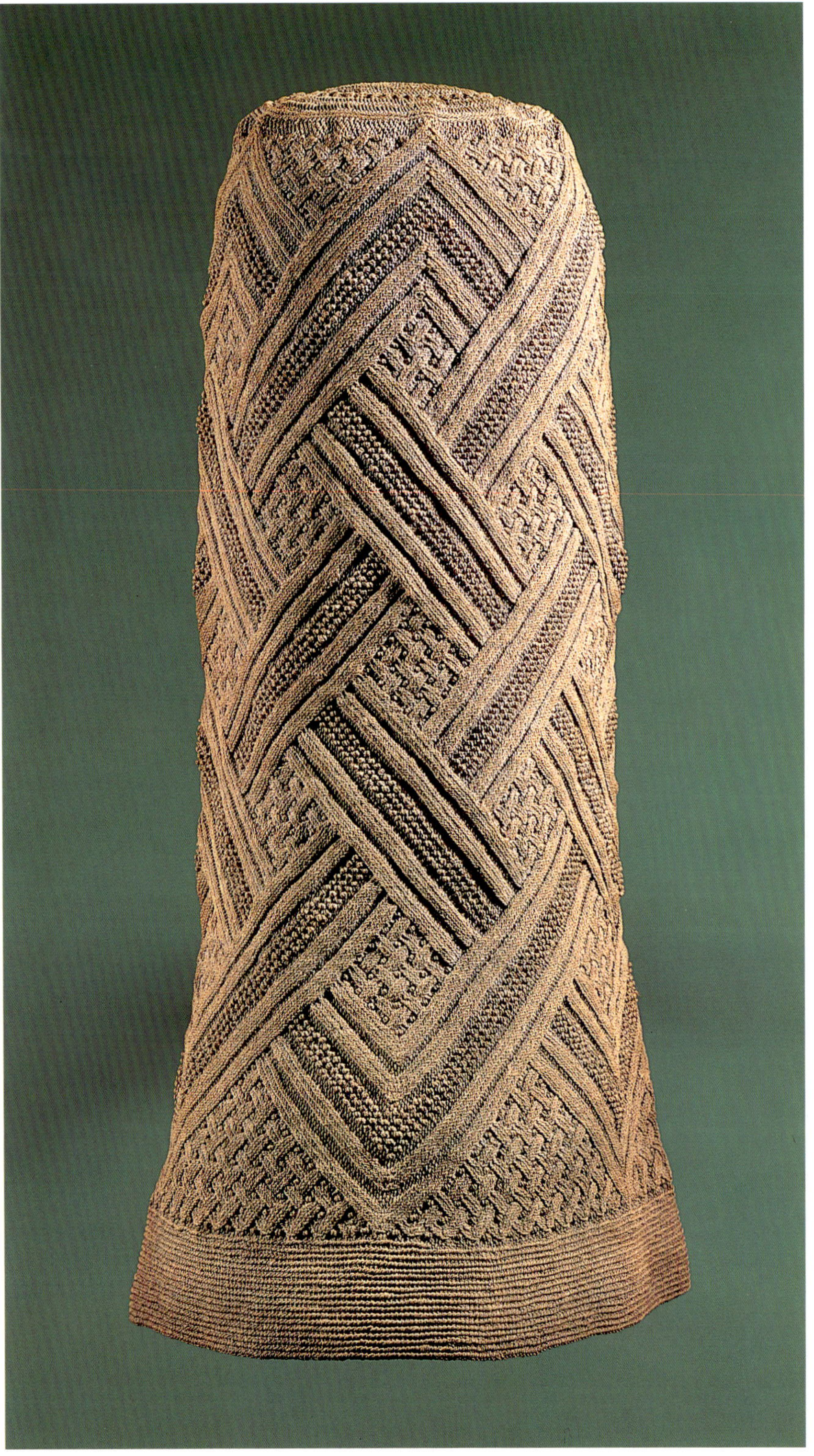

**Figure 2.15. Chief's hat *(mpu)*. Kongo, Republic of Congo and Zaire. Raffia palm fiber. H. 35.5 cm. Late nineteenth century. Neutrogena Corporation**

The Kongo people live along the coast and the lower Zaire River region of the Republic of the Congo, Zaire, Cabinda, and northwestern Angola. The kingdom of the Kongo was founded in the last half of the fourteenth century. When Portuguese traders reached the Kongo kingdom in 1482, they encountered a well-formed centralized political system that included a divine king and a cadre of governors, senior advisors, and village chiefs (Koloss 1990:12). Wood and ivory carving, funerary sculpture, raffia fiber weaving, pottery, iron-working, and other arts were well-developed. An important center of trade, the kingdom of the Kongo was influenced not only by European commerce but by Christianity which was introduced in the late fifteenth century. Although the Kongo remain a prominent people in present-day Zaire and the Republic of the Congo, the extent of the kingdom declined in the eighteenth and nineteenth centuries.

## OBJECT

Among the Kongo and related groups in Zaire, Angola, and the Republic of the Congo, caps *(mpu)* function as insignia of status and authority. The importance of the cap as a symbol of leadership is demonstrated by the Kongo word for village chief, *mfumu* or *mfumu a mpu,* "chief of the cap" (Gibson and McGurk 1977:73). At the lowest level of political hierarchy, the village chief *(nkazi)* is charged with overseeing the village's political, judicial, and economic activities. The chief is also seen as an important ritual leader responsible for maintaining proper spiritual relations with the ancestors for the benefit of the village population. The transfer of political office is signalled by the passing of the cap belonging to the late chief to his successor.

From the sixteenth to the early twentieth century, European visitors to the region provided fairly detailed descriptions and illustrations of royal attire including the hats. As early as 1491, the Portuguese explorer, Rui de Sousa, noted that in the Kongo capital, the king wore a mitre-like hat made of finely woven raffia palm cloth that gave the impression of being a luxury velvet (Fourneau and Kravetz 1954:5). Close-fitting woven raffia caps were reserved for men and women of noble rank and, like the tall hats, were ornamented with raised linear patterns and geometric designs. Figure carvings from the region, dating from the seventeenth century on include depictions of these intricately patterned caps.

## TECHNIQUE

Men make the caps and fashion them from palm leaves, pineapple fibers, and banana fibers, as well as cotton, grasses, and baobab fibers. The interior fibers of these plants are stripped, dried, and then shredded into thin "threads" (Gibson and McGurk 1977:80). Most caps are constructed in a spiral form, working from the center of the crown out to the edge of the hat border. Many caps are characterized by half and one-and-a-half twist constructions, where the fiber thread is wrapped or looped around itself one or more times creating tightly woven patterns (Gibson and McGurk 1977:83). Additional geometric designs are made using the overhand knot technique which gives the cap a raised knotted surface. Lateral loops along the border of many caps create a ribbed border design with either a rounded or angular braided appearance. Slip knots of various forms create openwork patterns that characterize the crowns of many Kongo caps. Leopard claws, tusks, feathers, shells, and other materials decorate some of the higher-status hats.

**Figure 2.16.** Woman and child figure, collected before 1914. Kongo peoples, Congo and Zaire. Wood, mirror, glass beads, fiber, metal, brass tacks. H. 25.7 cm. Purchased with funds provided by the Smithsonian Collections Acquisition Program, 83-3-6. Photograph by National Museum of African Art. The female figure wears a raffia cap associated with high-ranking men and women in Kongo society.

## COLLECTION

This hat was originally part of the James Hooper collection. Beginning as a young man, Hooper (1894–1971) actively collected art from Oceania, Africa, and the Americas. In 1957 he founded his own museum, the Totems Museum, at Arundel in Sussex. The museum closed in 1964, and after Hooper's death in 1971, the entire collection was catalogued and sold at a Christie's auction in London in 1976. Subsequently, the hat came into the possession of a Belgian dealer and then it was purchased by Mary Hunt Kahlenberg. She sold it to the Neutrogena Corporation in 1982.

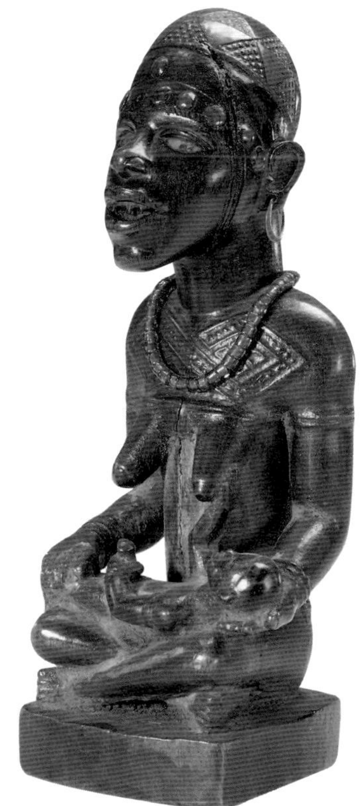

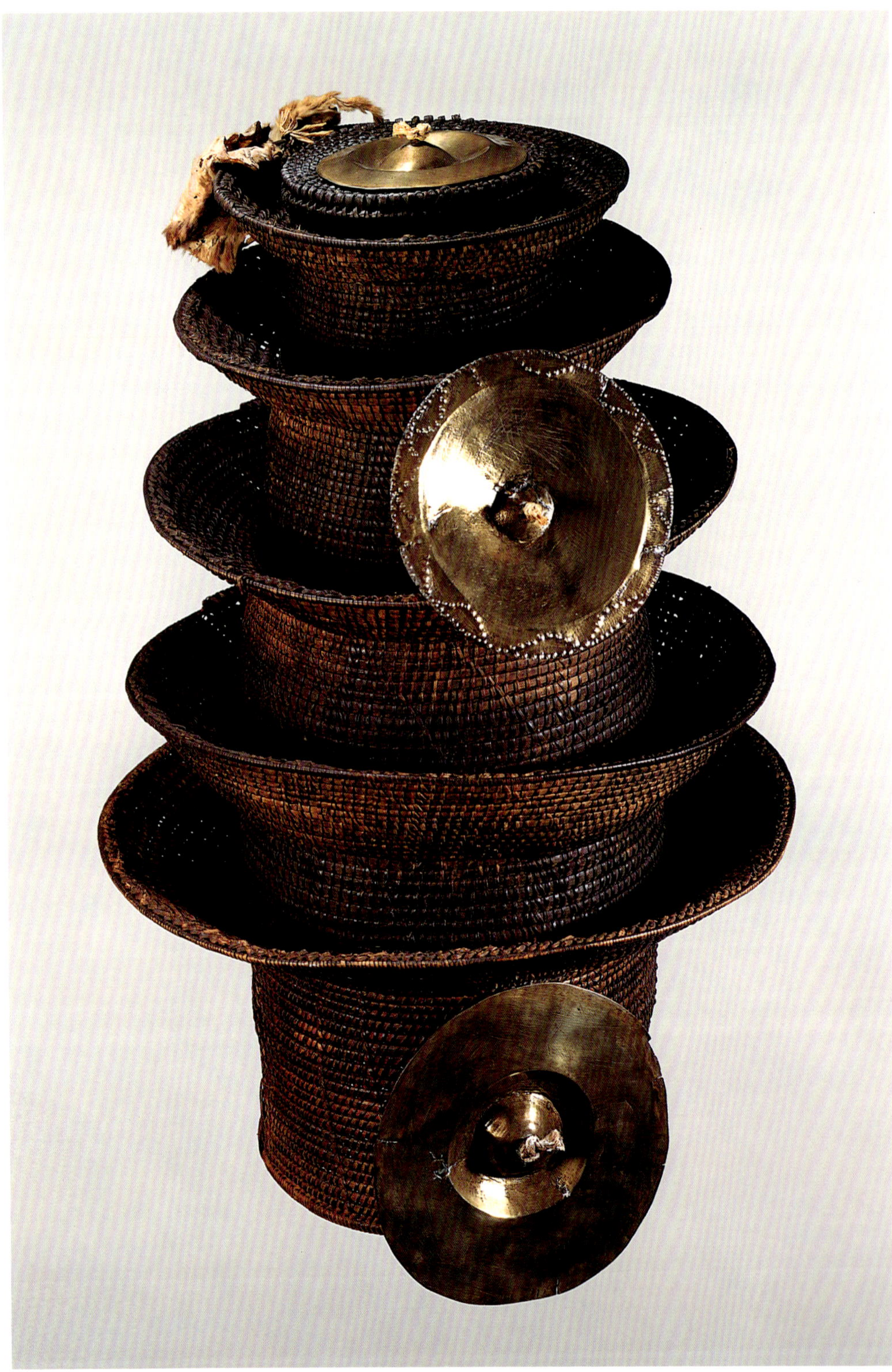

**Figure 2.17. Chief's hat *(botolo).* Ekonda, Zaire. Vegetable fiber, brass, fur, fiber cord. H. 45.0 cm. Nineteenth–twentieth century. FMCH X425.6.**

The Ekonda (also known as the Baseka) and related Bantu groups live in northwestern Zaire near the border with the Republic of the Congo as part of the great Mongo nation (Murdock 1959:84). They number under 500,000. Agriculture, hunting, and fishing are the primary occupations; manioc, bananas, yams, maize, peanuts, and sweet potatoes are the principal crops. Although there are secular political systems in place in the region, the village chief (*nkumu*) still features prominently in the socio-religious organization. The authority of the chief is conferred by the elders of the village and is associated with the powers of the ancestors, important ritual functions, and divination. The material objects that validate village-based chieftaincy are the *botolo* (or *montolo*), a special kind of raffia headwear, and a stool called *mbata* (H. Brown 1944:434).

## OBJECT

This Ekonda hat *(botolo)* is also worn by neighboring groups including the Ntumba, Bolia, Badia, Iyembe, Sengele, and some Sakata (Biebuyck and Van den Abbeele 1984:96). Among the Ntumba, for example, the hat is called *montolo* and is worn as an insignia of office by the *nkumu* (ritual chief) of the region. If a chief is the first in his line, he must purchase the hat; hats of deceased chiefs are safeguarded and passed down to their successors. The hat itself is brought out on the occasion when the chief is named and assumes office (H. Brown 1944:434–435).

The chief's hat is a critical part of his public dress. Propriety dictates that Ntumba men should appear during the day with their heads covered, and they may wear skin hats called *louku* which have long been part of the daily dress of men. It is the obligation of the chief, however, to always wear his *montolo* hat when in public during the day. For displays at certain public occasions, the chief's hat, including the brass disks or plates, may be smeared with camwood powder mixed with oil (H. Brown 1944:438–439).

## TECHNIQUE

The hat is made from woven raffia or cane fibers that are fashioned into a tall, cylindrical shape accented with horizontal bands along the top that project out from the surface of the hat. Burnished brass disks, which may be locally made or imported from a neighboring group, are attached to the hat using fiber thread. There is usually a disk at the front of the hat and others may be sewn to the top or back according to the taste of the hatmaker. In the 1940s, due to the scarcity of brass disks, it became fashionable to suspend a row of safety pins from the brim (H. Brown 1944:435). It is likely that the large brass disks that ornamented hats of this style functioned as items of wealth and prestige, enhancing the visual power of the hat and emphasizing the considerable prominence of the wearer.

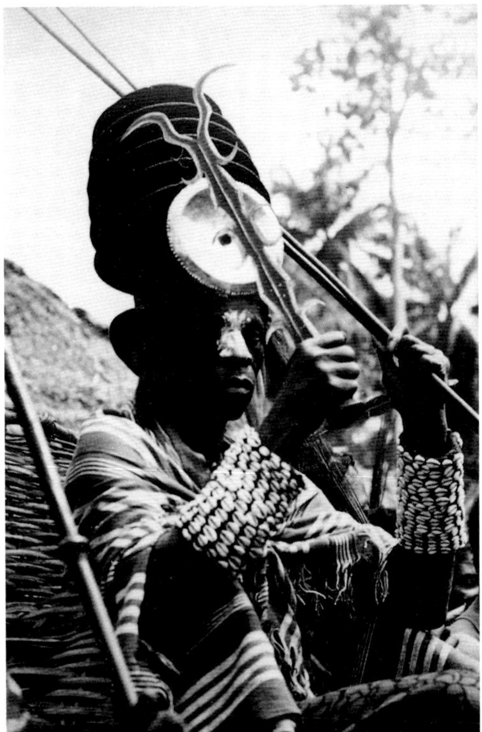

## COLLECTION

Jean Pierre Hallet was a Belgian colonial official who amassed a large collection of African art and subsequently opened the Central African Curio Shop in the former Belgian Congo. In 1961, he brought his collection to California and opened Congoland U.S.A. in Bakersfield. Through the initiative of former chancellor Dr. Franklin Murphy, UCLA purchased Mr. Hallet's collection of 5,000 objects in 1963 for $100,000. Hallet is well-known for his popular books *Congo Kitabu* (1966), *Animal Kitab*u (1967), and *Pygmy Kitabu* (1973), *kitabu* being the Swahili word for "stories."

**Figure 2.18**. Musée Royal de l'Afrique Centrale, Tervuren, Belgium. Photographer unknown.

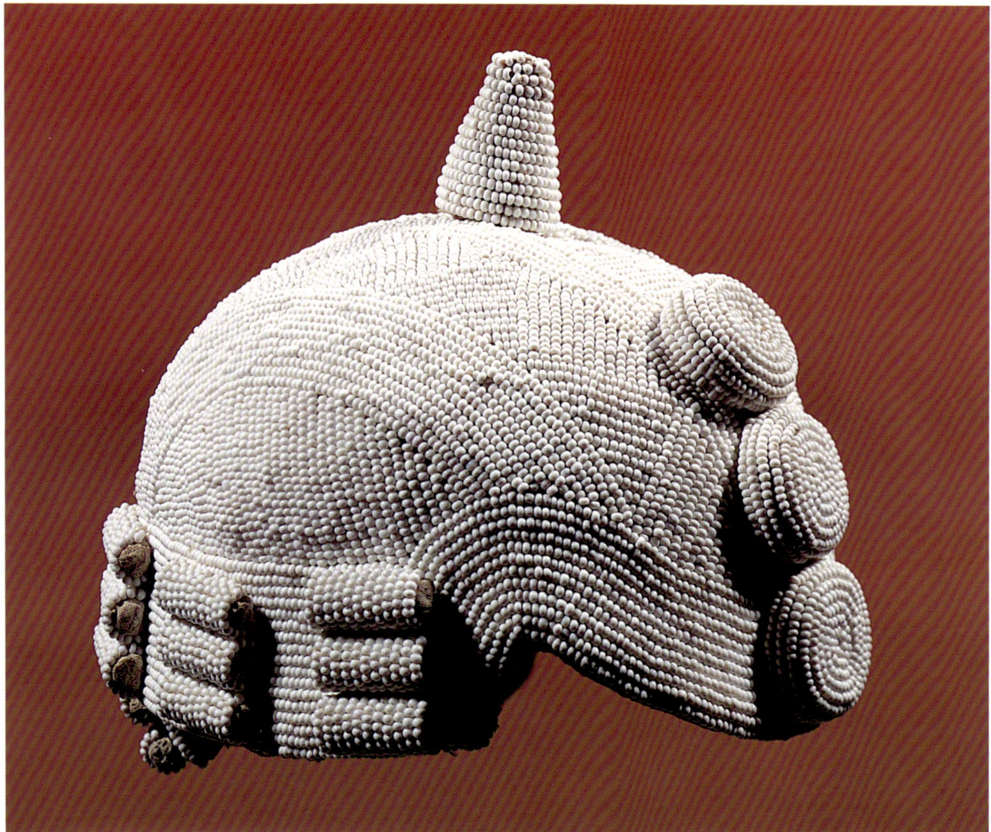

**Figure 2.19. King's crown *(orikogbofo).* Yoruba, southwestern Nigeria. Raffia, canvas, glass beads. H. 19.0 cm. Twentieth century. FMCH X91.8086.**

The Yoruba-speaking peoples live in southwestern Nigeria and number over twenty million people. They are the predominant ethnic group in Nigeria's Ogun, Oyo, Lagos, and Kwara states, and large communities of Yoruba people also live in the neighboring countries of Benin and Togo. Agriculture, craft specialization, and trade were once the mainstays of Yoruba society. Today, many Yoruba are also engaged in a variety of professions such as law, education, civil service, business, and manufacturing.

Historically, the Yoruba were divided into independent city-states that were ruled by Obas (kings), who owed their spiritual allegiance, if not their political allegiance, to Ife where according to myth, the world began. Within each city-state, the Oba is the focal point of Yoruba identity and unity. An Oba must be elected by consensus which involves complicated interactions between the royal family, kingmakers, women in the palace, and the Ifa oracle. The election of a new Oba can be fraught with many disputes and take years to resolve.

## OBJECT

As with other elements of royal regalia, Obas typically own more than one beaded crown. The Olokuku of Okuku, for example, has fifty-eight beaded crowns in his collection (Beier 1982:48). His ritual crowns are imbued with powerful medicines and all of them have *oriki,* or praise names. Obas also have other beaded headwear *(orikogbofo)* that are more casual royal hats worn for secular events (Thompson 1972:230, Euba 1985:4).

In the early 1980s, there were six beaded barrister wig crowns in the Olokuku collection. The Oba wears this type of crown when he presides over the opening of the legislature, the opening ceremonies for local courts, or numerous other social occasions (Beier 1982:85). Vestiges of the British legal system are apparent in Nigeria today. This Yoruba beaded hat in the form of a powdered barrister's wig makes an unambiguous link between Yoruba chiefly authority and the contemporary Nigerian judicial system where members of the judiciary still wear powdered wigs as part of their official attire. There is a marvelous sense of humor, playfulness, and political astuteness in choosing to imitate the barrister's wig, reminding everyone that the traditional power of the Oba clearly transcends the secular state power. While the conical ritual crowns with beaded veils *(ade)* are the central symbol of the divine king's authority, the beaded barrister-style crowns have a projection from the top that seems to allude to the sacredness of the Oba's head and his role as intermediary between his people and the gods.

## TECHNIQUE

Since *orikogbofo* are not sacred, the crownmaker is not bound by convention and can give free reign to his imagination both in creating the forms and choosing the colors and motifs (Beier 1982:85). These beaded crowns are made the same way as the ritual crowns. A wickerwork or cardboard frame is covered with cloth and then strands of beads are sewn onto the cloth that covers the frame. Glass beads were being used on Yoruba crowns by the middle of the seventeenth century, and today professional crownmakers use a variety of imported glass beads. Many glass beads were traded into Yorubaland during the period of the slave trade between the seventeenth and nineteenth centuries either from coastal trade with Europeans or from the North African trans-Saharan trade. Today, older beads are often recycled, but new ones continue to be imported. Some of the major bead centers in the Yoruba region are Efon-Alaye, Ile-Ife, Oyo, Ilesha, Abeokuta, and Iperu-Remo (Thompson 1972:229).

## COLLECTION

This crown can only be traced back as far as 1988 when it was in the possession of the late Alfred L. Scheinberg, a prominent New York City dealer who offered it for sale for $1,200. It was acquired by another New York dealer, Nobel Endicott, who sold it to the UCLA Fowler Museum for $2,000 in 1991.

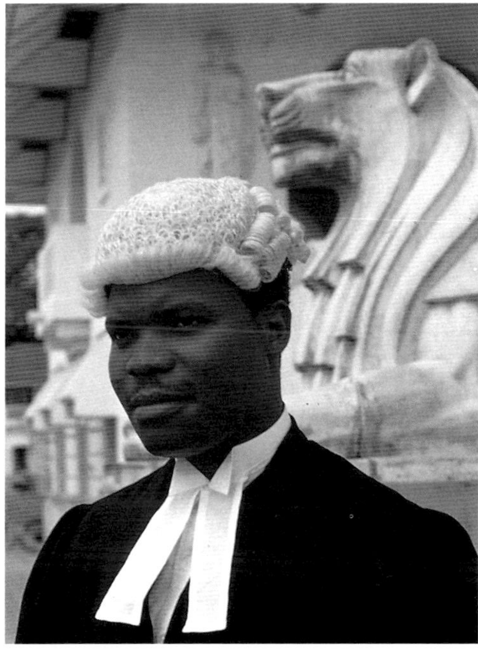

**Figure 2.20**. Barrister at High Court. Nigeria. Photograph by Eliot Elisofon, 1959. Slide no. C NIG 21.5 (1929). Eliot Elisofon Photographic Archives. National Museum of African Art.

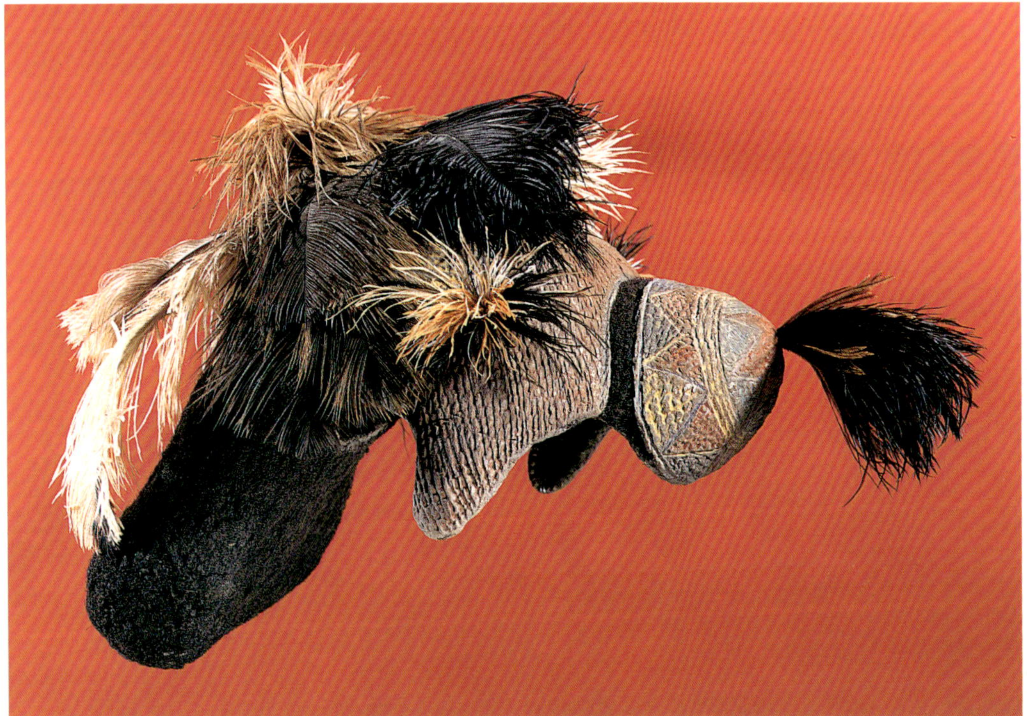

**Figure 2.21. Mudpack coiffure *(emedot)*. Karamojong, Uganda, Kenya. Earth, pigment, ostrich feathers, human hair, beads. H. 26.0 cm. Twentieth century. FMCH X94.25.1.**

The Karamojong belong to a cluster of ethnic groups who share a dialect and who have a common cultural heritage. According to oral history, the Karamojong are the original group from which the Jie, Dodoth, Turkana, Toposa, Jiye, and Donyiro are descended (Gulliver 1952:5). The Karamojong live primarily in eastern Uganda and in western Kenya. They have a mixed economy with women practicing agriculture and men taking primary responsibility for cattle-keeping. Karamojong move with their cattle to different pastures depending on the requirements of the herd and the season. Prior to the enforced peace in the mid-1920s, the Karamojong regularly raided other neighboring groups for cattle and other stock.

## Object

Among the Karamojong, mudpack coiffures *(emedot)* are worn by adult men. A man's hair style generally stays the same throughout his adult life, unlike the Pokot, for example, where some hair styles and decorations are restricted to certain age-sets and grades. A Karamojong man shows his status as an elder or a warrior by the addition of colored ostrich feathers to his coiffure. His hair style takes the form of a large bun of hair at the back of the head and an intricately designed plate in colored ochres above the forehead (Gulliver and Gulliver 1953:35).

Prior to the arrival of the British in the early 1920s, older men wore a bun of matted hair and mud that was detachable and might reach as far down the back as the waist. This style could still occasionally be seen in the early 1950s (Gulliver 1952:4).

## Technique

Creating this hair style is time-consuming and requires the help of friends. The front of the hair that forms the plate is mudded over with gray ochre. When dry, this base is divided into six or eight squares, each of a different color, with a contrasting color forming a border between two squares. The whole is stippled with a tooth comb (Gulliver and Gulliver 1953:35). Precious and highly valued ostrich feathers, which are signs of status, may be inserted into the crown of the coiffure, visually extending the height of the wearer and adding a touch of spectacle and drama to the coiffure.

An uninitiated adolescent wears quite a different hair style. Until puberty a boy's hair is cut short; then he begins to let it grow until it can be worked into a bun. Mud is applied to the bun and then a friend sews sisal string dyed red with ochre around it until the hair resembles a tall columnar hat, not unlike a fez in shape (Gulliver and Gulliver 1953:35).

## Collection

Mudpack coiffures were formerly maintained and repaired so that they could be worn for weeks before they had to be replaced. When the hair grew out and the mudpack became otherwise unserviceable, the mud was chipped away ,the hair was cleaned and cut, and a new hair style was created. Today, these coiffures are valuable commodities, sought out by museums and private collectors. Men take great care with their hair, shaving off the coiffures, and preserving them for sale.

This mudpack coiffure was purchased from an unidentified dealer in August 1994 by Ruth Schaftner, Director of Gallery Watatu in Nairobi, Kenya. It was purchased that same month by the UCLA Fowler Museum of Cultural History for $500.

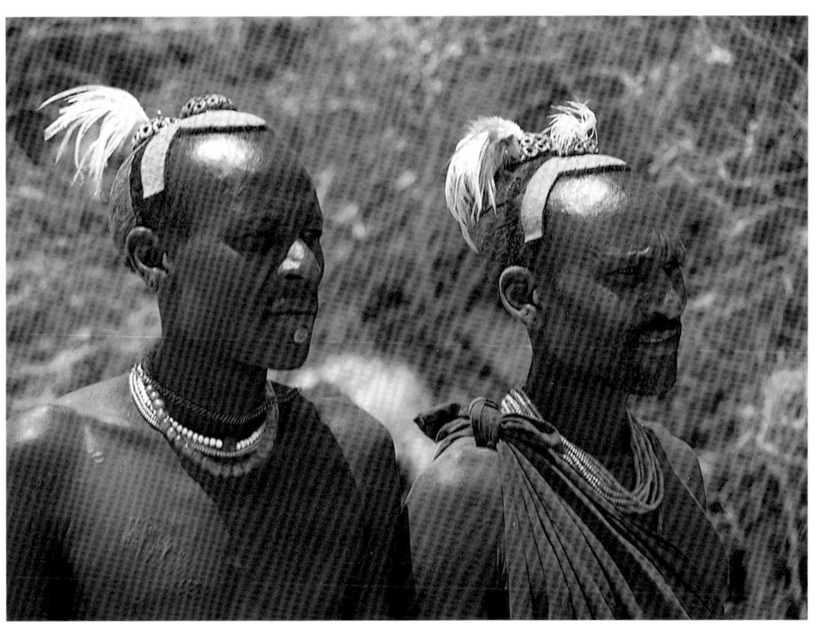

**Figure 2.22.** Pokot men's coiffure. Photograph by Herbert M. Cole, 1973. This Pokot hair style is similar to men's mudpack coiffures worn by the Karamojong, although the Karamojong examples usually include a section of densely matted hair that extends down from the back of the head.

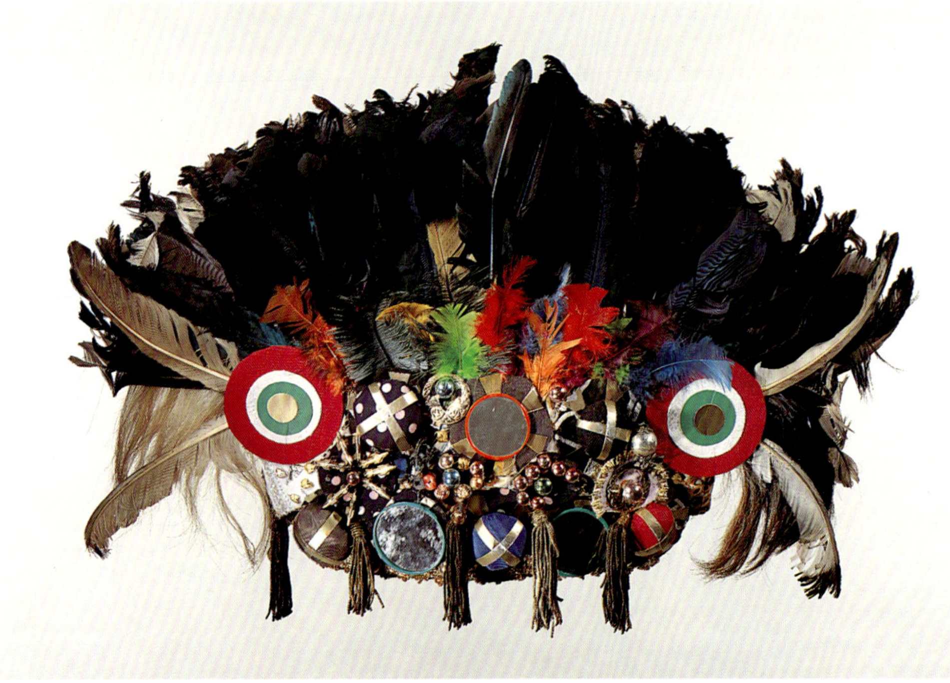

**Figure 2.23. Chief's hat *(ajibulu)*. Kalabari Ijo, Nigeria. Cloth, feathers, rams beard, mirrors, foil paper, plastic. H. 46 cm. Twentieth century. Collection of Joanne Eicher.**

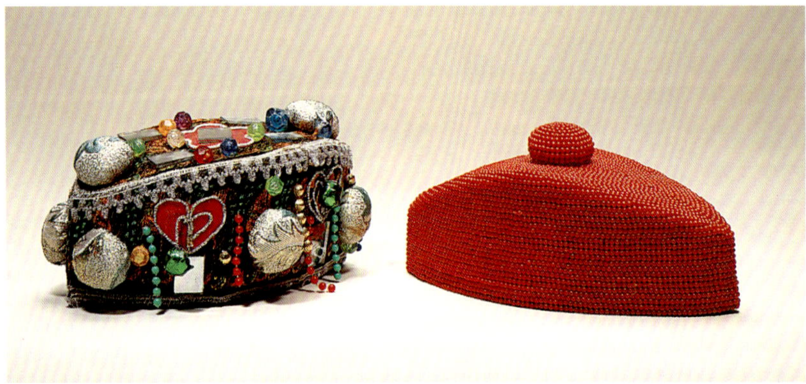

**Figure 2.24**, above. Women's hats *(angara sun)*. Kalabari Ijo, Nigeria. Cloth, beads, plastic, ribbon, braid trim. Twentieth century. Collection of Joanne Eicher. Women wear the hats for ceremonial occasions in their role as *iria bo*. They are worn during the "coming out" ceremony of public thanksgiving after the birth of a child and by the chief female mourners at the funerals of esteemed elders.

The Kalabari Ijo, numbering well over 500,000, live in the eastern Niger Delta in Nigeria. They inhabit a number of small communities on islands in the creeks and mangrove swamps of the area. Many now also live in the bustling city of Port Harcourt, but they often return to the smaller settlements for weekends and for major celebrations including festivals and funerals.

Ijo involvement in long-distance trade within the Delta and into the interior of West Africa was developed before the fifteenth century (Alagoa 1971:293), and increased between the fifteenth and nineteenth centuries when the Kalabari became pivotal in the trade between Europeans on the coast and groups further inland. During this period, communities began to be organized into corporate canoe houses which provided both the military personnel and the labor force necessary to support this trade.

For centuries, Kalabari Ijo society has been fluid and competitive, and an individual's status was achieved rather than ascribed by birth. Entre-prenurial skills and zeal were given a high value, but were always dependent on a leader's abililty to attract and maintain the support of his descent group and others.

### OBJECT

Kalabari believe that the head, specifically the forehead, houses personal will *(teme)* which controls a person's behavior (Horton 1965:4, Barley 1988:16). It is forbidden to casually touch the head of an older person as this would demean the elder. Doffing one's hat to another is not merely a polite gesture, but is understood as a sign of submission. Young men are not permitted to wear hats in the presence of elders, and when the king sits in council with his chiefs, only he may wear a hat (Erekosima 1988:36). In the nineteenth century in New Calabar state, sumptuary laws limited access of imported goods to chiefs and this included hats (Barley 1988:36). Erekosima suggests that the hat was adopted by the Kalabari as a material symbol of the person, and that hats worn by the central figures on ancestral screens depict personality rather than merely indicating status (1988:37).

Chiefs wear a distinctive crescent-shaped hat *(ajibulu)* decorated with feathers, mirrors, and rams' beards. The *ajibulu,* unlike other styles of men's hats (top hats, fedoras, and bowlers) is never worn by women (Daly 1987, Erekosima and Eicher 1981, Eicher and Erekosima 1987). The primary male mourners at the funeral of a chief often wear *ajibulu* hats to celebrate the achievements of their lineage.

### TECHNIQUE

The *ajibulu* are made by professional male hatmakers, and this example was made by Chief Johnny West of Buguma, who is considered to be the preeminent hatmaker in this area. He has transformed the European hat form into a distinctive Kalabari object by creatively reworking it and adding his own elements. Erekosima and Eicher (1981) describe this process as "cultural authentication."

An *ajibulu* must have three components: the *aji ebule* (ram's beard); feathers (both natural and dyed); and the *bia-ba*, the Kalabari symbol of concentric circles (Eicher and Erekosima 1988:2). Other elements, including a variety of plastic items and foil papers, are added to the hat and contribute to its total aesthetic effect. The hat symbolizes chiefly power and is worn as part of a proscribed ensemble that can include various types of prestige textiles, such as imported silks and embroidered velvets. The ensemble constitutes a category of appropriate dress for wealthy and powerful men and expresses Kalabari views about correct comportment and appearance (Eicher and Erekosima 1987:38).

### COLLECTION

This hat was collected by Joanne Eicher in Buguma, Nigeria in 1988. Dr. Eicher, an anthropologist, has conducted research in Nigeria for over three decades and, since 1977, has collaborated with Dr. Tonye Victor Erekosima, an Ijo scholar, on the social and aesthetic importance of Kalabari textiles and dress. This collaborative research has resulted in numerous professional papers, articles, and exhibitions.

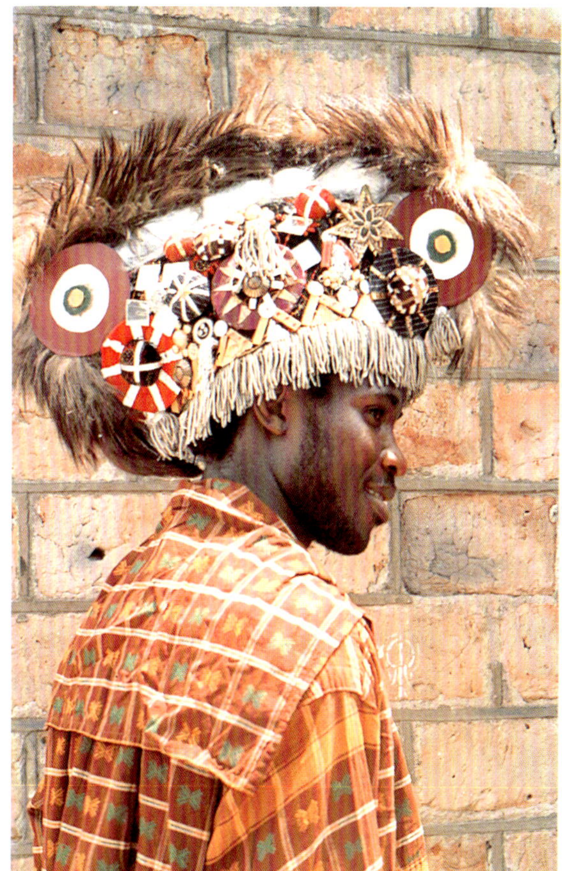

**Figure 2.25**. Young man modeling an *ajibulu*. Buguma, Nigeria. Photograph by Joanne Eicher, 1988.

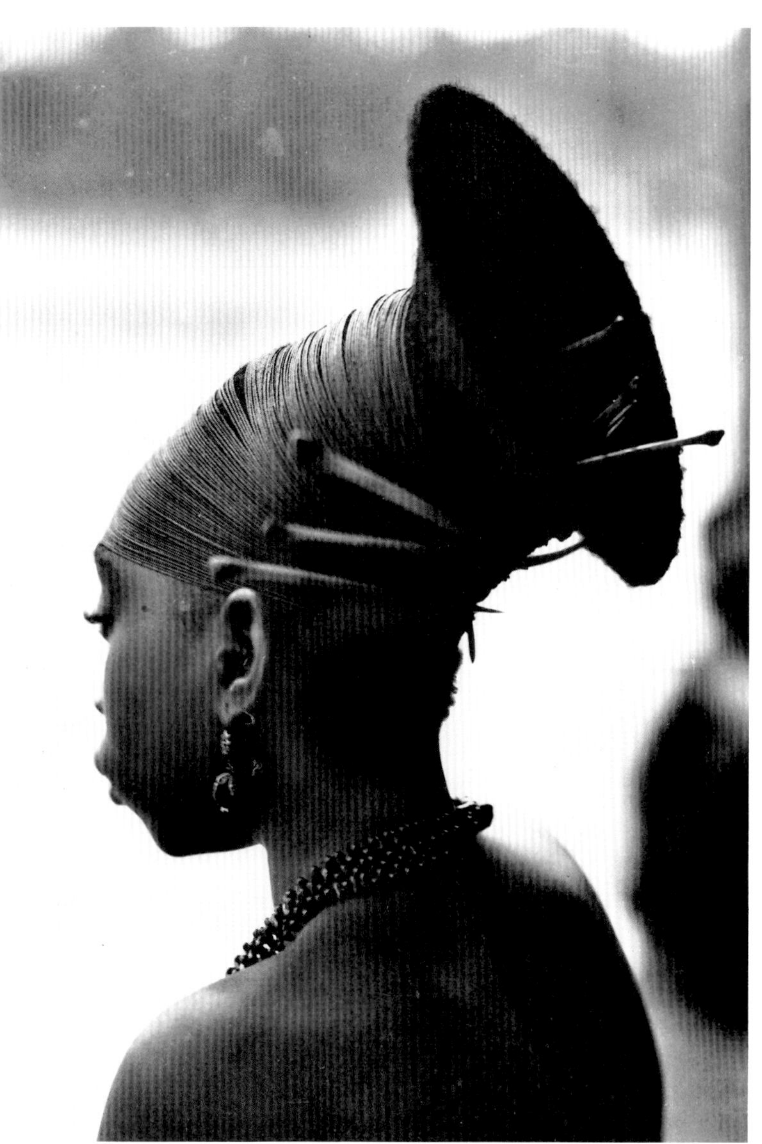

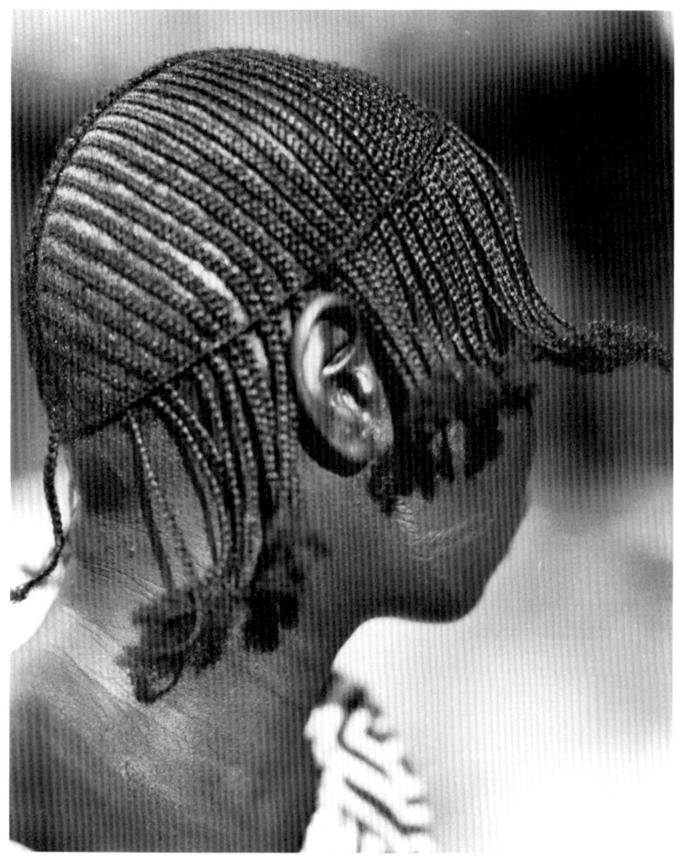

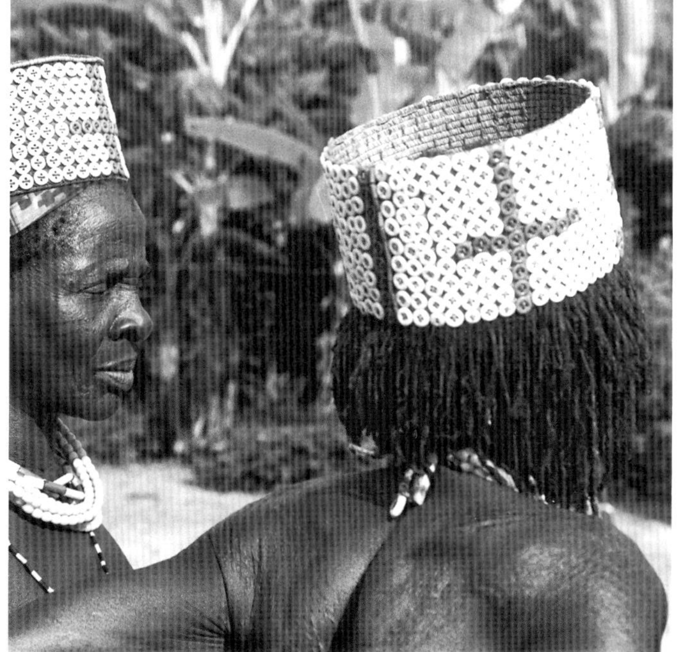

A B

C

# 3 CROWNING GLORIES: THE HEAD AND HAIR

## MARY JO ARNOLDI

Human hair can be fashioned and manipulated in a seemingly endless variety of ways. Styling, tressing, shaving, uncovering, or covering the hair with hats and headgear, are cultural practices through which multiple identities are expressed. These identities may be based on personal values, gender, age, religion, or ethnicity. Some hair styles have endured over centuries, others have changed significantly and undergone multiple permutations over time. Popular hair styles respond to the accelerated tempo of contemporary fashion, gaining prominence for a short period of time and then fading into obscurity, quickly replaced by new creations or updated versions of older forms.

In many African societies, hair, as an extension of the head, is an especially potent material and special precautions often surround its manipulation and disposal. Among the Tuareg, hair is considered to be the outer manifestation of intelligence, and abundant hair is linked to noble status (Rasmussen 1994:85–6). A Yoruba child born with curly hair is thought to be sacred and is given the name of the curly-headed god, Dada. The hair of these children is considered to have supernatural or divine powers (Houlberg 1979:376).

Distinctive hair styles are often reserved for special segments of society including royalty, religious specialists, hunters, and warriors. In many African societies, key participants in critical rites of passage, including coming of age, marriage, and funerary rituals wear special hair styles. Among the Yoruba, Mangbetu, Luba, and Chokwe, for example, distinctive hair styles were once the exclusive prerogative of high-ranking men and women. For Mangbetu men and women of the ruling class, the shape of the head (they practiced head elongation), elaborate hair styles, hats, and prestige ornaments to decorate the hair were an important aesthetic preoccupation (Fig. 3.1). Schildkrout and Keim note that women's hair styles changed significantly from the time that Schweinfurth first visited the Mangbetu in 1871 and Lang arrived in 1910. They described the 1910 hair style for royal women: "First string was wrapped around the forehead and much of the head. The long hair was then drawn around a basketry frame to produce a halo-like shape. Numerous hairpins of ivory, bone, or metal completed the style" (1990:126). Lang wrote of this hair style, "The basket like type, however, if once adopted is seldom abandoned. It needs rather long hair and women are proud of it" (Lang quoted in Schildkrout and Keim 1990:127).

Many historical hair styles are no longer worn today, but are known from early drawings or photographs or are preserved in sculptural forms. In nineteenth-century

**Opposite. A.** "Mangbetu coiffure." [Mangbetu headdress], Northeastern Zaire. Photograph by Casimir d'Ostoja Zagorski, 1926. "L'Afrique qui disparait," Series 1, no. 55. Eliot Eliosofon Photographic Archives. National Museum of African Art.

**B.** "Province de l'Equateur. Coiffure." [Equator province, Hairstyle], Zaire. Photograph by Casimir d'Ostoja Zagorski, 1926. L'Afrique qui disparait," Series 2, no. 32. Eliot Elisofon Photographic Archives. National Museum of African Art.

**C.** *Kanyamwa*-grade wives in *bwami* society at a dance for a member reaching the fourth level (of five). Photograph by Eliot Elisofon, 1966. Neg. no.OA 71264, C-11,24A. Eliot Elisofon Photographic Archives. National Museum of African Art.

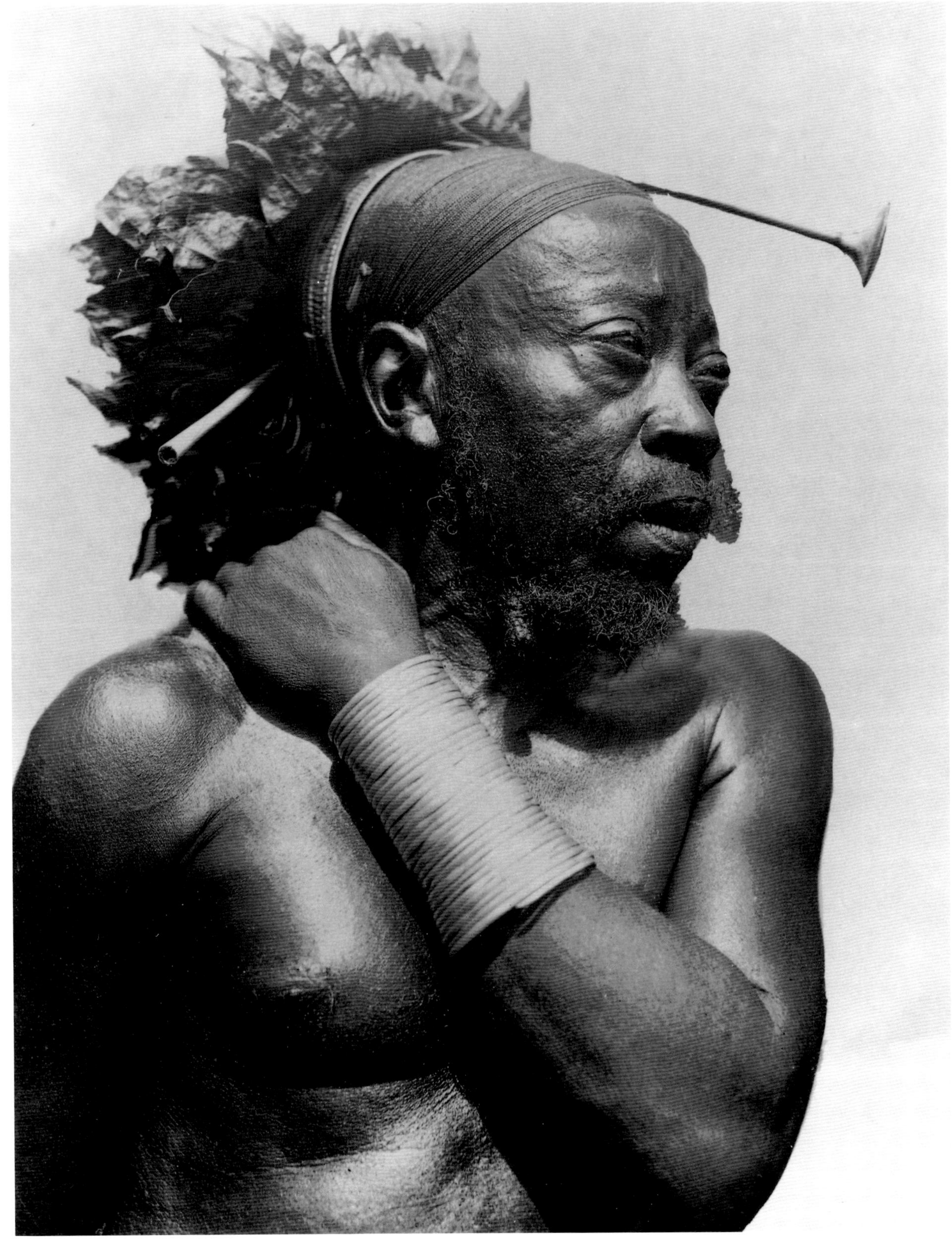

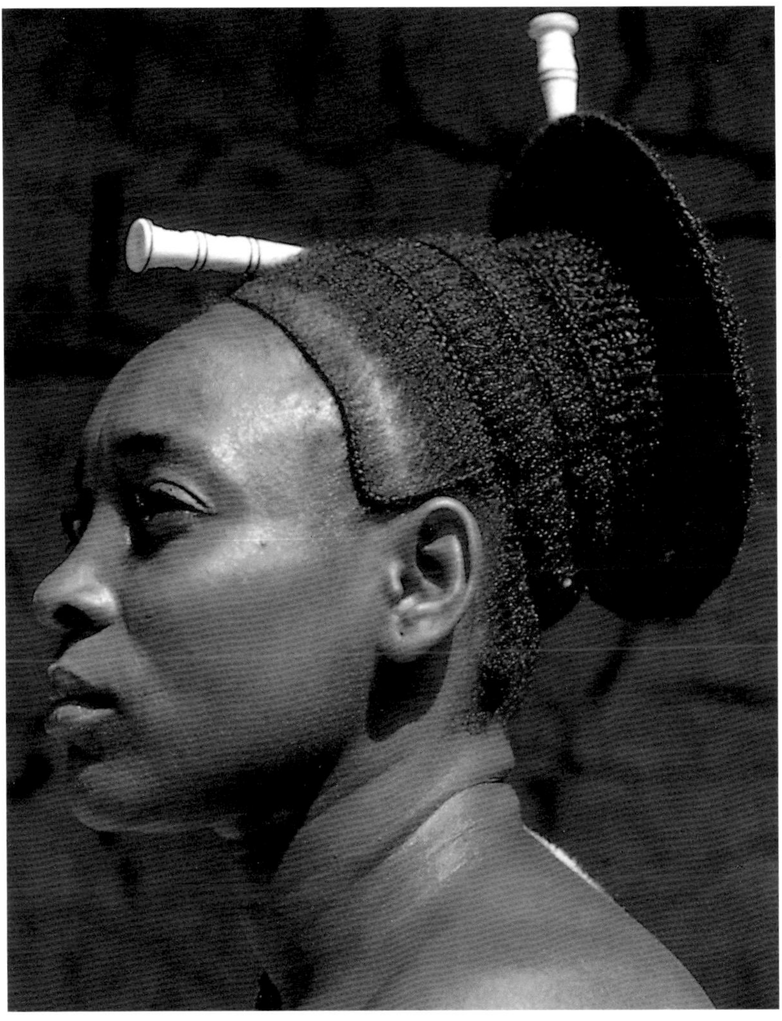

Zulu society, married men wore a head ring *(isicoco)* to signify their social status. It was the Zulu king who gave permission for an individual to assume the head ring. It consisted of a fiber or sinew circle into which the man's own hair was woven. When the hair grew out, the head ring was cut off and replaced with a new one. In the early nineteenth century, married women among the Zulu wore a hair style equivalent to the men's called *isicholo*. Women shaved their heads leaving a small oval or circular patch on the crown which they greased and colored with a mixture of animal fat and red ochre. This tuft of hair was worked into a top knot that resembled a truncated cone.

Sometime in the mid-nineteenth century, this top knot became more elaborated and the tuft was lengthened by adding grasses which were worked into the hair and bound with fiber to create a more extended cone (Fig. 3.3). Covering the head was a sign of a woman's respect for her in-laws, and married women wore a band *(umnqwazi)* across the forehead as a material sign of this respect. Later, in the twentieth century, this hair style was replaced by a hat. Hats were constructed from a woven fiber base that was covered with either human hair or string dyed with a mixture of fat and red ochre. The requisite headband was attached to the hat itself or worn as a separate piece in addition to the hat (Fig. 3.4; Kennedy 1978, Conner and Pelrine 1983).

**Figure 3.1**, opposite. "Magnifique indigène de race Mangbetu (District de l'Uele — Province Orientale" [Magnificent Mangbetu man Uele District — Oriental Province]), Zaire. Photograph by G. de Boe, 1936. C. I. D. Belgium. Eliot Elisofon Photographic Archives. National Museum of African Art.

**Figure 3.2.**, above. Mangbetu chief's principal wife with traditional hair style, Medje village, Zaire. Photograph by Eliot Elisofon, 1970. Slide no. D MNG 29 (3026). Eliot Elisofon Photographic Archives. National Museum of African Art.

In Nigeria an elaborate Ejagham hair style with curling extensions was formerly worn by young women in "coming out" ceremonies which announced their status as adult women and proclaimed their eligibility for marriage. While these elaborate hair styles are no longer worn today, they do still appear on skin-covered masks that are used in performances by men's societies in southern Nigeria (Fig. 3.5). In the Grassfield kingdoms of Cameroon, high-ranking men formerly wore wrapped, tufted hair styles. This specific hair style appears on carved wooden masks and figures from the nineteenth and twentieth centuries and was the inspiration for the cotton prestige caps *(ashetu)* that are worn today by ranking men at non-Islamic festivals (Fig. 3.6). On ceremonial and ritual occasions, Fante royal wives and female priestesses wear distinctive horsehair wigs *(tekuwa)* fashioned into elaborate hair styles decorated with gold ornaments (Fig. 3.7). These wigs seem to have been inspired by actual Fante women's hair styles worn in the nineteenth century in this region (Fig. 3.8; Cole and Ross 1977:fig. 29).

Yoruba hunters wear a distinctive braided hair style that falls down the back or

**Figure 3.3**, below. Zulu woman's hair style *(isicholo)*. During the latter half of the nineteenth century, women grew a tuft of hair several inches long to facilitate the creation of a truncated cone. To give the hair cone the desirable volume, grass or false hair was sometimes woven into the hair and the cone was smeared with fat and ochre. Photographic postcard. Photographer, undetermined. "A Zulu woman, Copyright L.692." Publisher, date, and printer undetermined. The Metropolitan Museum of Art, New York. Department of the Arts of Africa, Oceania, and the Americas. The Photograph Study Collection.

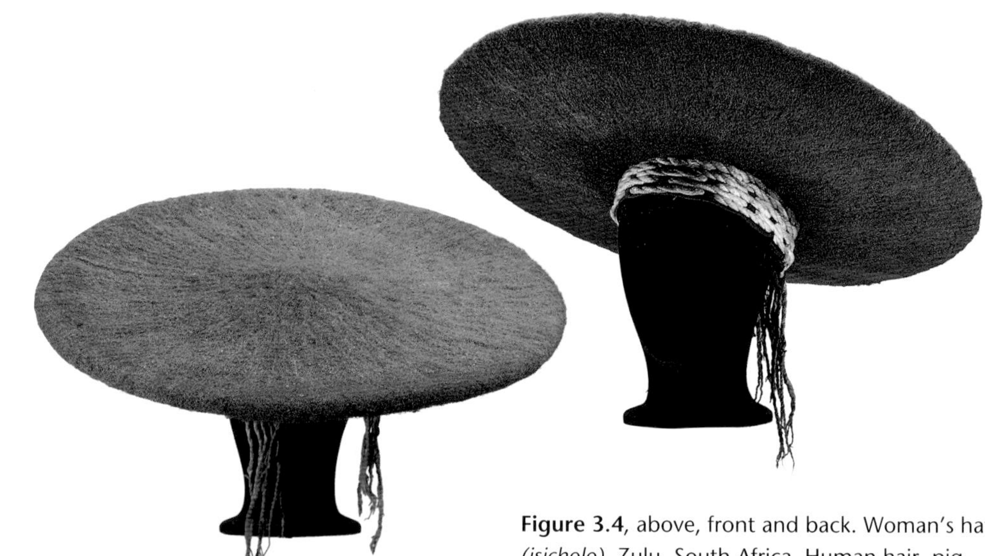

**Figure 3.4**, above, front and back. Woman's hat *(isicholo)*. Zulu, South Africa. Human hair, pigment, twine, cloth. H. 29.0 cm. Private collection. Human hair is worked into the woven fiber base of this hat and then the whole is dyed with a red ochre and fat mixture. A braided headband of commercial white yarn is attached to the hat.

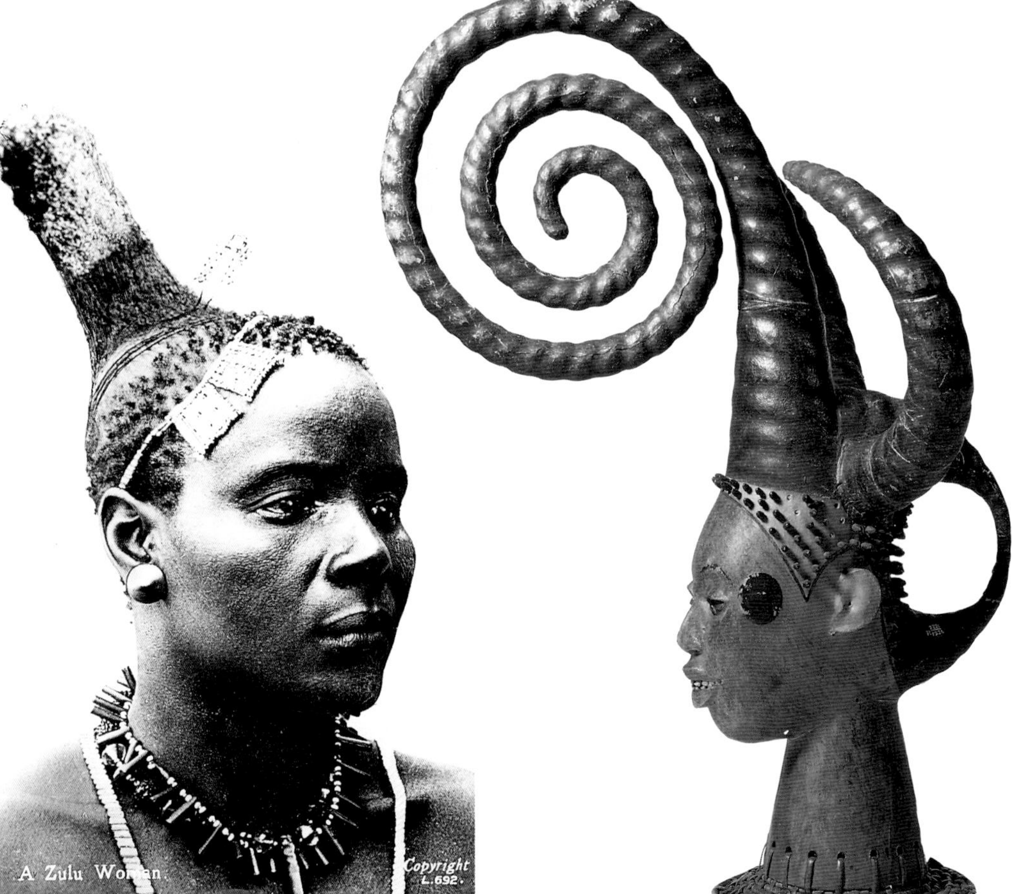


**Figure 3.5**, left. Headdress. Ejagham, Nigeria. Wood, paint, metal, bone, rattan, leather. H. 67.0 cm. FMCH X65.9043. Gift of the Wellcome Trust. The coiffure on this mask represents an older version of a young woman's hairdo that was worn in coming-of-age rites prior to marriage. Today these headdresses are worn for initiation and for funerals of members of certain men's associations.

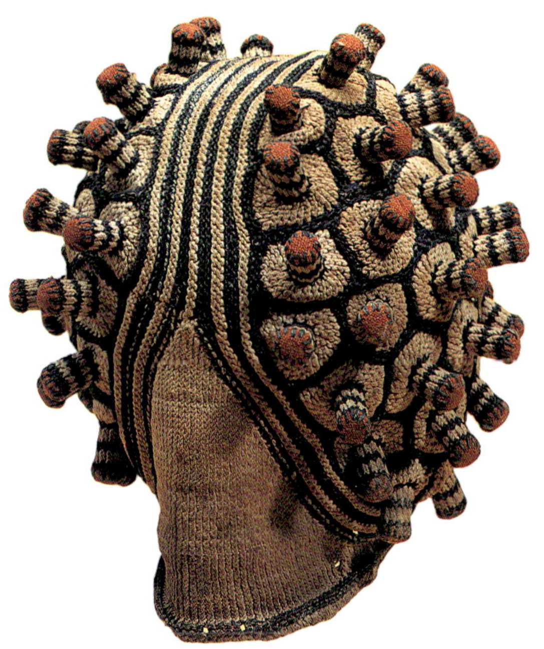

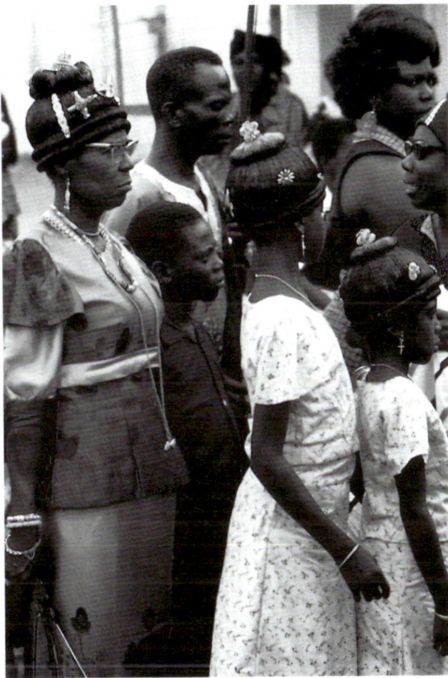

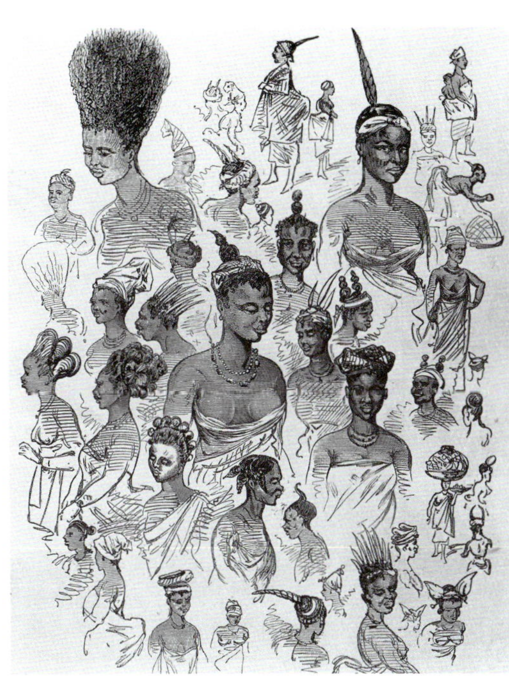

**Figure 3.6**, above left. Man's hat *(ashetu)*. Bamileke, Cameroon. Cotton, wood. H. 25.0 cm. FMCH X94.29.1. Museum purchase, Jerome L. Joss Endowment Fund. These cotton prestige hats have burls reinforced with wood and are reminiscent of an elaborate hair style once worn throughout the Grassfields area. This hair style is also carved on wooden masks from the area.

**Figure 3.7**, above middle. Fante women wearing elaborate wigs *(tekuwa)* with gold ornaments in a procession at annual state festival *(Fetu Afahye)*. Cape Coast, Ghana. Photograph by Doran H. Ross, 1979.

**Figure 3.8**, above right. Nineteenth-century Fante women's hairdos from southern Ghana. The *Illustrated London News*, April 4, 1874.

**Figure 3.9**, right Egungun mask. Yoruba, Abeokuta, Nigeria. Wood, paint. H. 44.5 cm. FMCH X65.9051. Gift of the Wellcome Trust. This ancestor mask represents a hunter who wears a distinctive braided hair style. Hunters wear this braid either down the back or, as in this example, over the left shoulder.

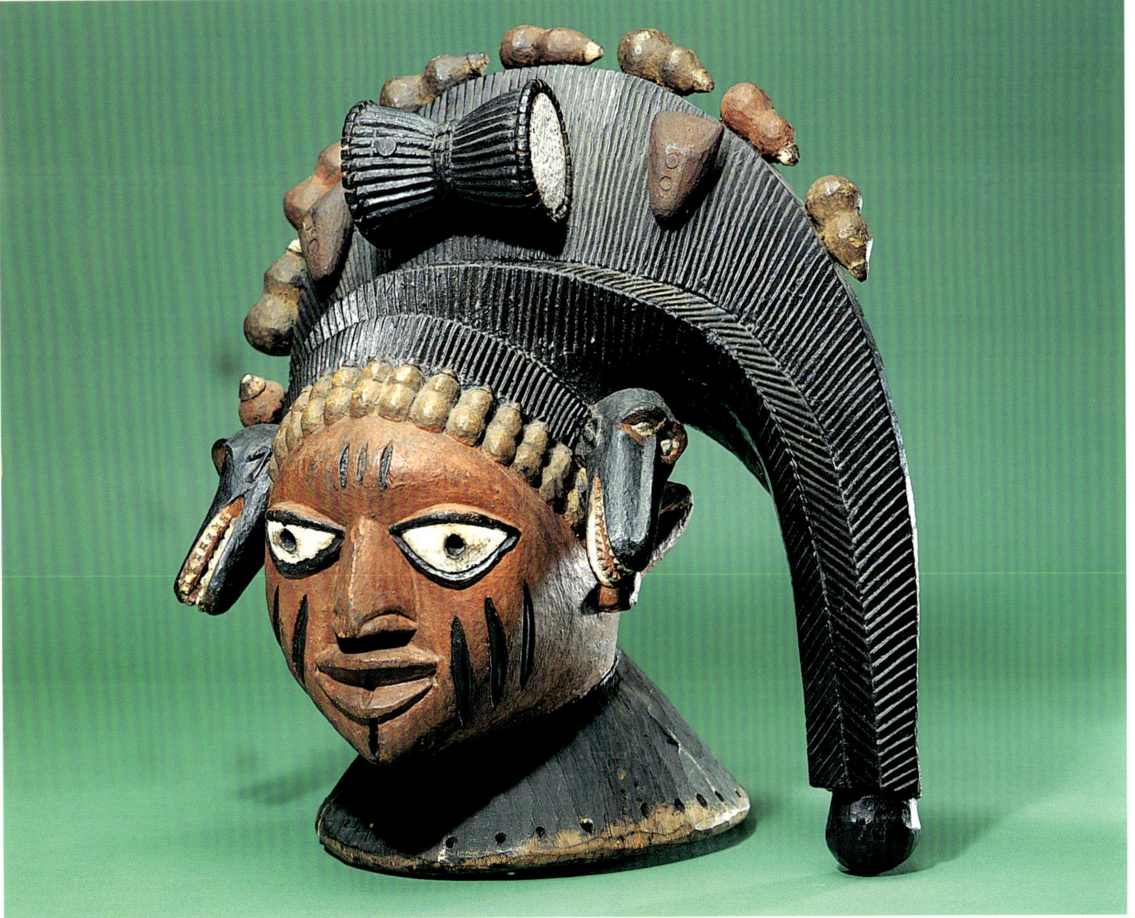

on the left side of the head. Their hair is associated with strength and along with the medicine pouches they attach to their hats, it serves to protect them from the forces of the bush (Houlberg 1979:374). The same hair style and medicine pouches are often depicted on Egungun masks that celebrate ancestral hunters (Fig. 3.9).

Historically hair styles could also indicate religious affiliation. Moslem men in Mali wore their hair cropped short, while their non-Moslem neighbors, especially hunters and warriors, often wore their hair long and braided. Slaves among the Tuareg, Bamana, Yoruba, and in the Grassfield chiefdoms of Cameroon often had their heads shaved as a sign of their status. In Cameroon slaves were not allowed to wear hats, which were the sign of free adult men in these chiefdoms. Priests and priestesses among the Yoruba still wear distinctive hair styles today that distinguish them as members of particular *òrìṣà* cults.

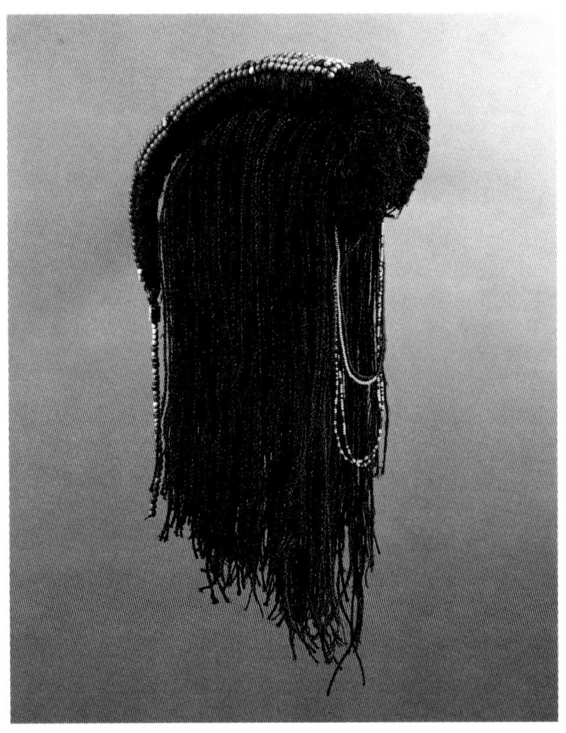

**Figure 3.10**. Wig. Zulu, South Africa. Fiber beads, leather. H. 44.0 cm. FMCH X76.877. Gift of Mr. and Mrs. Donald Brody. The donors have identified this wig as a Zulu female shaman's wig, but its origins have not been independently confirmed.

In Akan areas in Ghana, certain religious specialists of both sexes regularly appear with long unkempt hair to which they add various spiritually potent objects such as gold pieces, coins, cowries, and bone (Cole and Ross 1977:22). Their unkempt hair is more remarkable when compared to the carefully braided and styled hair of most Akan women and the short cropped hair styles of Akan men. Contemporary male adherents to the *Bay Fal* Muride Islamic sect in Senegal wear their hair long imitating the dreadlock hair style of precolonial *cedo* warriors in the service of the Wolof kings (Colvin 1981). This *Bay Fal* hair style stands in sharp contrast to other Islamic Senegalese men who keep their hair cropped short. Among the Zulu of South Africa, most men and women keep their hair cut relatively short, however fiber wigs that imitate long twisted locks are worn by women diviners, a class of religious specialists (Fig. 3.10).

Among the Pokot, Karamojong, Turkana, Maasai, and Samburu in East Africa, young men of the warrior age-grade *(moran)* spend hours grooming their hair (Fig. 3.11). Intricately coiffed hair is a sign of masculinity, courage, and strength. Among the Pokot, mud-plastered coiffures are worn by young men, and the colors and the shape of these hair styles are prescribed and identify the wearer's age-set. If an individual or group violates these rules by wearing colors, styles, or decorative elements to which they are not entitled it can lead to serious interage-set or intergenerational conflict. Jean Brown notes "These conflicts are ostensibly over personal ornaments, but actually express a thwarted desire for promotion" (1986:28). Individuals are, however, free to create decorative designs in their coiffures at will. Patterned striations are made in wet clay with a special spatula, color is applied, and feather holders and other decorative items are embedded in the mudpack before the clay dries. The blue mud-plastered hair style, achieved with commercial laundry blueing, identifies a man as a member of the junior age-set (Fig. 3.12; Cole 1974).

Maasai and Samburu warriors do not create mud-plastered hair styles, rather they twist their hair into hundreds of small braids, saturate them with fat and red

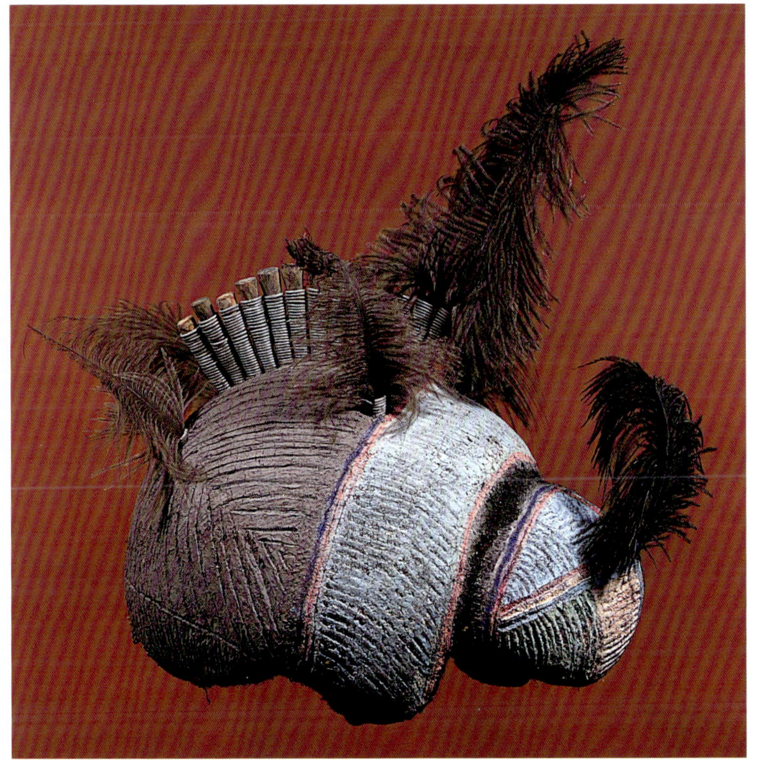

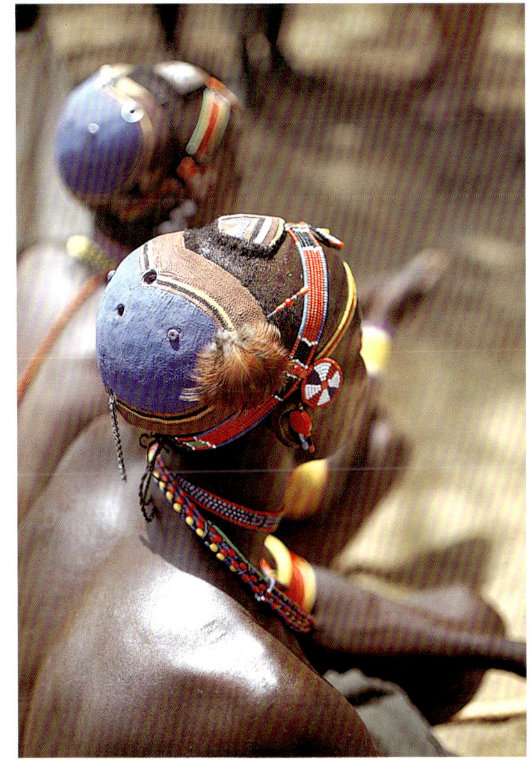

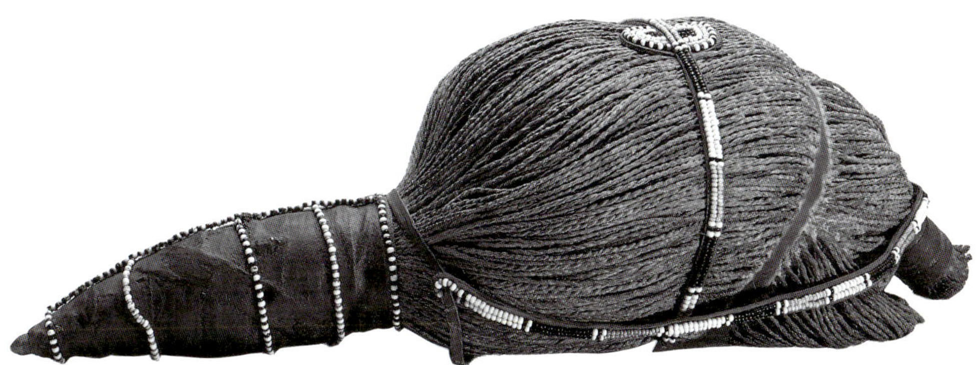

**Figure 3.11**, above left. Mud cap. Pokot, Kenya. Mud, paint, ostrich feathers, wood, aluminum, human hair. H. 26 cm. FMCH X89.366. Promised gift of Jerome L. Joss.

**Figure 3.12**, above right. A recently initiated Pokot man with feathered blue mud cap. His ochred frontal hair reflects his junior status. The hairdo has an old zipper imbedded spirally. Photograph by Herbert M. Cole, 1973.

**Figure 3.13**, left. Wig. Maasai, Kenya. Hide, fiber, beads, wood. H. 32.0 cm. FMCH X81.1255. Gift of Mrs. Paquita Machris. Wigs of twisted fiber sewn onto a fiber cap and twisted over wood forms are fashioned in the style of the plaited coiffures worn by the warrior age-grade *(moran)*. On important ceremonial occasions these wigs might be donned by men who had abandoned the practice of wearing the distinctive plaited hair style on a daily basis.

ochre (obtained from iron-rich stones), and then they pull these braids forward and backward securing them to wooden pendants or wrapping them into a larger braid (Cole 1974, 1979). The Maasai fiber wig imitates the splendid braided hair styles worn by members of the warrior age-grade on a daily basis (Fig. 3.13). Warriorhood lasts about twelve to sixteen years beginning when a boy is initiated and ending when he marries as a man in his late twenties or early thirties. Once he marries, he ceases to participate in *moran* activities and dances, and he generally cuts his hair short as an indication of his new status in the community. Women in these ethnic groups either keep their hair cropped short or wear only short twisted braids from the time they are adolescents until they reach old age. Rather than hair styles, the focus of their aesthetic and symbolic elaboration is decorative headbands, metal and beaded earrings, and massive accumulations of beaded necklaces (Cole 1974, 1979).

Throughout much of Africa, most children's hair is kept short, is periodically shaved, and remains relatively unadorned. However, in urban and rural areas in Mali, Senegal, and elsewhere in the region, many young girls today wear modest versions of the tressed and braided styles of their older sisters. Among the Igbo of Nigeria, children's heads are often shaved in bold asymmetrical patterns (Cole and Aniakor 1984:39, pl. 64). Himba boys' heads in Namibia are also shaved into decorative patterns, and line drawings are created in the shaved areas (Gustaaf Verswijver, personal communication 1994).

Combs to style and decorate the hair are widespread throughout Africa and come in a variety of different woods, plant fibers, metal, and ivory (Figs. 3.14). Metal studs and ivory hair pins, porcupine quills, cowries, and glass beads were used in the past, and some continue to be used today to decorate the hair (Fig. 3.15). Among the Mangbetu, long ivory pins ending in flat discs were highly prized by both men and women (Figs. 3.1, 3.2). It is said that it took a full elephant tusk to make a single one of these hairpins and that only a master artist was capable of creating them (Schildkrout and Keim 1990:130). Elsewhere in Central Africa the use of iron and copper nails inserted into elaborate coiffures is an ancient practice documented in a Kisalian-period grave dating from the eighth to the thirteenth century A.D. The nails excavated from this grave site have the same shape as more recent examples used by the Luba. People claim that the nails were used in the coiffures to symbolically lock in the power of chiefs and kings, who are associated with the introduction of iron technology into the area (Dewey 1993:21).

Headrests were used by many groups in eastern, central, and southern Africa (Fig. 3.17a-d). Among the Luba, many of these headrests were carved with a female figure as the central caryatid (Fig. 3.17b). Special attention seems to have been given to the rendering of the coiffure and the body scarification of these female figures, suggesting the importance of bodily adornment in Luba culture. While these head-

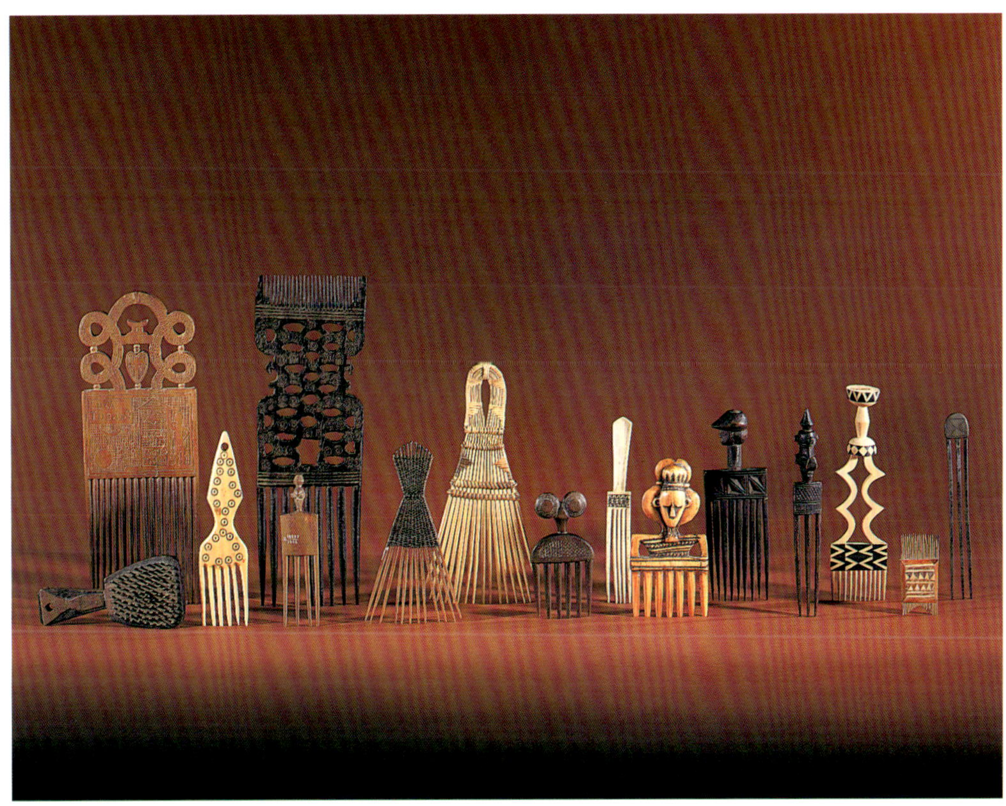

**Figure 3.14**, left above, a–o. An assortment of African combs from the Fowler Museum of Cultural History collections. Longest, 27.5 cm. Museum purchases unless other wise noted (see materials and catalogue numbers in Note 1 for this chapter). Combs made from a variety of materials are used in styling the hair and are sometimes worn as decorative additions to both men's and women's coiffures. A number of these combs are carved with figures with elaborately styled hair.

**Figure 3.16**, left below, a–x. An assortment of African hairpins from the Fowler Museum of Cultural History. Longest, 39.5 cm. Gifts of the Wellcome Trust unless otherwise noted (see materials and catalogue numbers in Note 2 for this chapter). Hairpins made from a variety of materials are found throughout Africa. They are used both to style and to decorate men's and women's finished coiffures.

**Figure 3.15**, below. Late-nineteenth-century hairdressing scene from southern Ghana (Akuapem?) showing plaited hair and wood comb. Photograph courtesy of Basel Mission.

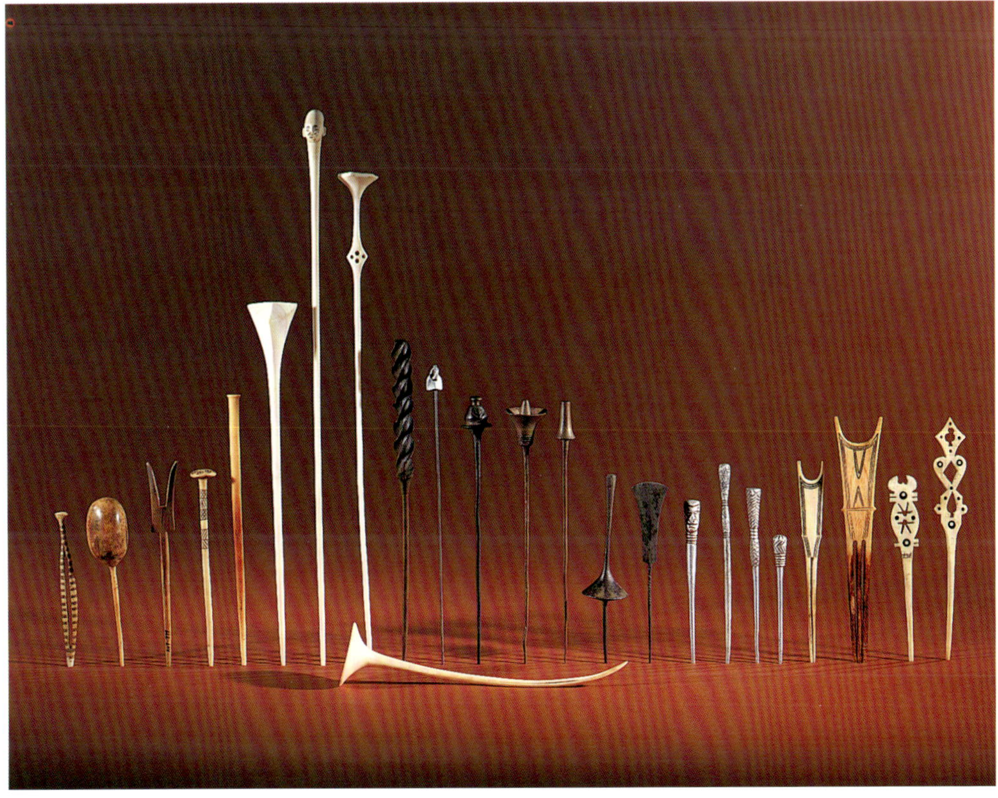

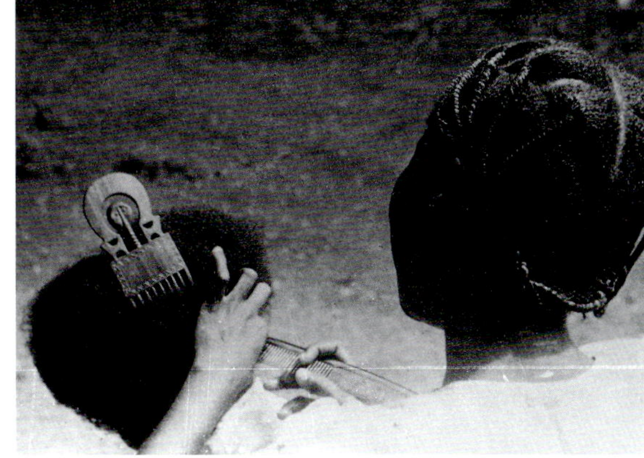

rests certainly protected elaborate coiffures while sleeping, some were also used ritually. For example, Maesen reported that among the Luba the headrest could substitute for the body of the deceased, if the body itself was not retrievable (Nooter 1984:62–63). Shona spirit mediums and chiefs sometimes used their headrests to induce dreams about the ancestors as a means of acquiring knowledge (Dewey 1993:102). Dewey suggests that the Yaka headrest with the caryatid of the European merchant riding an ox might have served a similar purpose (Fig. 3.17d). Among the Songo and Chokwe there was a cult that employed images of European merchants to symbolize the wealth that an initiate would gain from participation in the cult. The Yaka owner of this headrest might well have been an initiate of the cult and have used the headrest in order to induce dreams about wealth (Dewey 1993:56).

Manipulation of the hair is often the focus of ritual activities (Leach 1958). In many rites of passage, for example, the hair is shaved as an expression of an individual's transformation from one social status to another. Among the Bamana, during the naming ceremony of a newborn, an animal is sacrificed, the child's head is shaved and anointed with blood, and the name is pronounced. This ritual act authenticates the reincarnation of a specific ancestor in the person of the newborn child (Zahan 1960:333). Among the Yoruba, a newborn's head is also shaved (except for sacred children) at the naming ceremony. This act is said to separate the newborn from the world of the spirits and to incorporate the child into the world of the living. The shaved hair is endowed with power and is incorporated into an amulet to ensure the good health of the child (Houlberg 1979:368).

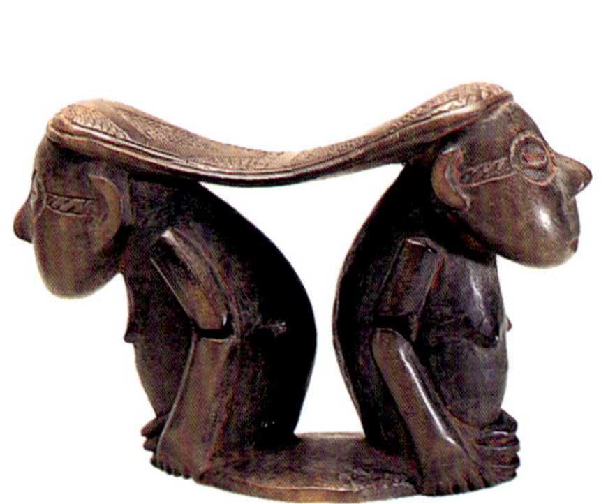

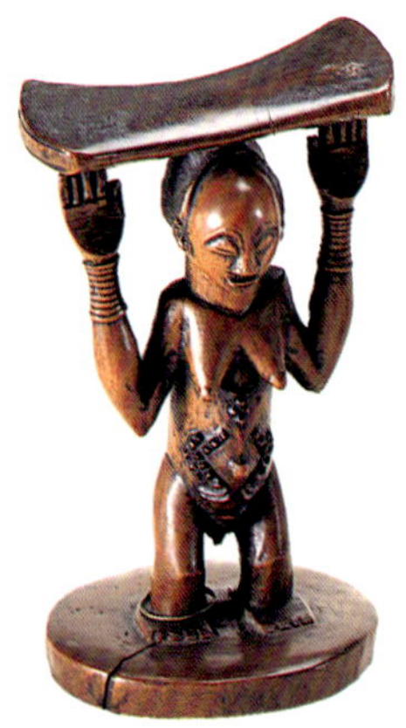

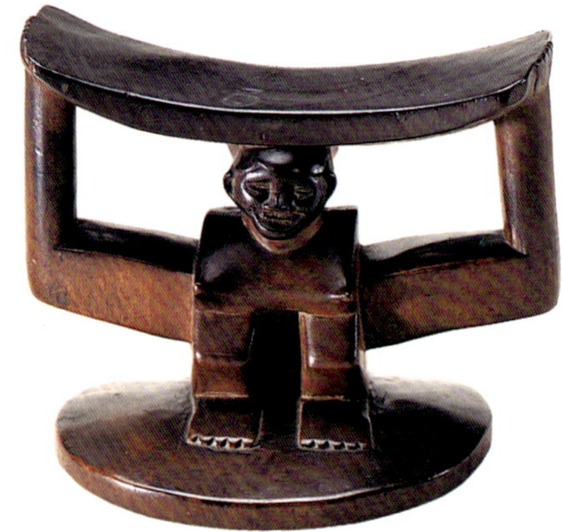

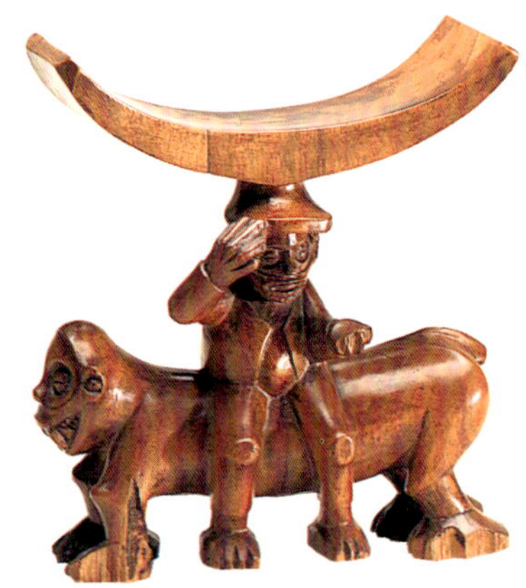

**Figure 3.17.** Headrests. a. Twa, Zaire. FMCH X92.464; b. Luba, Zaire. FMCH X91.60; c. Mbala, Zaire. FMCH X90.453 d. Yaka, Zaire. FMCH X87.612. Greatest height: 23.8 cm. Both figurative and nonfigurative wooden headrests are found in many societies in Zaire and elsewhere on the continent. While all types protect elaborate coiffures when sleeping or resting, the figures on the headrests, carved with elaborate headgear or coiffures, demonstrate the creative play of head imagery. Gift of Jerome L. Joss.

One of the first ritual acts performed in many coming-of-age ceremonies involves shaving the initiates' heads in order to accentuate their present state of childhood and to mark the beginning of their movement to a new adult status. Among the Okiek and the Maasai, both girls and boys undergo this head-shaving ritual. During this one-day ceremony, which may precede the final initiation rites by many years, the child's and the mother's heads are shaved in the morning, and later in the evening the child is given a new name (Kratz 1993:93).

Funerary rituals were often occasions for special practices regarding the hair. In many cultures close relatives of the deceased shaved their heads or went ungroomed during the period of mourning. Spencer (1965:74) notes that among the Samburu

> it is believed that when a man dies, the contamination of his death infects the hair of his age-mates within a certain range of kinship, and in order to rid themselves of this contamination and avert misfortune, they must all shave off their hair soon after death: they are said to "share their hair" *(kong'ar lpapit).*

Formerly, among the Yoruba the head of the deceased was shaved as a rite of separation (Bascom 1969:66).

In Africa and in its diaspora, hair styles for both men and women are part of the ever-changing face of fashion. Contemporary African hair styles, as a popular art form, comment upon society and on the changing attitudes and values that shape people's lives. Some hair styles are created as social commentary, others celebrate topical events, others are inspired by popular music and other forms of media. Houlberg documented a number of examples of older Yoruba hair styles that have been given new names based on more topical events and were then repopularized. She also found that certain older styles that had once been restricted to particular segments of Yoruba society (for example, royal wives) were now being worn by ordinary women. Her study suggests that the names for hair styles tend to change more rapidly than the hair styles themselves (1979:354–5).

In both African and African-American communities, there have been rapid shifts in hair fashions from the Afro styles of the sixties to the elaborate weave and shaped hair styles of the eighties and nineties. These hair styles convey a variety of different messages. First they serve as statements of individual creativity and indices of personal notions of presentation and aesthetics. Some, like the Afro styles of the sixties in America, communicated critical political ideologies. Often when this same style was adopted in Africa, it was viewed as a symbol of modernity and high fashion. Men's shaped cuts, popular among adolescents and young adults in African-American communities in the late eighties, were quickly embraced by African urban youth. In much the same way, the elaborately braided women's hair styles of the eighties and the nineties were worn simultaneously by women in Africa and in America, and these styles underscore the profound cultural links between African-American and African culture and the dynamic nature of con-

**Figure 3.18.** Wig stand with hair extensions. China. Plastic, synthetic hair. H. 34.0 cm. FMCH X94.28.21a-d. Museum purchase. Purchased at the 1994 African Marketplace in Los Angeles from "Shugar International Hair Extensions, Creator of Breece Weave, Treece Weave, and Shugar Rolls."

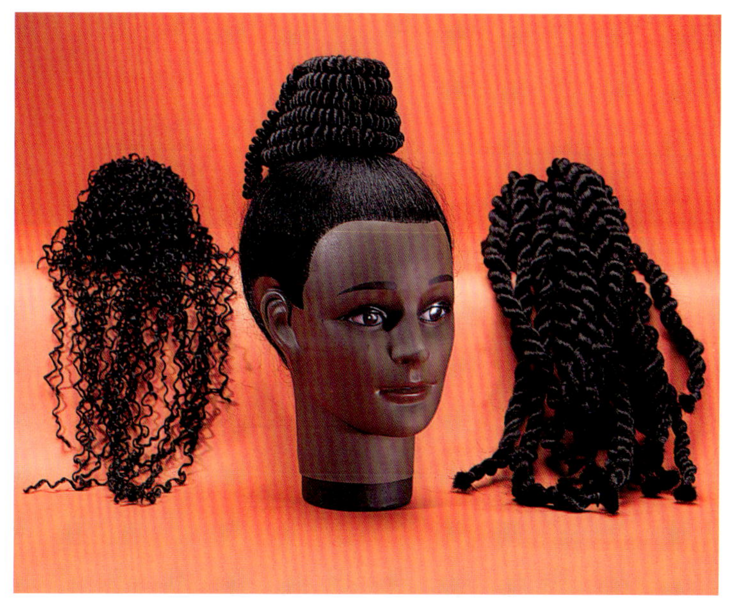

temporary transcultural exchanges.

Most of the very intricate tressed and braided women's hair styles and the sculpted and shaped men's styles are created by professional hairstylists and barbers. In cities and towns in Africa and in America, hairstyling salons have sprung up to meet specific local demands. These popular hair styles are often labor-intensive and require a substantial investment of time and money by the client. Human and synthetic hairpieces and hair extenders, and a multitude of hair products designed specifically for the African and African-American markets, constitute a growing business (Fig. 3.18). Human hair extenders are sold in specialty stores, while packages of synthetic hair are available from salons and in local markets and shops (Jones 1994:277–297).

In African towns and cities, professional hairstylists and barbers often advertise and attract their clientele by commissioning painted signs displaying current fashions. Next to the painted signs, they may also present options to their customers through assemblages of images drawn from various national and international magazines. The paintings are generally rendered on wood with enamel paints. Names for the different hair styles are often printed directly on the signs, and this conjunction of images and words tends to establish the styles, as both signs and fashions circulate in and out of the urban center.

Barber shop signs and other forms of hand-painted commercial art have been part of the vibrant urban landscape in Africa for at least half a century. Several different dates have been proposed for the origin of this commercial art form; the earliest suggested time is between the 1930s and 1940s and the latest in the 1950s (Lerat 1992:8). Many commercial barber shop signs are painted by self-trained artists, and the prices for signs continue to be based on the number and size of the painted heads. More recently in Bamako, Abidjan, and elsewhere, academically trained artists will sometimes produce these signs to supplement their incomes. The prices are, again, generally based on the number and size of the painted heads (Lerat 1992:14).

Sign-painting ateliers have been established in many urban centers from Bamako to Libreville. Many of the painters sign their names or a nickname, or use the name of their atelier on the paintings. In Kumase, there are several ateliers including "Almighty God Art," "Unity Best Art," and "Messian Art" (Kristen 1980:38, Lerat 1992:73). A Ghanaian barber, a recent immigrant to Bamako, brought several of the Kumase-produced signs with him. He told me in 1992 that he felt that the styles represented on the signs ("Fades" and "Box" cuts, which were popular in the 1980s in America) had been instrumental in attracting a younger clientele (Fig. 3.19). The paintings themselves are also rendered in a much more sophisticated manner than are the locally produced signs. The Kumase figures seem to have been originally copied from photographs in magazines or other media sources.

In Libreville, one of the most popular sign painters is Bikok T. Pierre, who was

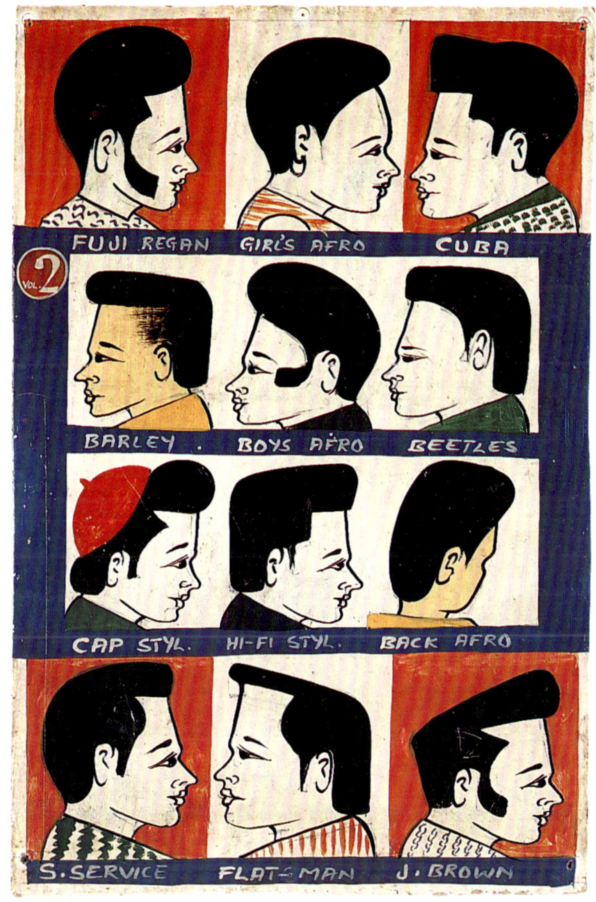


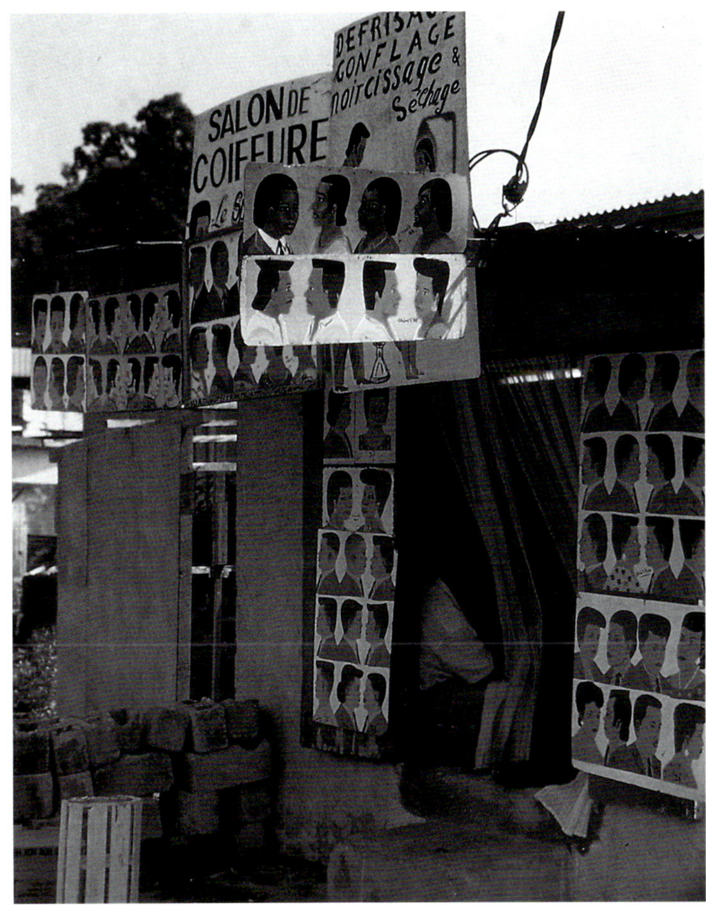


Figure 3.19, above. Barber sign. Iperu, Nigeria. Masonite, paint, H. 61.0 cm. FMCH X89.301. The men's hair styles on this sign were popular in West Africa in the 1970s.

Figure 3.20, above right. Men's barber shop with painted signs by Bikok T. Pierre in Libreville, Gabon. Photograph by Philip Ravenhill, 1989.

Figure 3.21, right. Women's hairgrooming salon in Libreville, Gabon. Photograph by Philip Ravenhill,1989.

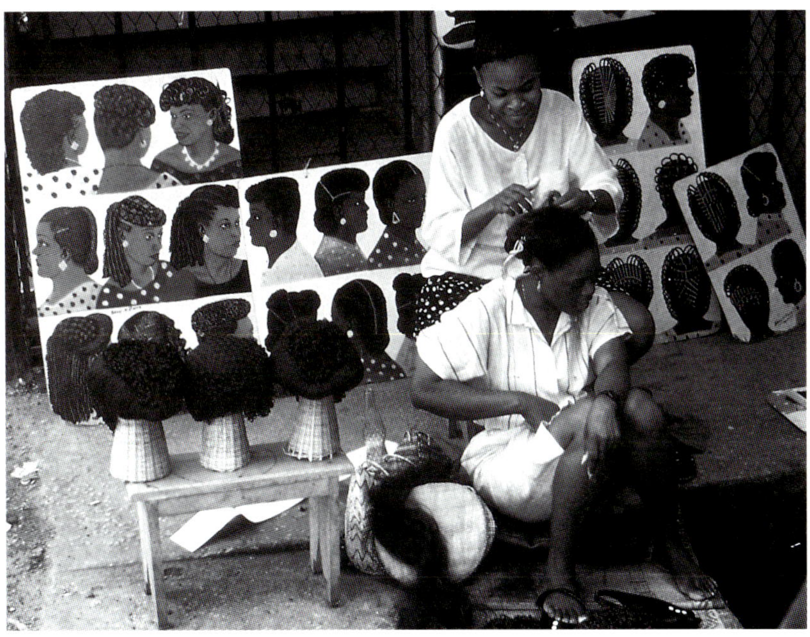

born in Cameroon in 1940. In the late 1960s, Bikok came to Libreville as a young sign painter and in 1969 he received his first commission. Between 1977 and 1986, the number of salons in Libreville grew from about fifteen to about one hundred (Lerat 1989:51). Today, there is hardly a barber shop or hairdressing salon in the city that does not display multiple paintings by Bikok (Figs. 3.20, 3.21). Like sign painters in other parts of Africa, Bikok now regularly copies photographs from a variety of fashion magazines and other publications in order to keep current with the latest styles (Fig. 3.22). Working directly from photographs has changed how he renders his figures. In his early work he concentrated on relatively flat profiles which he outlined in black. In his more recent work, he has moved to three-quarter poses, as well as paintings of full figures which he renders in a more realistic manner (Lerat 1992:87–104; Fig. 3.23).

Today in Bamako, barbers not only commission signs painted on wood, but they buy paintings on cotton sheeting. The images on the cotton sheeting are in the same style as those on the wood signs and are clearly being produced by the same group of local artists. Many barbers who set up their temporary stalls in residential quarters, near markets, and in taxi and bus depots now commission paintings on sheeting. The sheets may be tacked up as banners stretching across the entrance of the stall or, in some cases, they are used to form the actual sides of the shop. More and more barbers also display large, commercially printed color posters as advertisements. Most of these posters are of African-American music groups, like High Five and Troop, who were popular in America in the late 1980s. The question remains if these commercial posters become more widely available and affordable, will they begin to replace the demand for hand-painted signs?

## CONCLUSION

Much time and attention is paid to hair throughout Africa and its diaspora, and culturally specific beliefs and values associated with the head and hair underlie people's notions of propriety, appropriateness, good grooming, beauty, fashion, and modernity. These beliefs and values, which have clearly been subject to modification over time, profoundly shape the manipulation of hair by men and women of different ages in everyday, ceremonial, and ritual contexts. The regenerative quality of hair and the emphemeral nature of hair styles, like hats that can be put on and taken off, make hair an excellent and dynamic vehicle for the visual expression of diverse and changing individual and social personae.

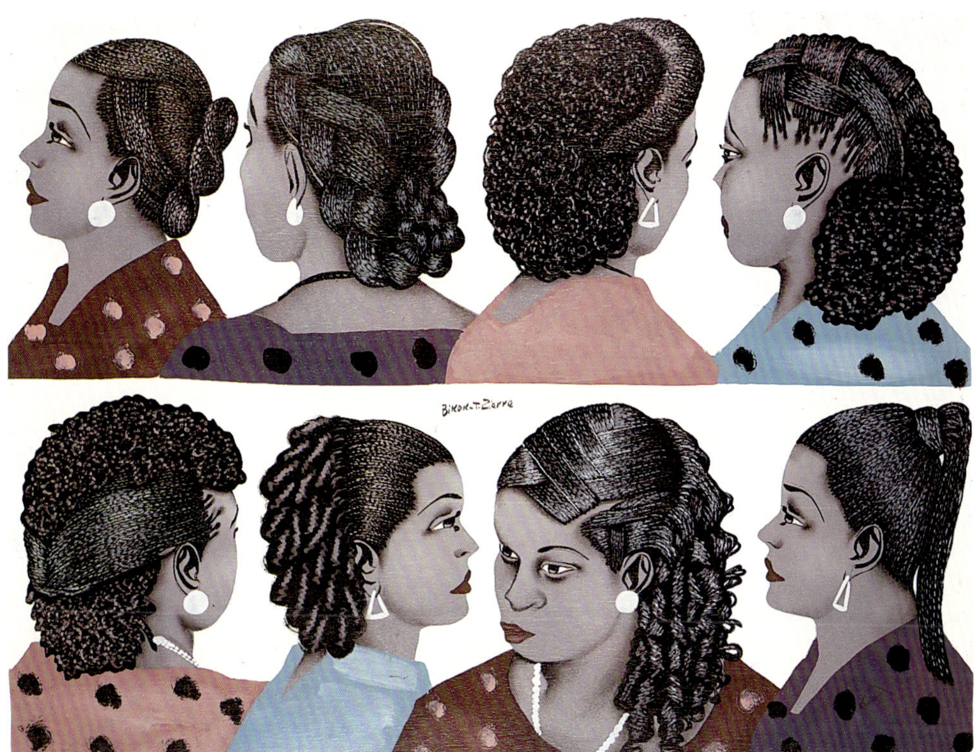

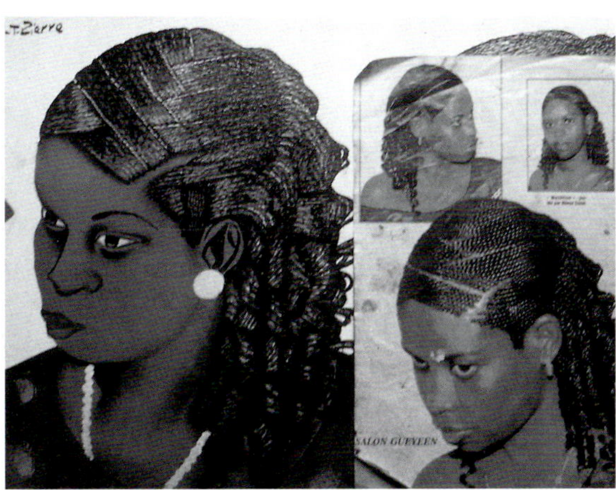

**Figure 3.22**, left. Detail of a hairdresser's sign by Bikok T. Pierre next to the fashion magazine that was its inspiration. Photograph by Philip Ravenhill, 1989.

**Figure 3.23**, above left. Barber sign. Bikok T. Pierre, Libreville, Gabon. Wood, paint. H. 62.0 cm. FMCH X90.0. Museum purchase, Manus Fund. The women's hair styles on this sign were popular in Libreville in the 1980s.

DEFRISAGE, GONFLAGE, NOIRCISSAGE & SECHAGE
SALON DE COIFFUR
C'EST CHIM'S
UN SPECIALISTE EN MODELES DE COIFFURES AFRICAINES & EUROPEENNES' COIFFE HOMMES, FEMMES, ENFANTS et vous offre ses meuilleurs services, à votre bon vouloir il vous coiffe à domicile. CONSULTEZ VOS PROFESSIONNELS
B.P. 4102 CARREFOUR LEONMBA. TEL..........
Soyez Chic, Produisez Un Effet De Choc. COIFFEZ VOUS Chez CHIM'S
la coiffure c'est mon métier.
Pour être chic sans trop user sonchèque c'est CHIM'S biensûr
Les personnes exigentes se coiffent chez CHIM'S.
MADO
OIFFURE

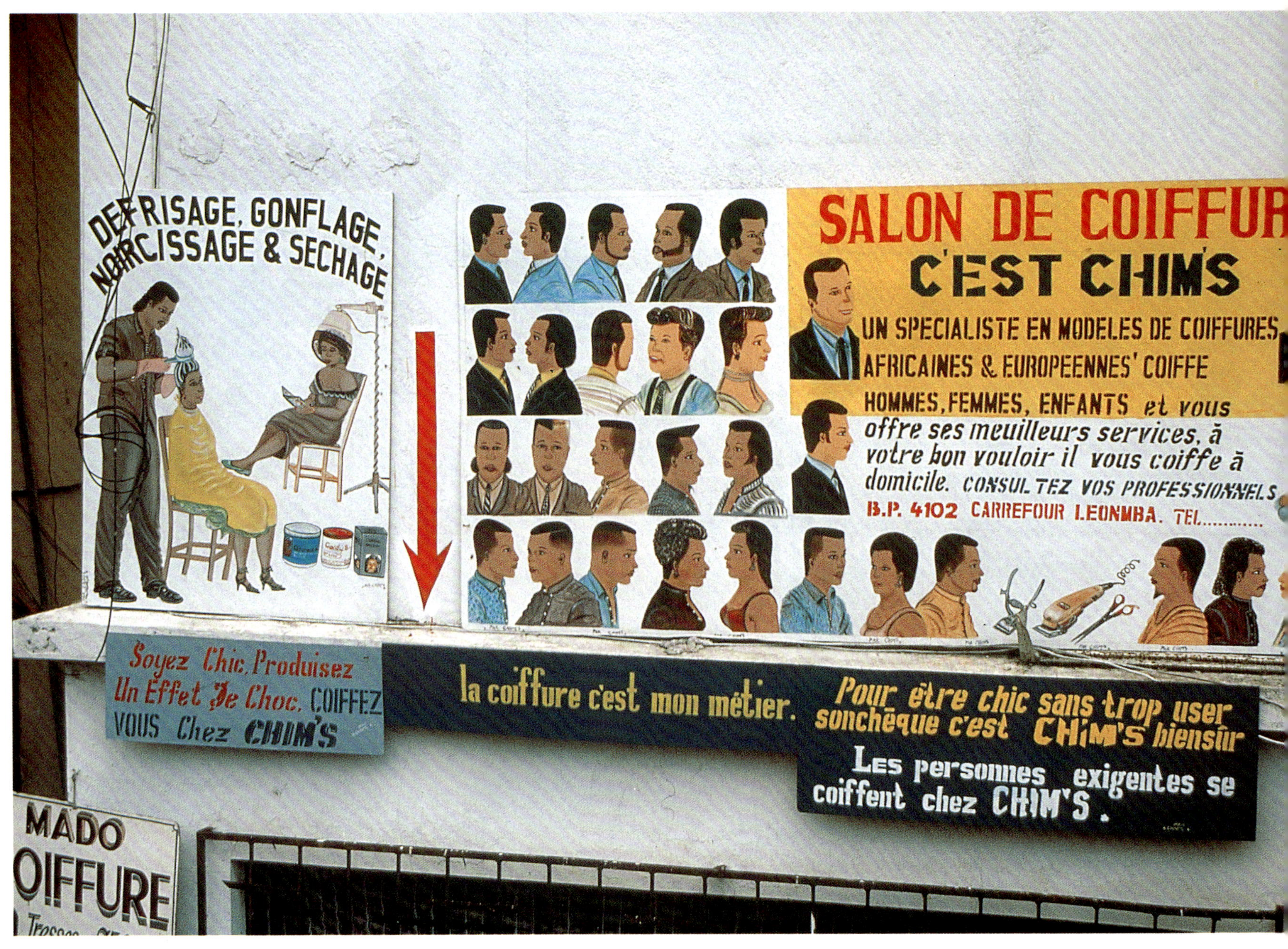

Signage above large barber shop in Libreville, Gabon. Photograph by Philip Ravenhill, 1989.

# COIFFURE MODERN

## A GALLERY OF AFRICAN HAIR STYLES

## 1970 – 1990

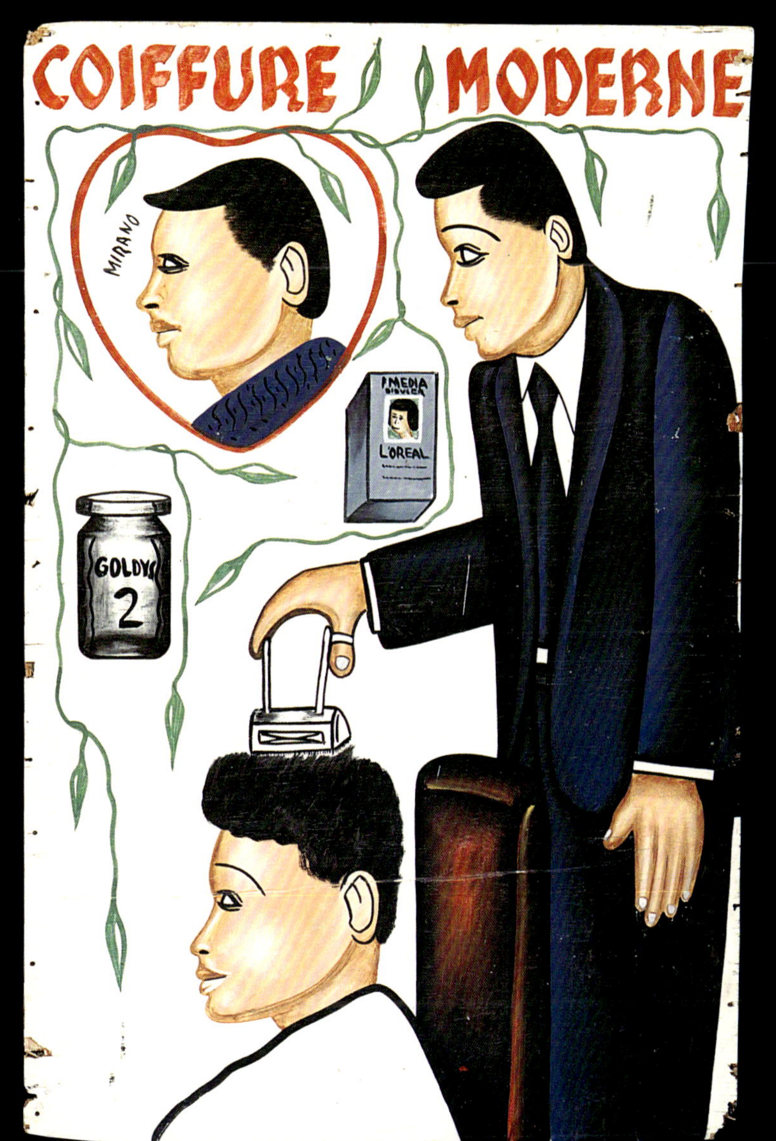

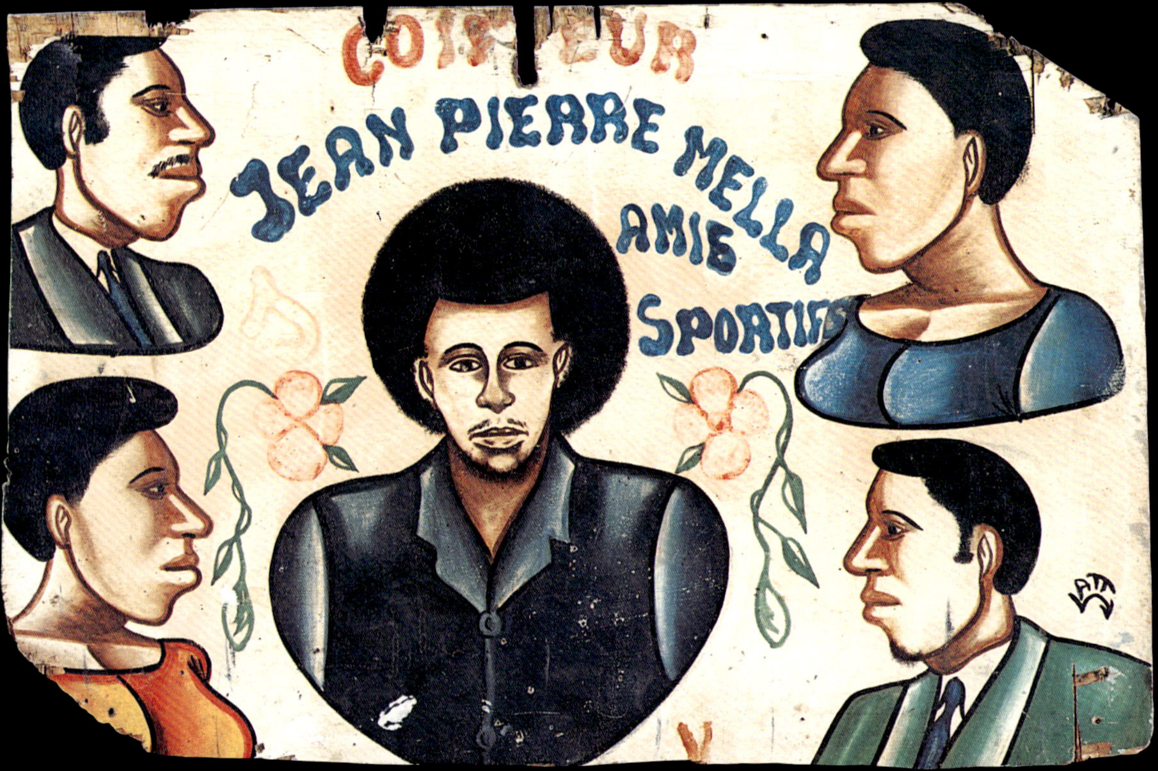

COIFFEUR
JEAN PIERRE MELLA
AMIS
SPORTIFS

B

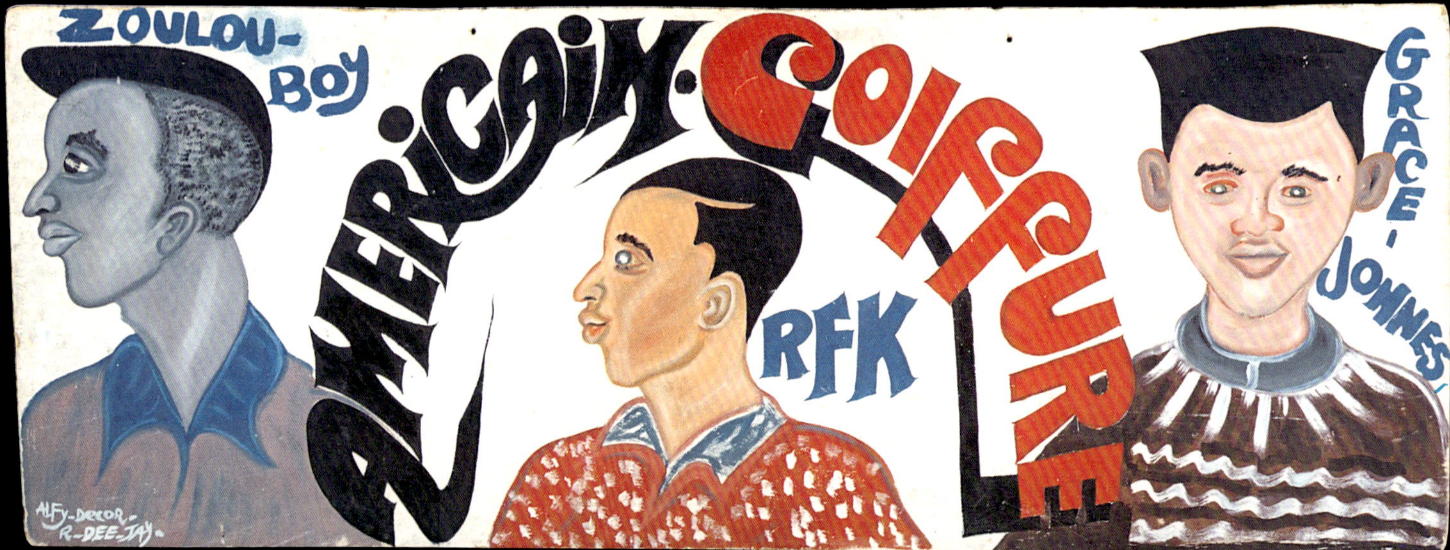

ZOULOU-
BOY
AMERICAIN.
COIFFURE
RFK
GRACE-
JOHNNES
ALFY-DECOR-
R-DEE-JAY.

ABIDJAN, CÔTE D'IVOIRE

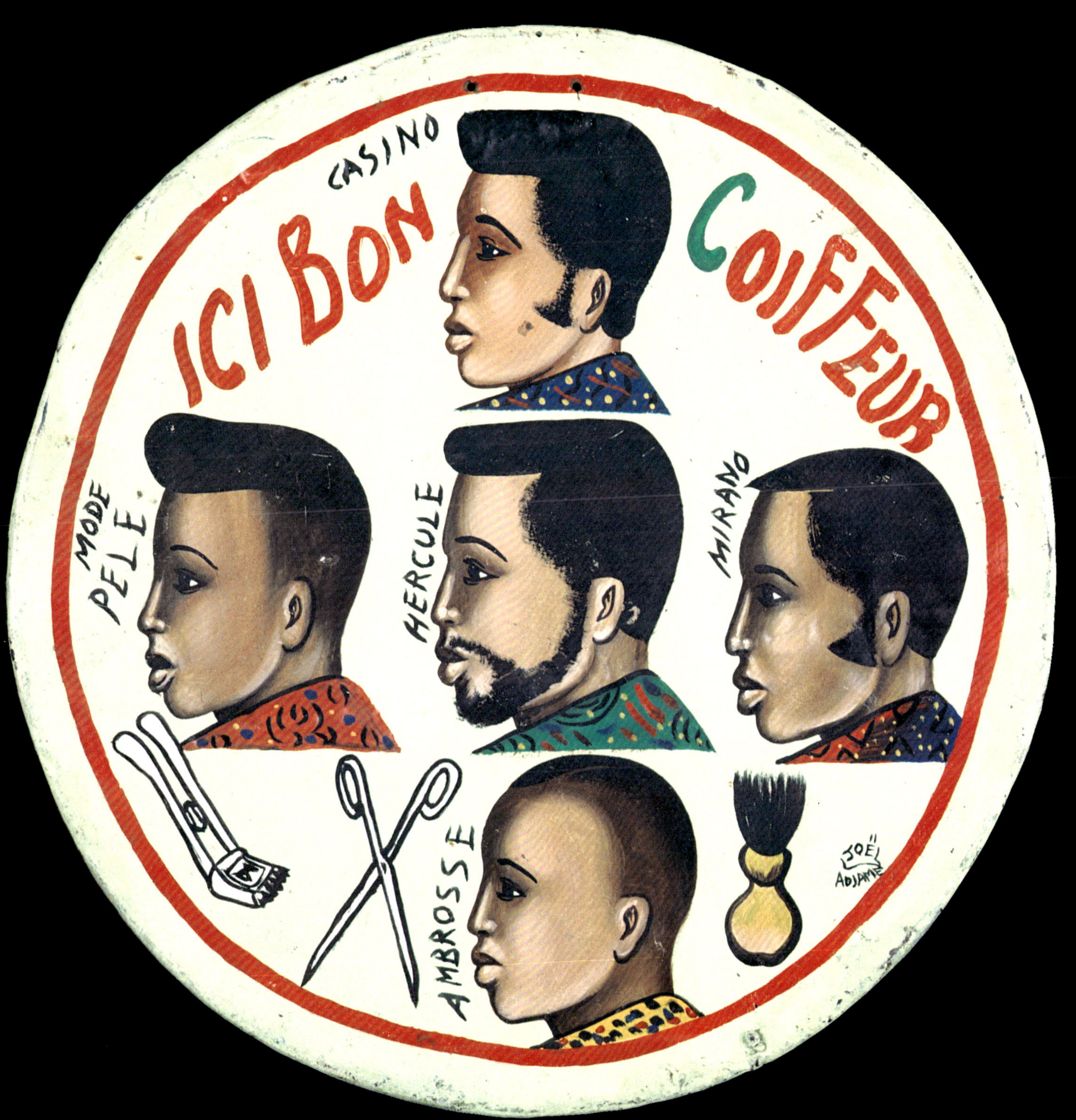


D

SALON DE
COIFFURE
DéFrisage-GonFlage
Noircissage
Bikok-T. Pierre

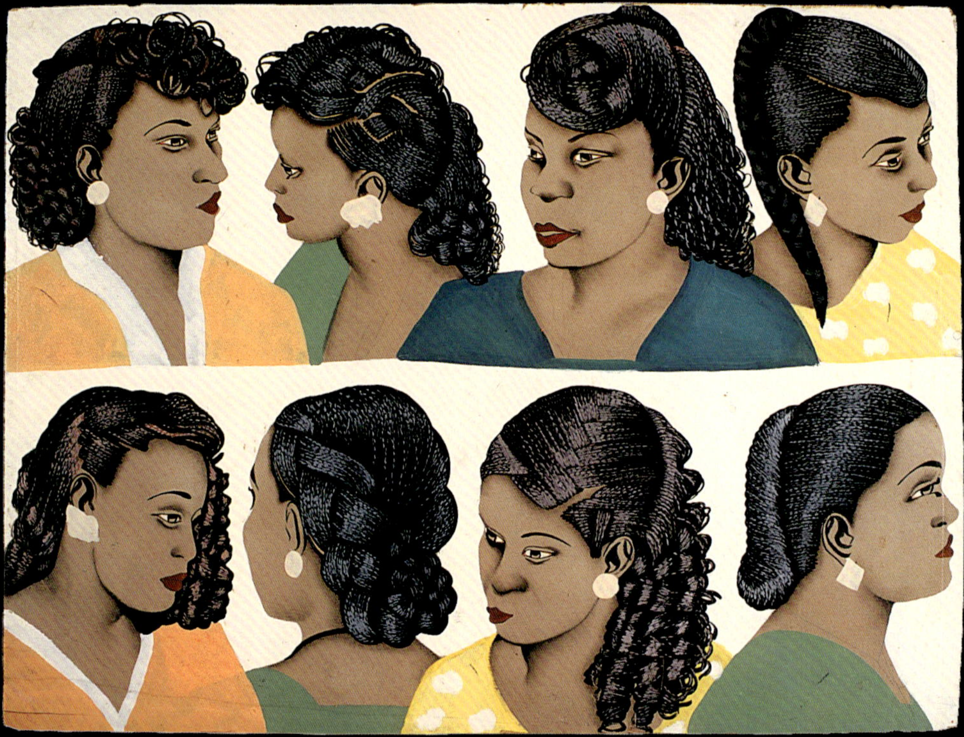

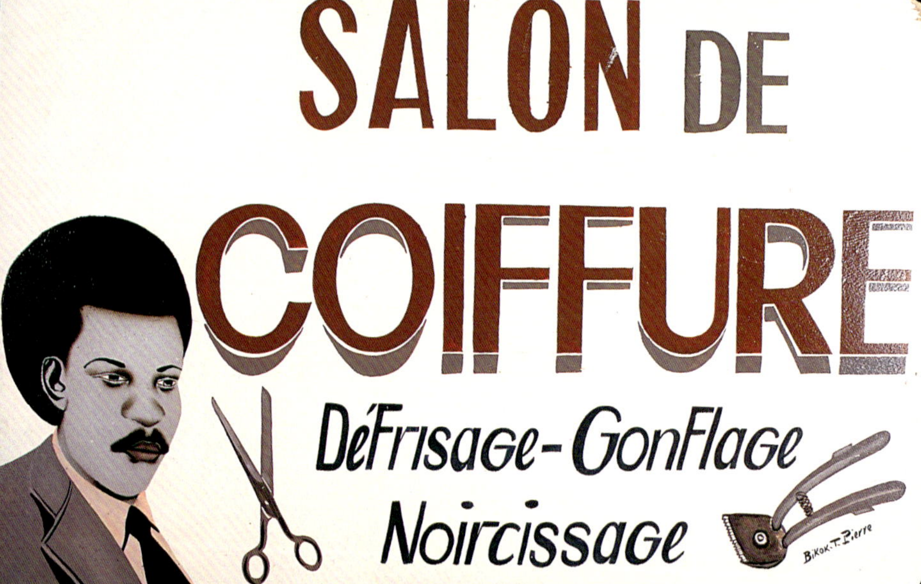

BiKoK J. Pierre

G

Retrouvez-votre
Ancien Coiffeur
Adamou
Akébé-Ville

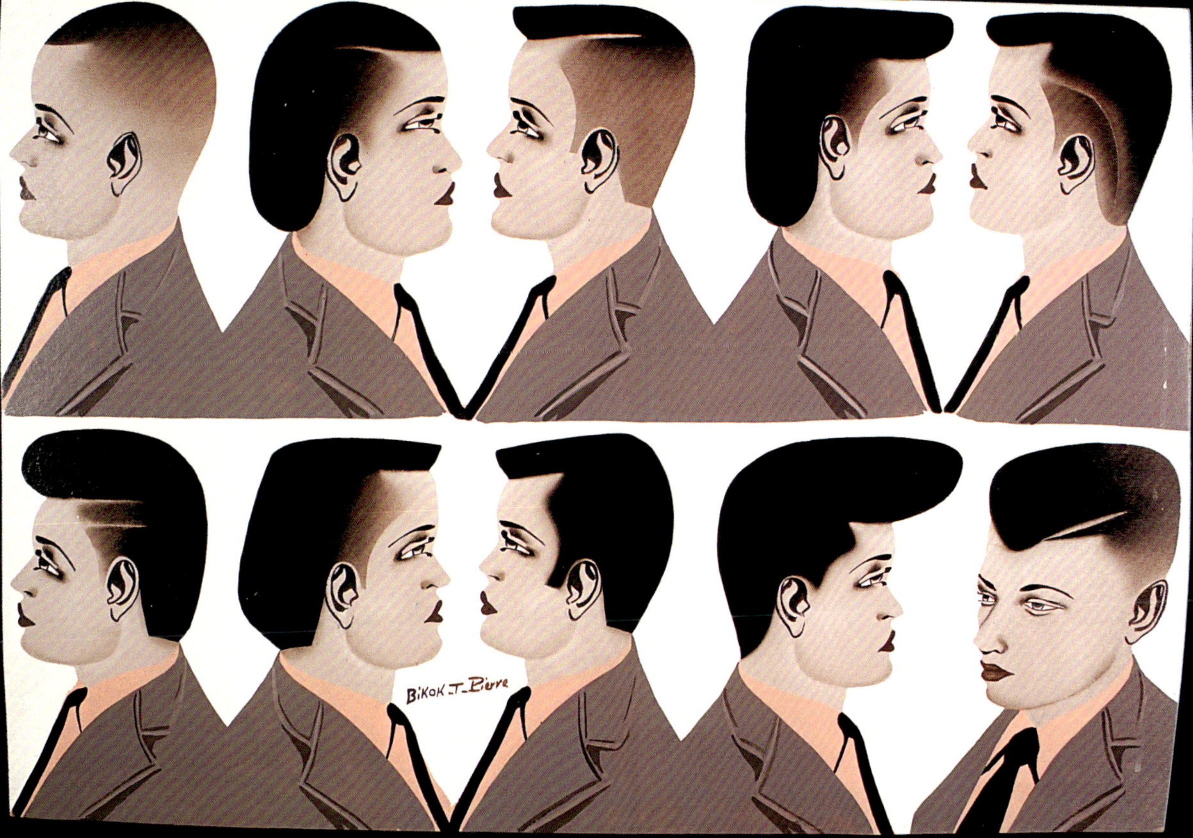

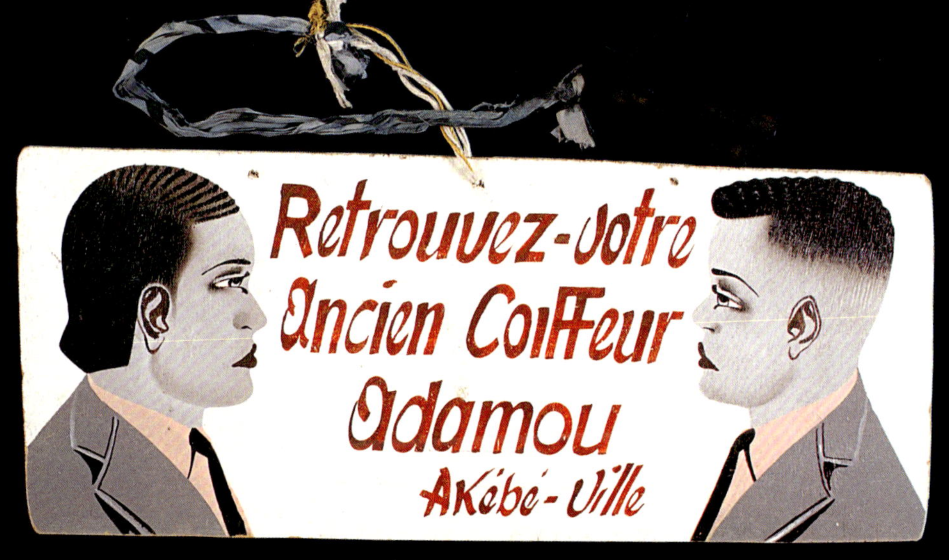

H

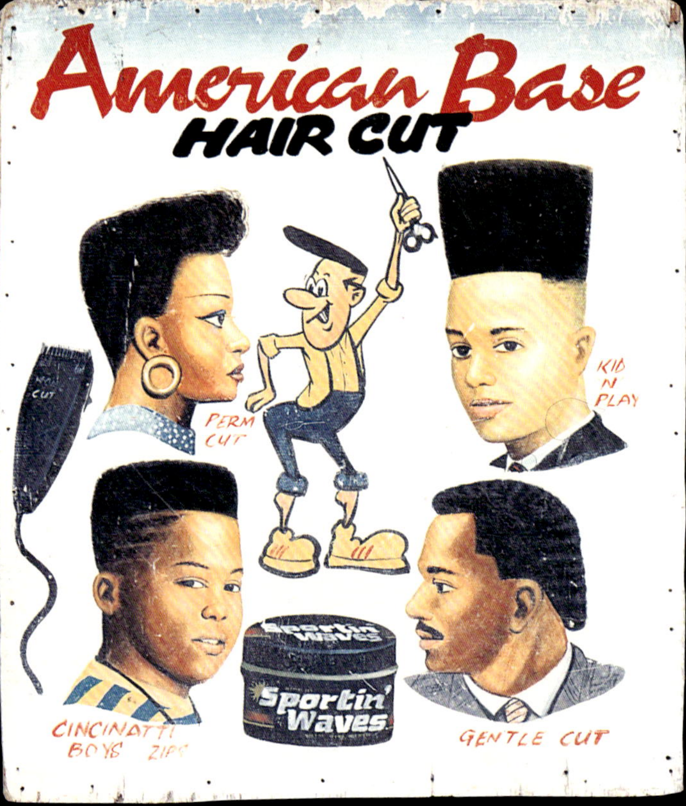

American Base
HAIR CUT

PERM CUT

KID N PLAY

CINCINATTI BOYS ZIPS

Sportin' Waves

GENTLE CUT

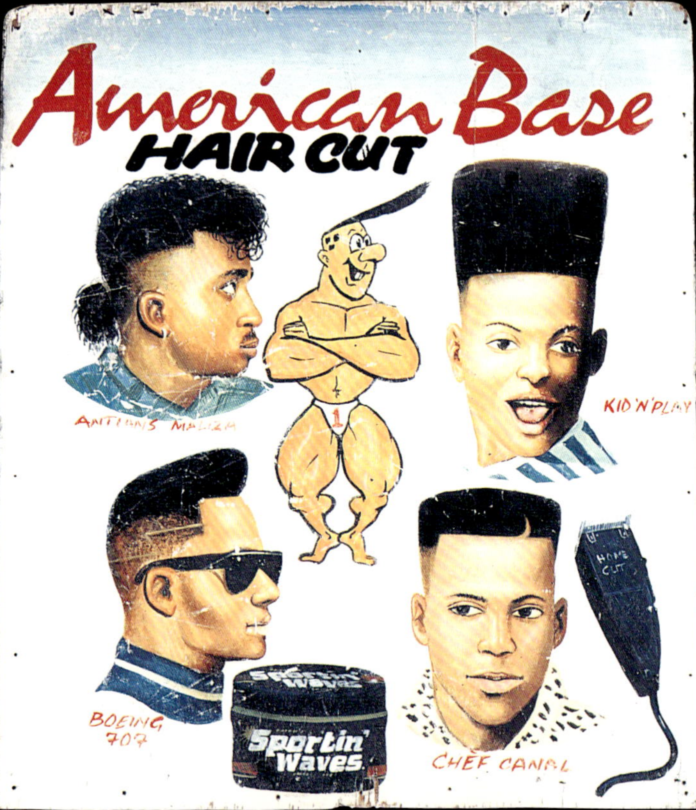

American Base
HAIR CUT

ANTHANS MALIZA

KID'N'PLAY

BOEING 707

Sportin' Waves

HOME CUT

CHEF CANAL

DIPLOMATIC
HAIR CUT

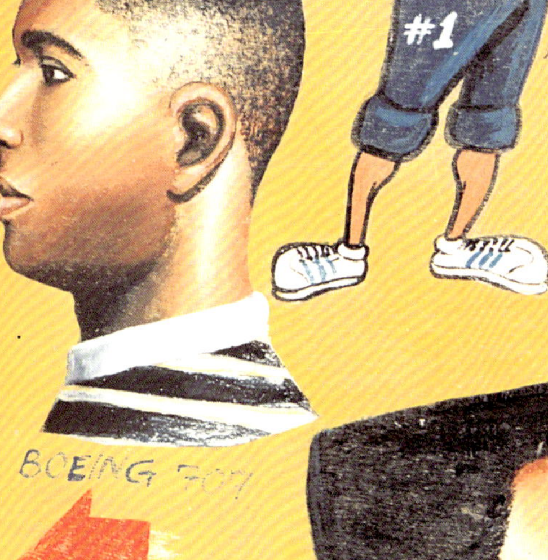
#1
BOEING 707

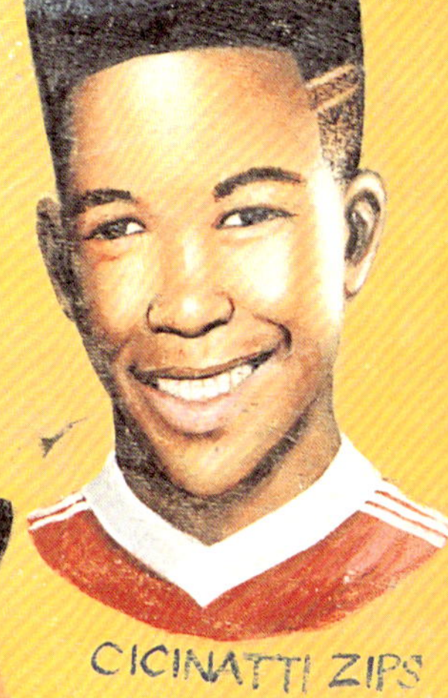
CICINATTI ZIPS

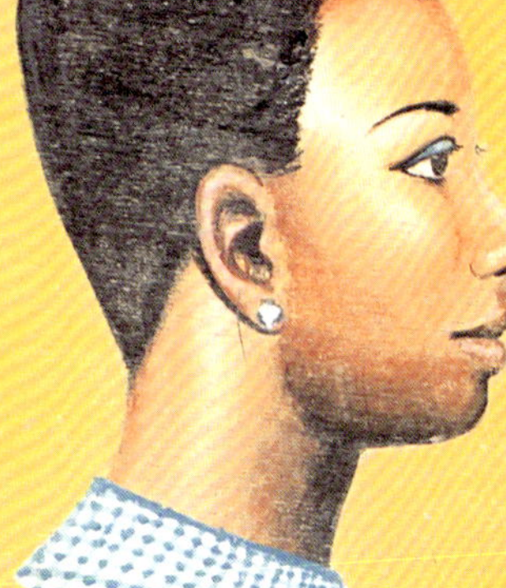
COCAINE CUT
U.S.A. TRAINED SPECIALIST FROM NEW YORK CITY
MURPHY MODELLE CURRENCY

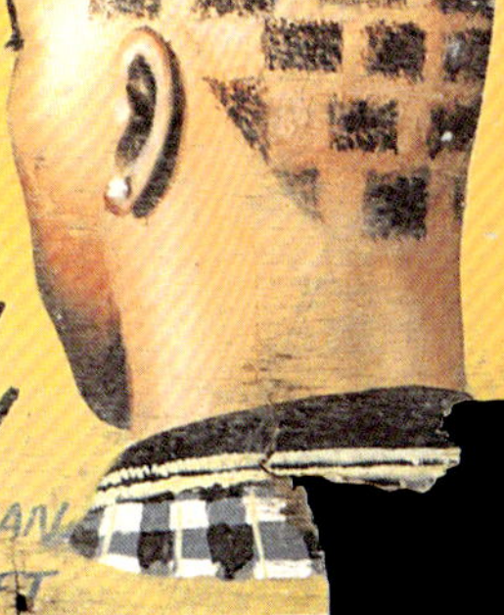
ITALIAN DRAFT

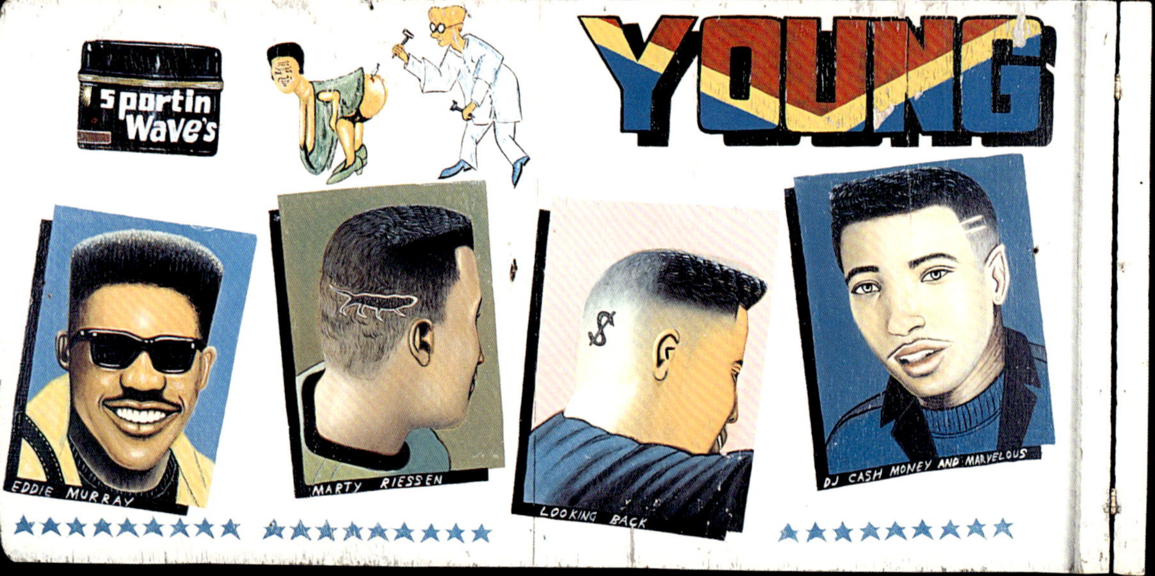

sportin Wave's

YOUNG

EDDIE MURRAY

MARTY RIESSEN

LOOKING BACK

DJ CASH MONEY AND MARVELOUS

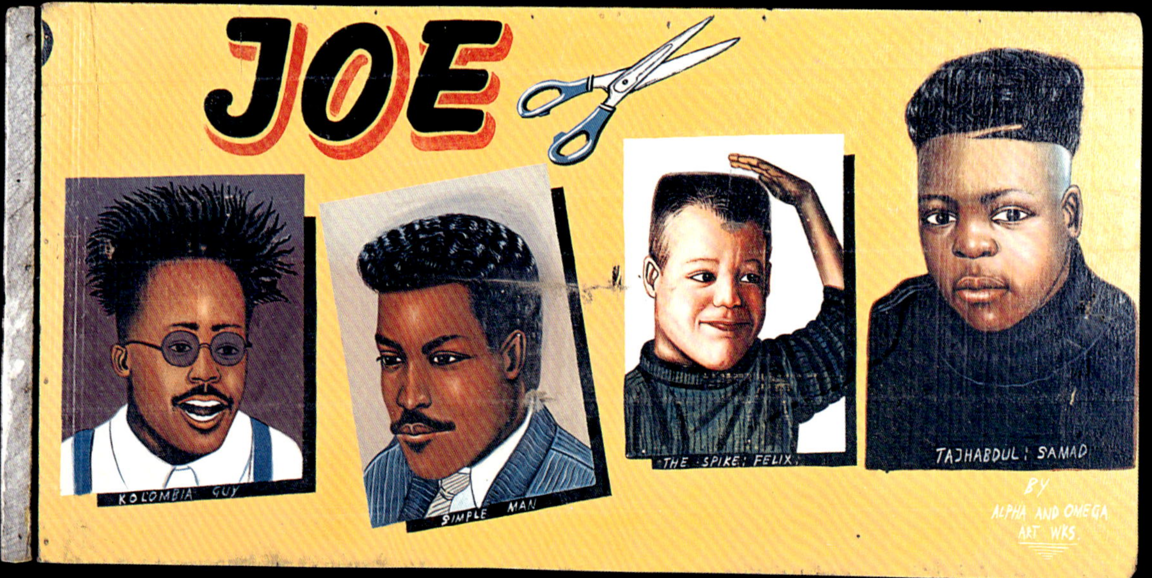

JOE

KOLOMBIA GUY

SIMPLE MAN

THE SPIKE: FELIX

TAJHABDUL: SAMAD

BY
ALPHA AND OMEGA
ART WKS.

YOUNG JOE HAIR CUT
AO
ALPHA & OMEGA
ART WORK
TECH-JUNCTION
KSI.
Sportin' Waves
AMERICAN +
U.S.A. +
LAOX
Wee!
COCAINE MODELLE
CONCORD UP
OBOYE CUT
GENTLE CUT

M

YOUNG JOE HAIR CUT
Expensive
No1
PERM CUT
GENTLE CUT
PLAY+-BOY+-PLAY+

N

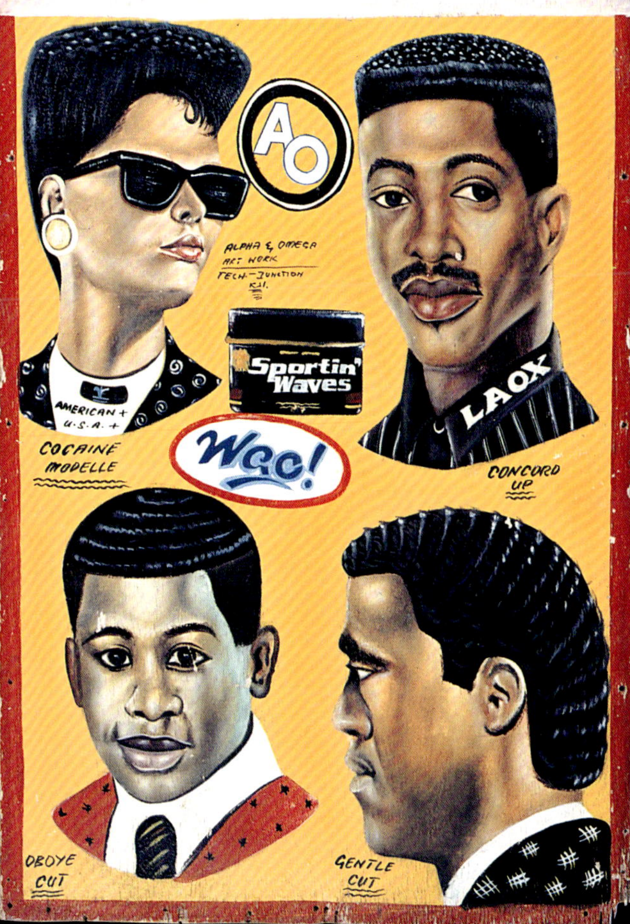

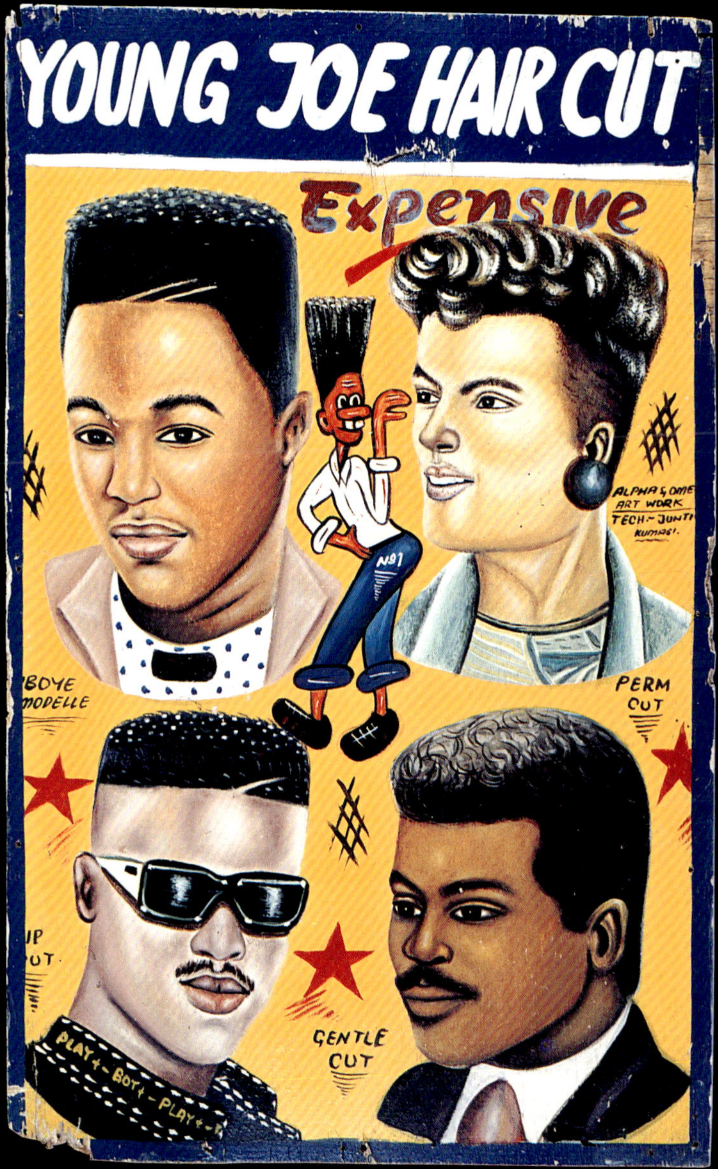

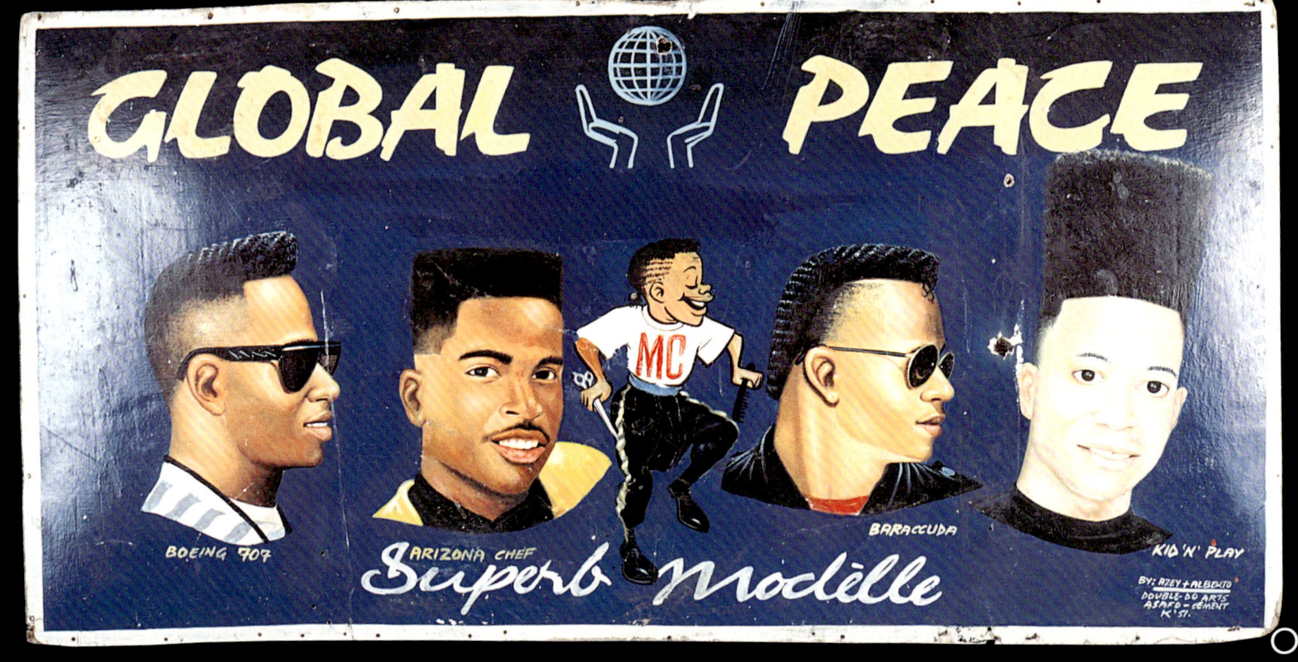
GLOBAL PEACE
MC
BOEING 707
ARIZONA CHEF
BARACCUDA
KID 'N' PLAY
Superb Modèlle
BY: AZEY + ALBERTO
DOUBLE-DO ARTS
ASAFO-CEMENT
K'SI.

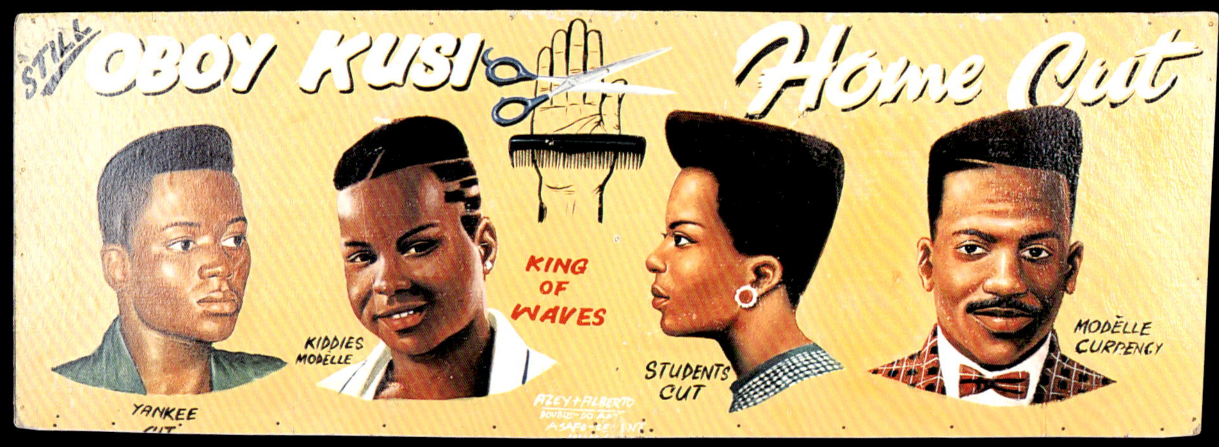
STILL
OBOY KUSI
Home Cut
KING OF WAVES
KIDDIES MODELLE
YANKEE
STUDENTS CUT
MODÈLLE CURPENCY
AZEY + ALBERTO

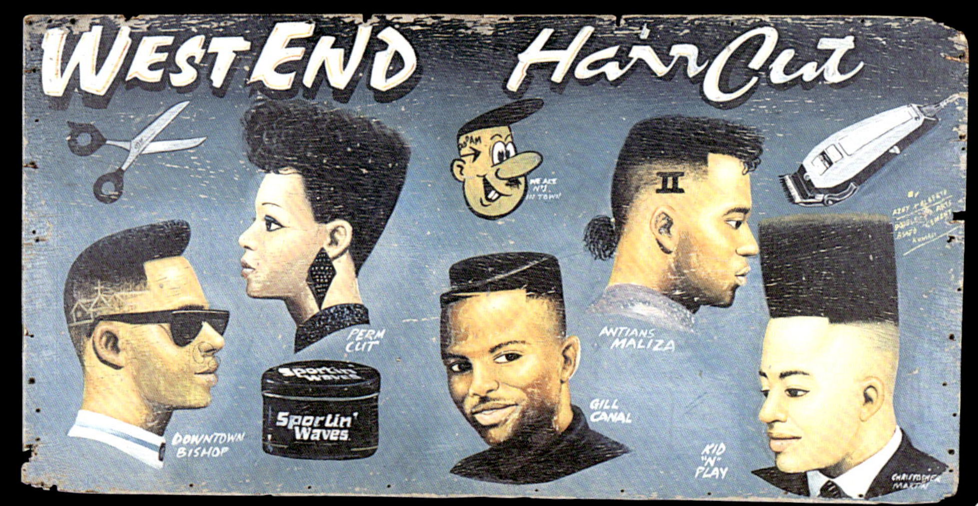
WEST END HairCut
PERM CUT
Sportin' Waves
DOWNTOWN BISHOP
ANTIANS MALIZA
GILL CANAL
KID "N" PLAY

SALLON DE
GOD'S TIME
UNITED STATE OF AMRICANO
BY OKALA AFLAO
GENTLE-USE
SPORTING-WAVES
I THANK GOD
AGONA BE LOVE
RESPECT
BOIENG-707
YOU THIS WOMAN YOU GET AIDS, SO. I WENT HELP YOU
AGYEI YOU WENT KILL ME
DR. J

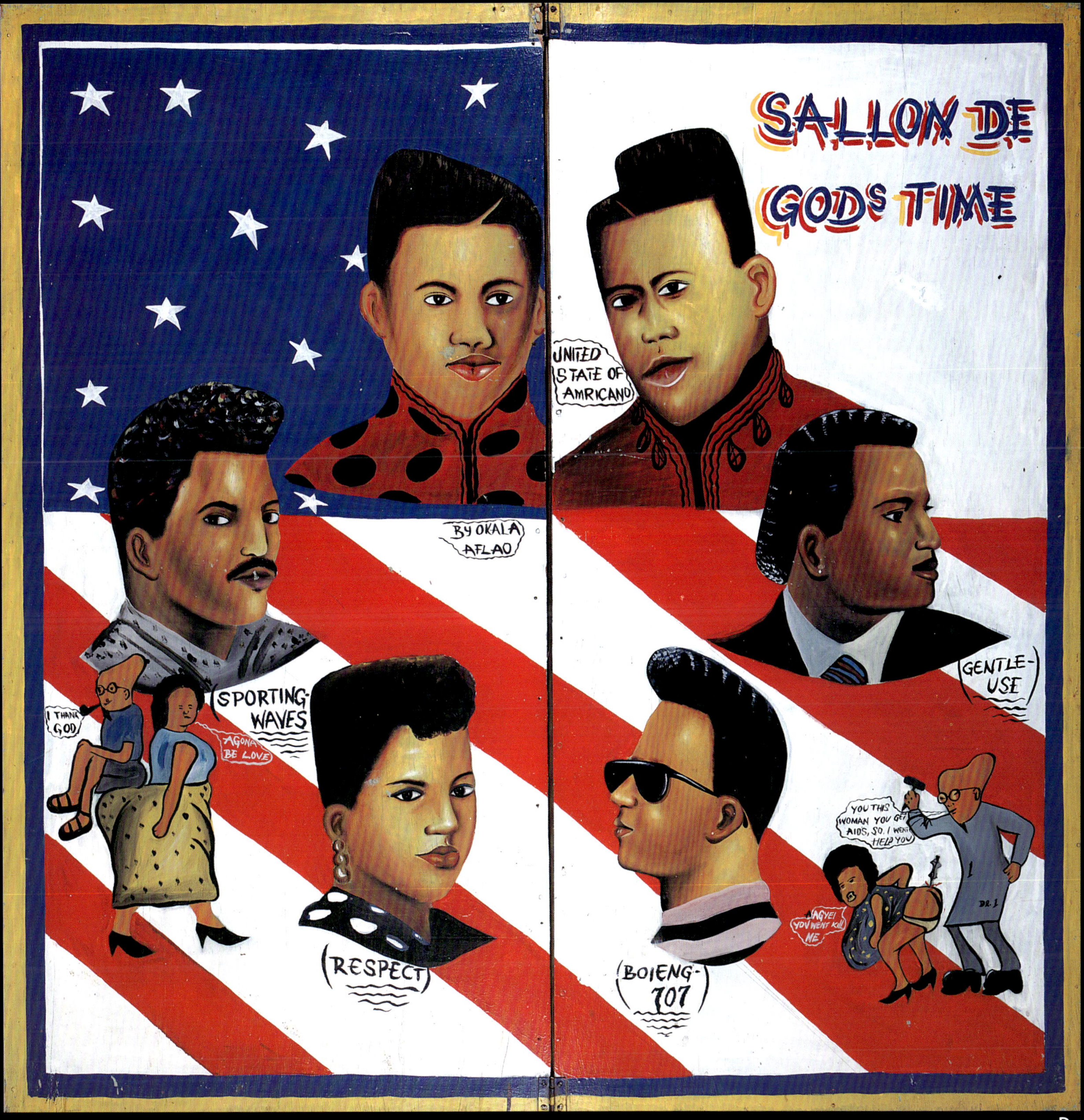

R

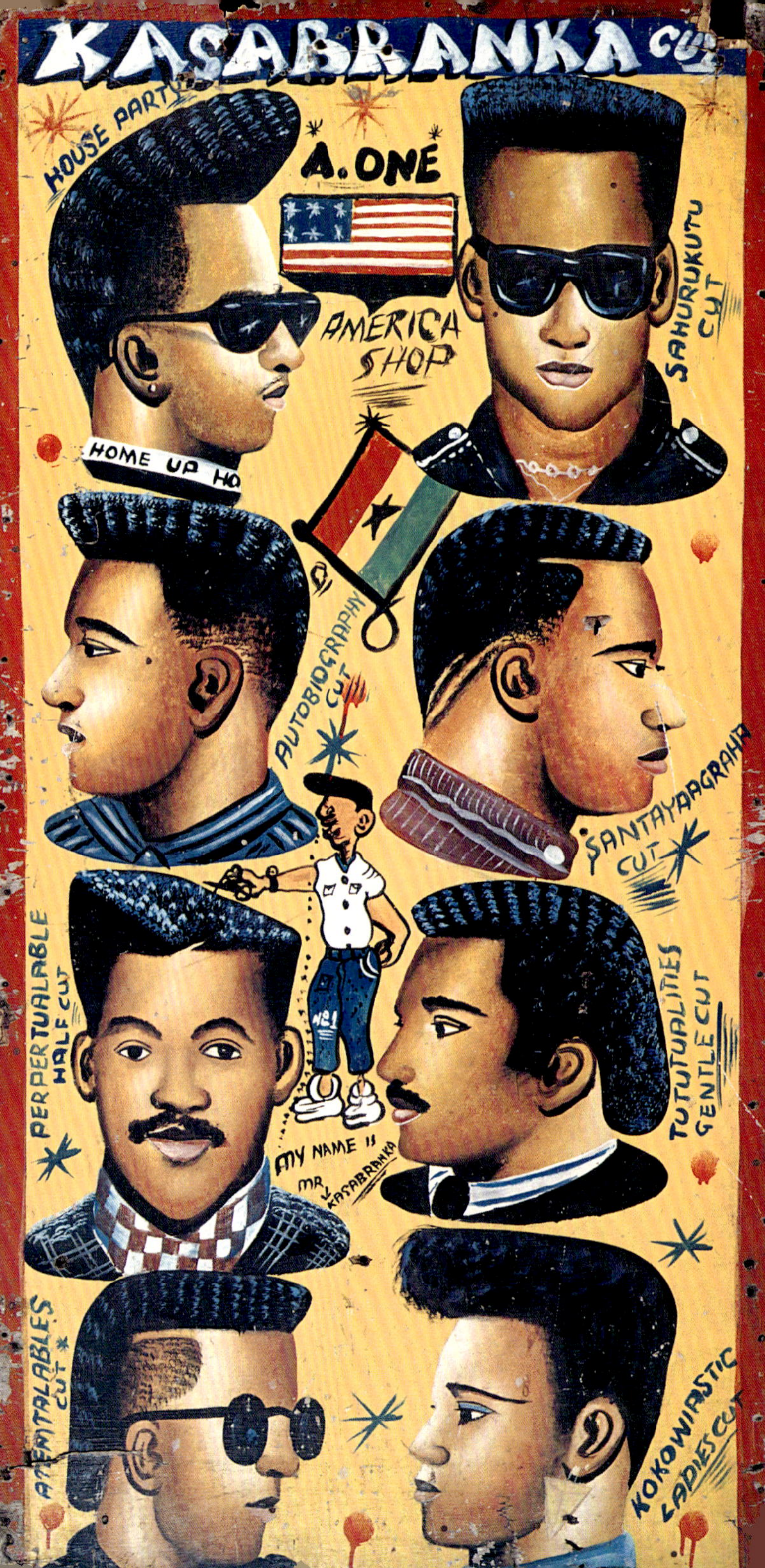
KASABRANKA CUT
HOUSE PARTY
A. ONE
AMERICA SHOP
SAHURUKUTU CUT
HOME UP HO
AUTOBIOGRAPHY CUT
SANTAYAAGRAHA CUT
PERPERTUALABLE HALF CUT
TUTUTUALITIES GENTLE CUT
MY NAME IS MR. KASABRANKA
AMERITALABLES CUT
KOKOWIASTIC LADIES CUT

KUMASE, GHA

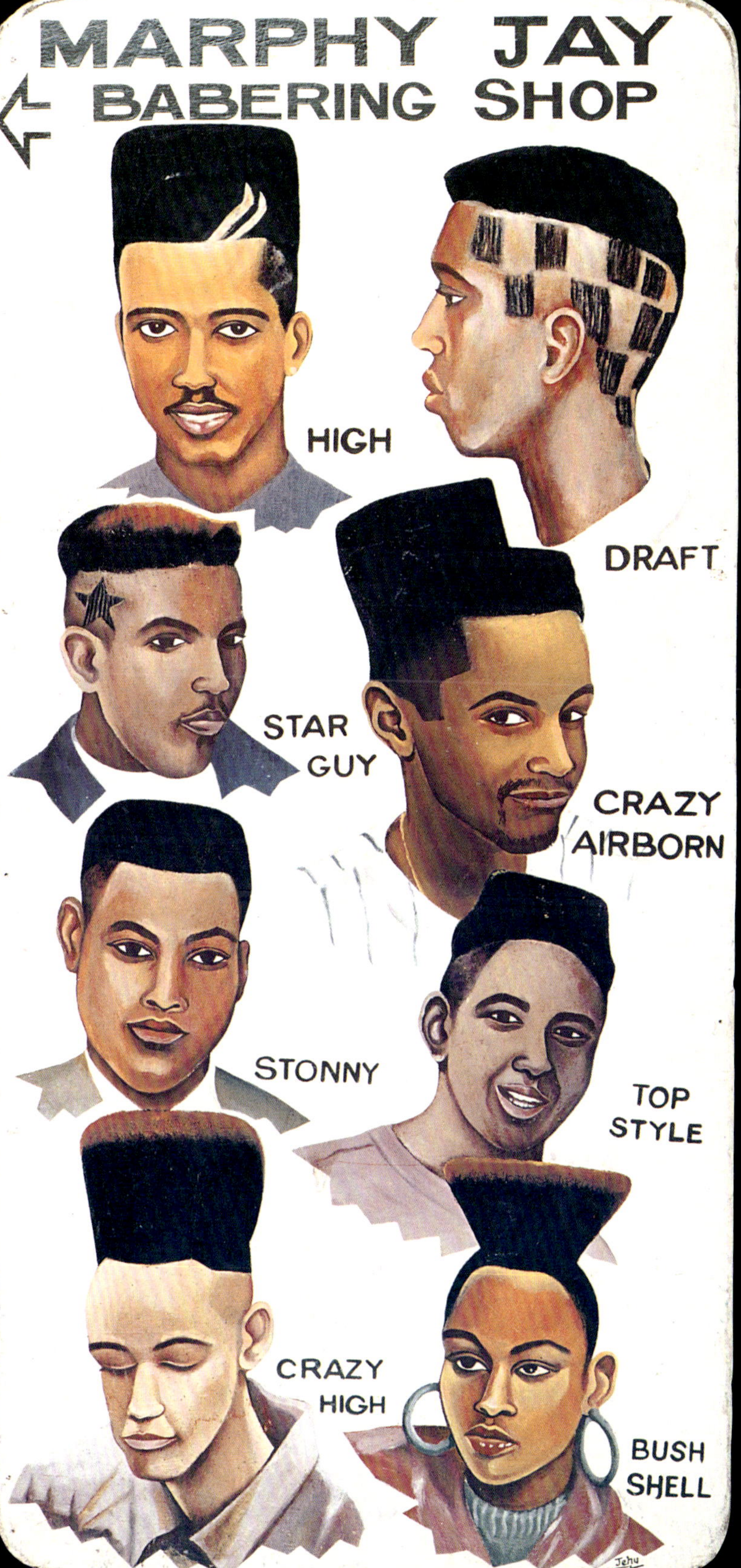


T

## COIFFURE MODERNE

Barber signs from Abidjan, Côte d'Ivoire. Collection of Ernie Wolfe, III and Diane Steinmetz.

A. Height, 105 cm
B. Height, 59.5 cm
C. Height, 42.8 cm
D. Height, 58.5 cm

Barber signs painted by Bikok T. Pierre, Libreville, Gabon. Fowler Museum of Cultural History. Museum purchase, Manus Fund.

E. FMCH X90.6,height 62 cm
F. FMCH X90.11, height 61cm
G. FMCH X90.10, height 25 cm
H. FMCH X90.4, height 68 cm

Barber signs from workshop of Alpha & Omega Artwork, Kumase, Ghana. Collection of Ernie Wolfe, III and Diane Steinmetz

I. Height, 68 cm
J. Height, 68 cm
K. Height, 114 cm
L. Height, 61 cm
M. Height, 89 cm
N. Height, 89 cm

Barber signs from workshop of Double-Do Arts, Kumase, Ghana. Collection of Ernie Wolfe, III and Diane Steinmetz

O. Height, 61 cm
P. Height, 43 cm
Q. Height, 61 cm

Barber signs by Okala, Aflao, Ghana. Collection of Tom Patchett

R. Height, 131 cm

Barber signs from Kumase, Ghana. Collection of Ernie Wolfe, III and Diane Steinmetz

S. Height, 119 cm
T. Height, 123 cm

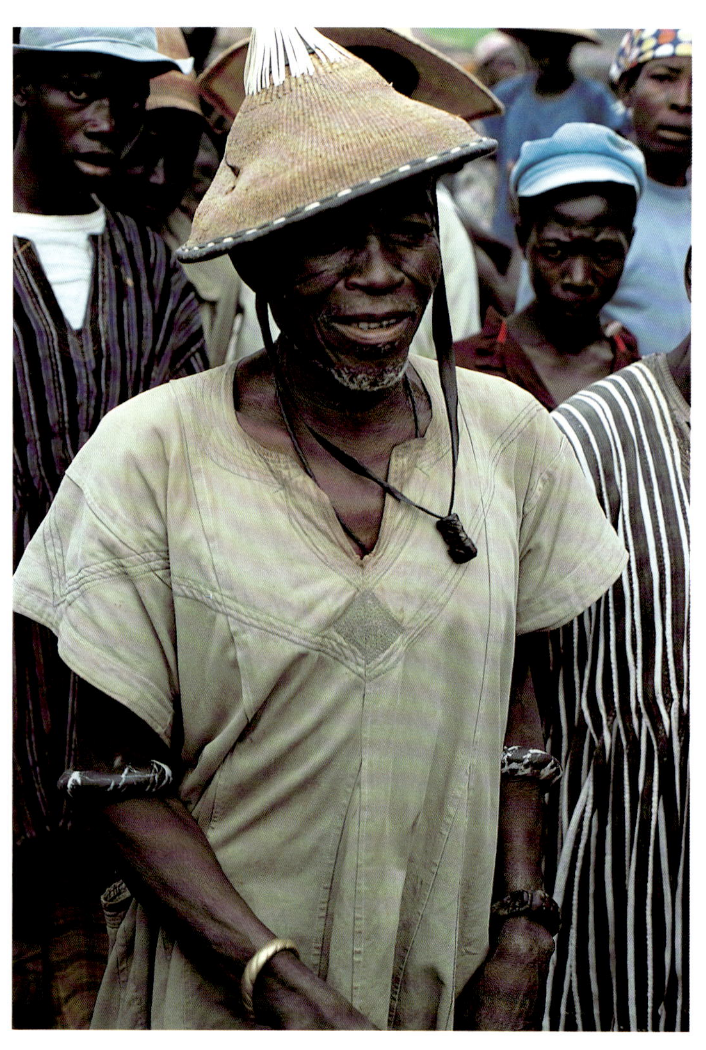

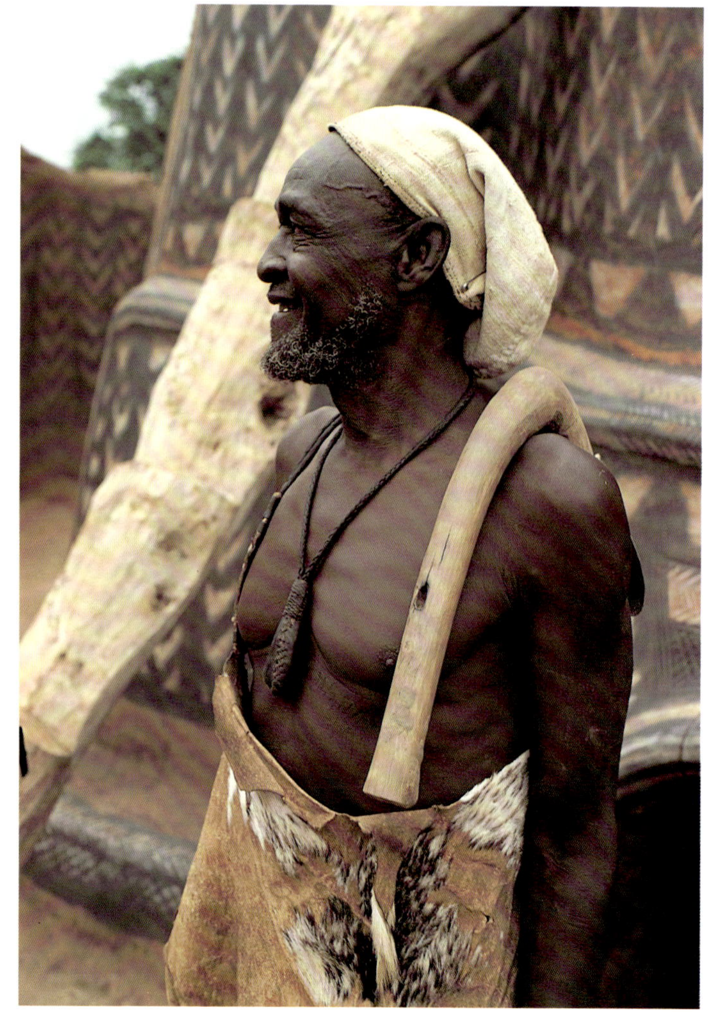

# 4 PRACTICAL BEAUTY: HEADGEAR FOR DAILY WEAR

CHRISTINE MULLEN KREAMER

Hats, caps, and headties are worn by men and women in the course of everyday activities. They function as effective shields against sun and rain. In addition to protecting the wearer from the elements, they also fulfill society's requirements of decorum and modesty, for among many groups, wearing a hat is "de rigueur" when one is outside the home. As a vital part of everyday wear, hats can also be vehicles for expressing individual and commonly held aesthetic preferences.

While not disregarding artistry or form, it is necessary to seek out durable and affordable solutions in the creation of everyday headwear. The functional demands of daily wear preclude the use of fragile materials that could deteriorate with extensive use. An appropriate response is to place greater reliance on locally available materials and to limit decorative elaboration.

## THE ENVIRONMENT AS A SOURCE

The natural environment provides a wealth of practical and economical raw materials for the fabrication of daily headwear. The !Kung of southern Africa create an impressive variety of fiber and ostrich shell-jewelry, including delicate headbands worn by both men and women as part of daily dress (Fig. 4.1). Ostrich shells are highly valued among the !Kung, who collect them for use as water containers and as a principal material in body ornamentation.

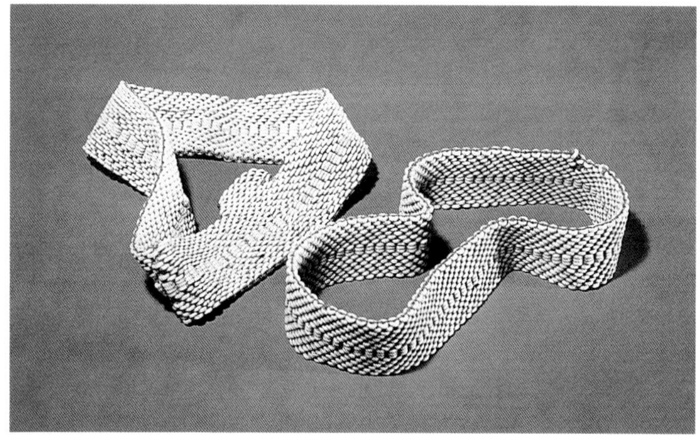

**Figure 4.1**, above. Headband. !Kung, Botswana. Ostrich egg shell, fiber. H. 3.5 cm. FMCH. Anonymous gift. On occassion, decorative beaded pendants, in triangular and other geometric shapes, are suspended from the simple band to create a colorful fringe around the forehead.

**Opposite.** Northern Ghanaian men wearing hats. Sirigu, Navrongo. Photograph by Herbert M. Cole, 1976.

### DECORATED CALABASHES

With minimal preparation, gourds can be used as functional headgear. Decorated with incised and pyro-engraved linear and curvilinear designs; or embellished with beads, cowrie shells, leather, or pigments; or surmounted with the horns of antelopes or bush cows, a simple gourd can be transformed into headwear of astonishing beauty. The Goudor cap from northern Cameroon (Figs. 4.2, 4.3) is a combination of the natural beauty of the calabash and decorative curvilinear designs, resulting in a functional and beautiful headdress. This cap is worn by women on a daily basis and for ceremonial occasions.

The horned helmet from northern Ghana (Fig. 1.15; called *ipiedza* among the Konkomba) is another excellent example of calabash headgear (Tait 1961:91).

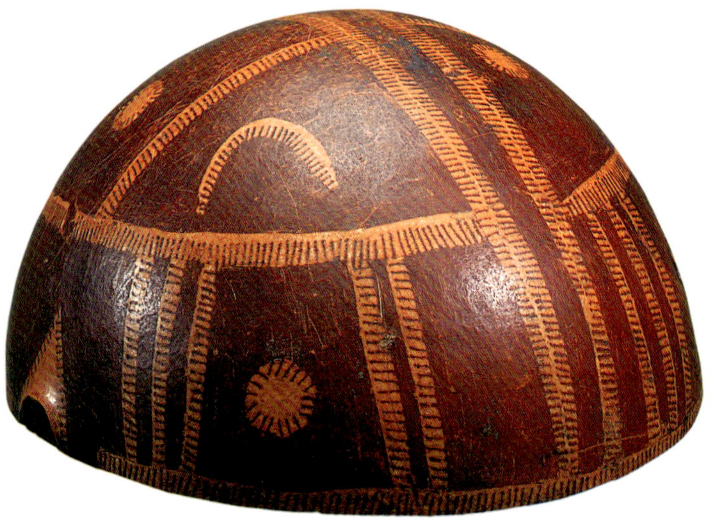

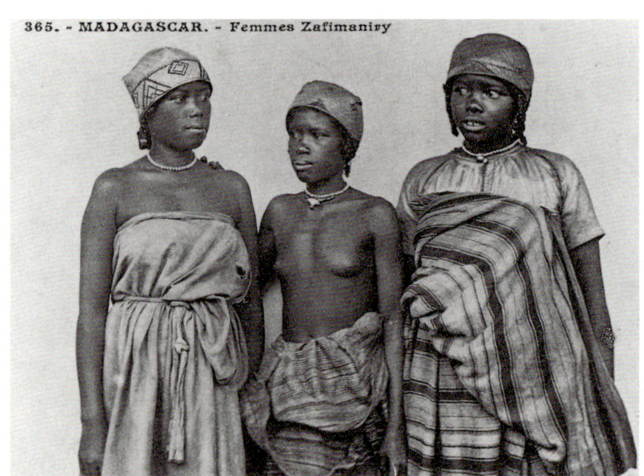


Figure 4.2, above. Woman's hat. Goudour, Cameroon. Gourd, pigment, paint. H. 12.0 cm. FCMH X94.29.3. Museum purchase, Jerome L. Joss Endowment Fund.

Figure 4.3, right. Hide Women in northern Cameroon wearing gourd hats. Photograph by René Gardi, 1953.

Figure 4.5, above right. "Femmes Zafimaniry" (Zafimaniry women), Madagascar. Photographer unknown, ca. 1910. Postcard collection. Eliot Elisofon Photographic Archives. National Museum of African Art.

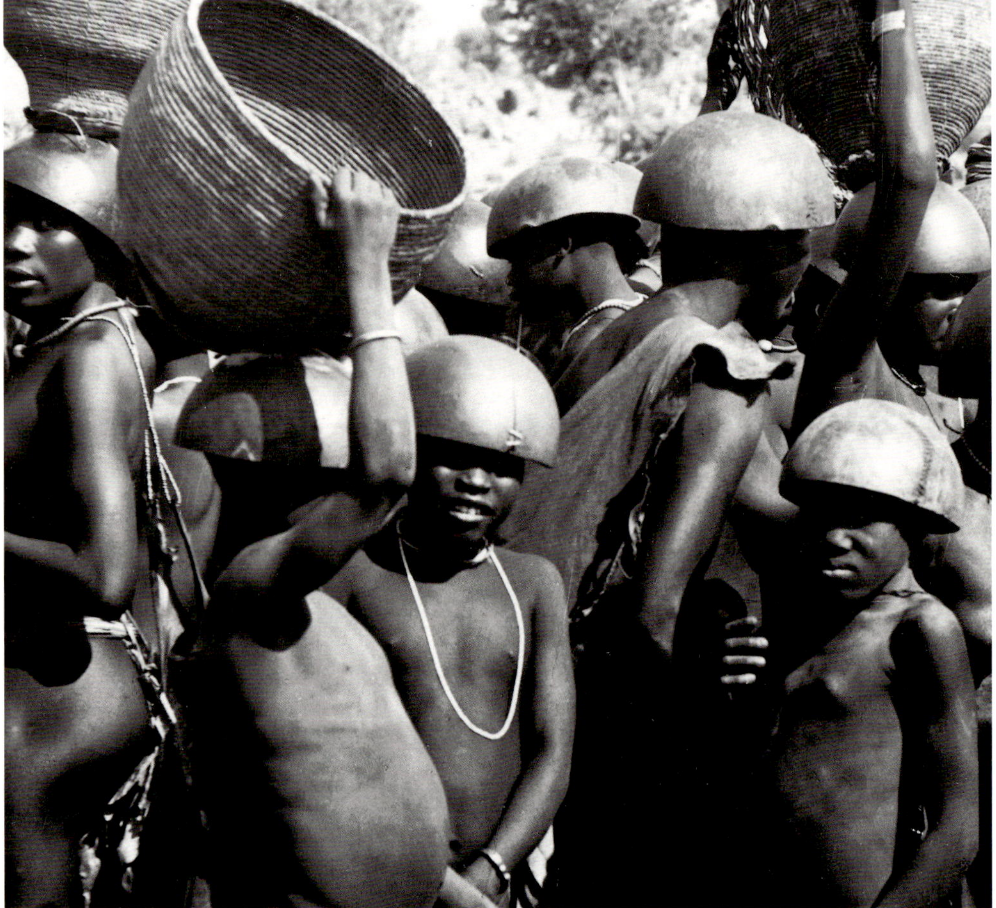

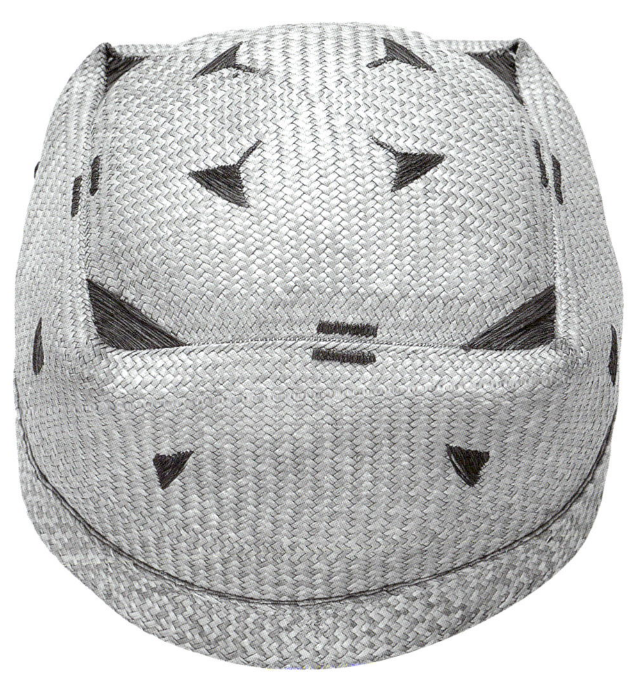

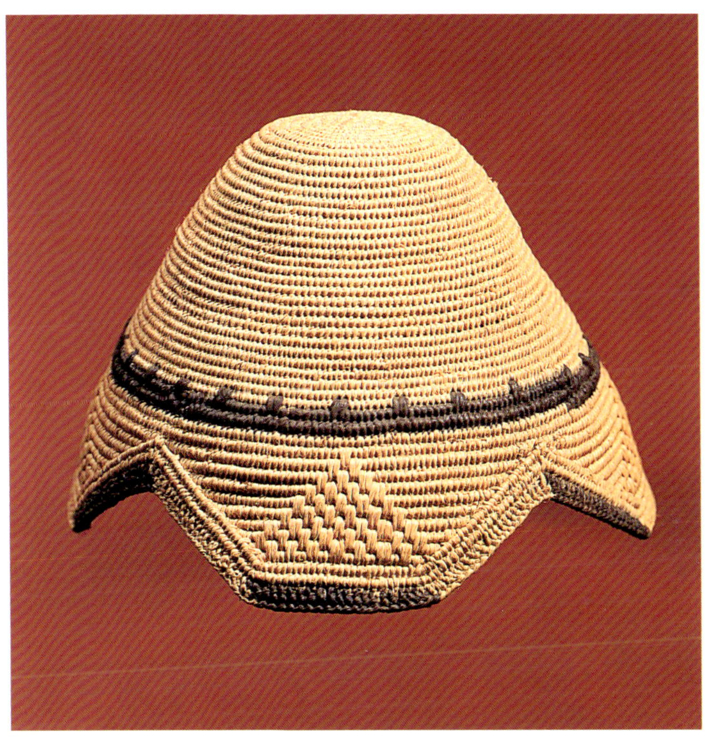

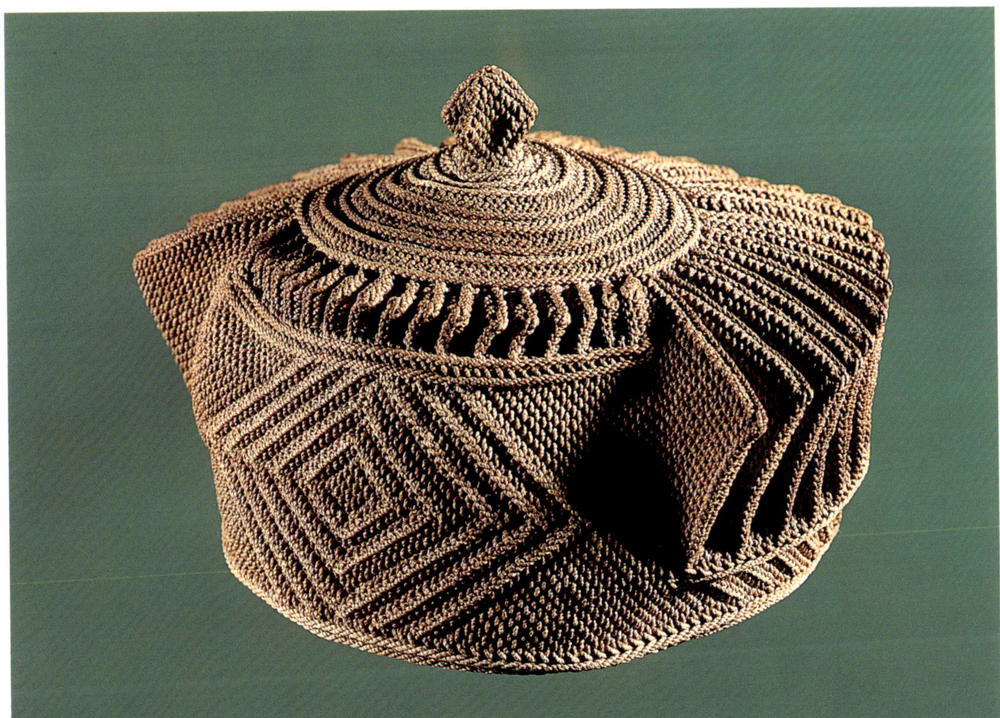

**Figure 4.4**, above left. Woman's hat. Tanala, Madagascar. Fiber. H. 13.0 cm. Department of Anthropology, Smithsonian Institution NMNH E175,412a. Photograph by Diane L. Nordeck.

**Figure 4.6**, above right. Man's cap *(laket)*. Kuba, Zaire. Raffia. H. 10.5 cm. Anonymous loan.

**Figure 4.7**, left. Nkutcu, Zaire. Raffia palm fiber. H. 10.0 cm. Neutrogena Corporation.

Calabash or basketry horned helmets were once fairly common forms of male headgear reserved for ritual occasions (funerals, annual agricultural rites) and commemorated the roles of men as hunters and warriors. Although they are still used in similar contexts among a number of groups in northern Ghana and Togo, such as the Moba, Konkomba, Kabye, Tamberma, and others, they have become increasingly rare — in part because the roles of hunter and warrior are largely symbolic nowadays. Furthermore, hunting bans and the scarcity of large game animals reduce the availability of animal horns and skins for use in ceremonial regalia (Fig. 1.16).

## BASKETRY TECHNIQUES

A variety of basketry techniques are employed to transform reeds, grasses, and tree fibers into beautiful, durable, and affordable headwear. At times the shapes and styles of basketry containers are faithfully replicated in headwear. The tightly woven grass fiber hat from Madagascar (Fig. 4.4) resembles an overturned basket in construction and decoration. Hats of this style have been worn daily by Malagasy women since at least the early twentieth century (Fig. 4.5). Deceptively simple in form, the technique is fairly sophisticated; the hat begins as a rectangular form for the crown, then changes to a circular construction for the body. Perched on top of the head and minus a wide brim, the hat probably serves less as a practical covering from the ele-

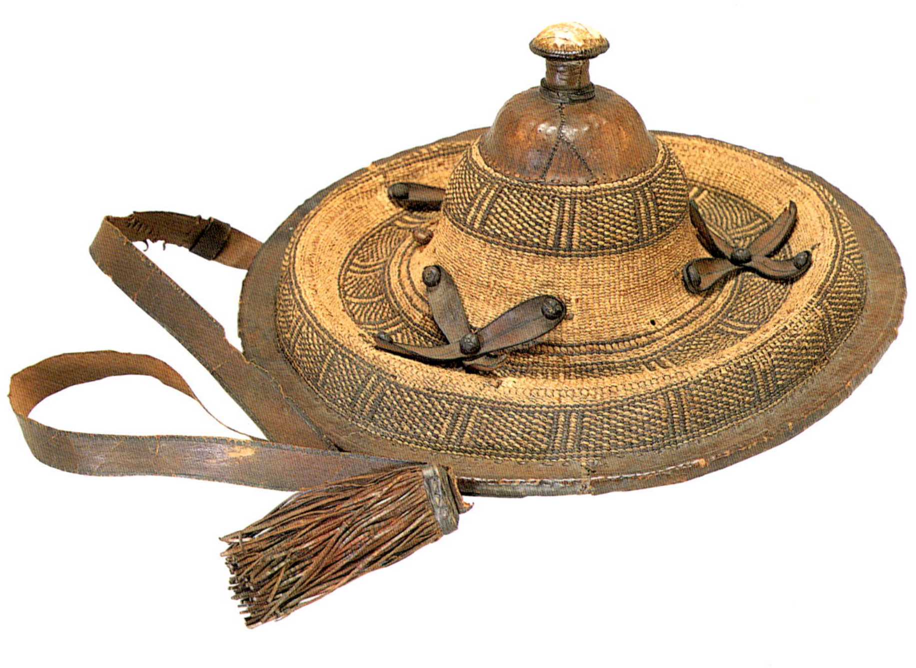

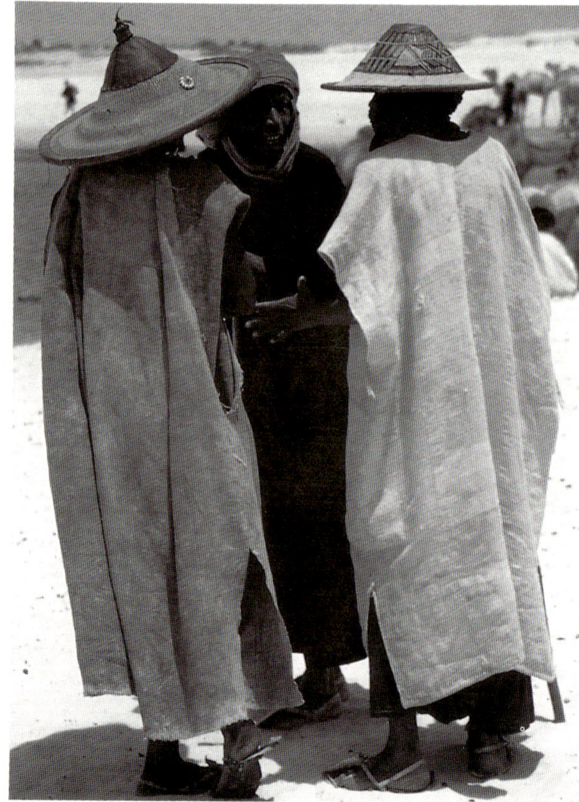

**Figure 4.8,** left. Man's hat. Fulani, Nigeria. Fiber, leather. H. 22.5 cm. Department of Anthropology, Smithsonian Institution NMNH E400,603. Photograph by Diane Nordeck.

**Figure 4.9,** right. Three men, two wearing Fulani-style hats, near a market in Goundam, Mali. Photograph by Eliot Elisofon, 1970. Slide no. D MAL 2 (2646). Eliot Elisofon Photographic Archives. National Museum of African Art.

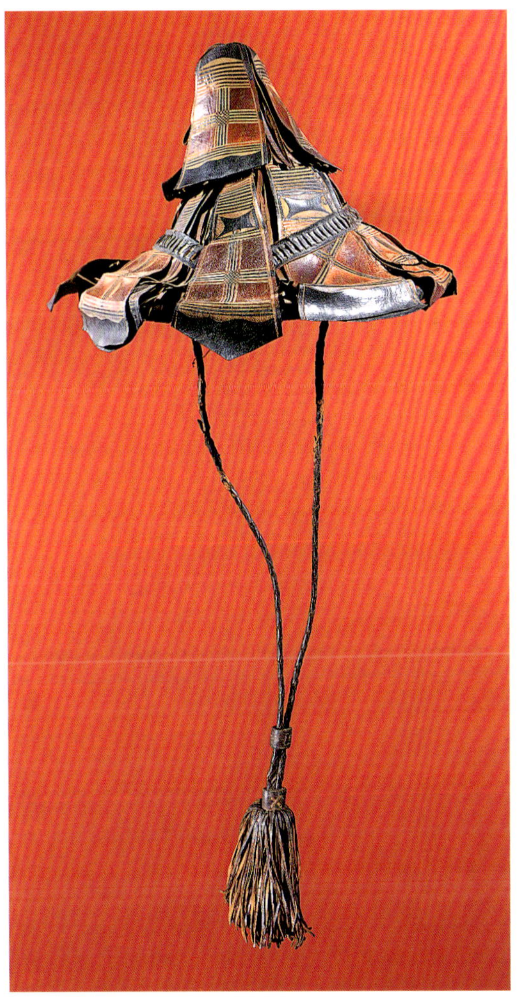

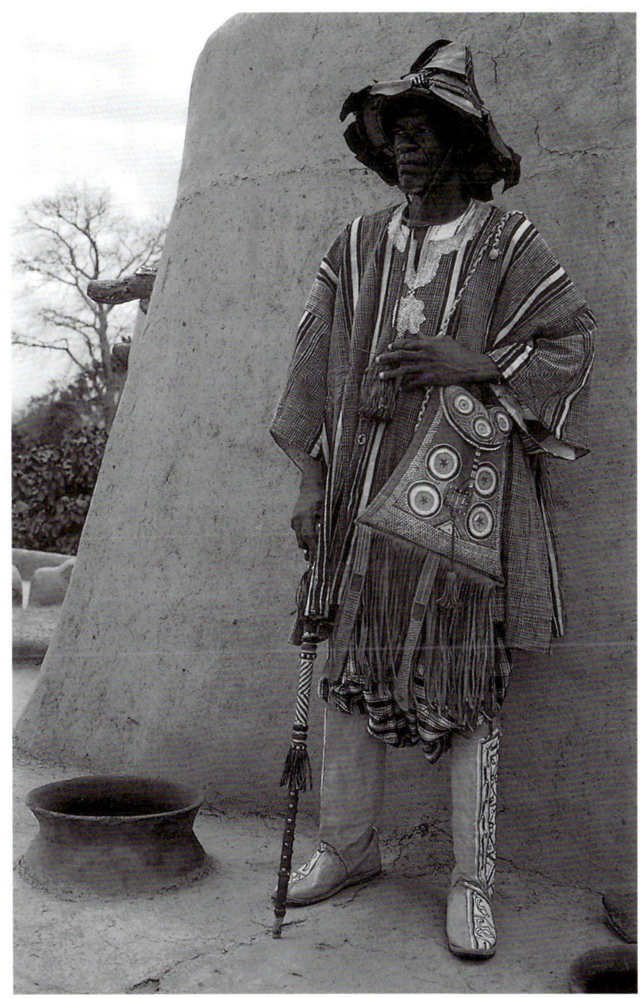

**Figure 4.10**, left. Man's hat. Bolgatanga, Ghana. Basketry, leather, straw. H. 76.0 cm. FMCH X76.666. Museum purchase. This hat was collected from Nikara, a Lobi man and the ex-regent of Birifu in northern Ghana. He originally purchased it in the market in Bolgatanga, Ghana.

**Figure 4.11**, right. Nikara, a Lobi man from Birifu, Ghana, in formal attire. This Lobi elder was very proud of the ten decorated leather hats he had in his wardrobe. Photograph by Herbert M. Cole, 1976.

ments and more as a statement about appropriate female dress.

The same can be said for the Kuba basketry caps (Fig. 4.6) that are worn by men as appropriate dress in the hierarchically ranked titled society. As Darish and Binkley point out in this volume ("Headdresses and Titleholding Among the Kuba"), variations and decorative embellishments on the basic form of the basketry cap indicate movement up the ranks of the titled men's association. The absence of bead, hide, and feather embellishments suggests that these hats are for daily rather than ritual wear and are probably worn by men of lower rank. Unembellished, however, the exquisite fiber cap reveals the high degree of technical expertise necessary to achieve the subtle, decorative linear and geometric patterns.

Similar mastery of the basket-weaving technique is demonstrated in the complicated patterns that embellish hats woven by the Nkutcu of Zaire. A mixture of plaiting, tying, and knotting combines to create tightly woven caps ornamented with surface and raised linear and geometric designs (Fig. 4.7). Woven fiber hats are worn

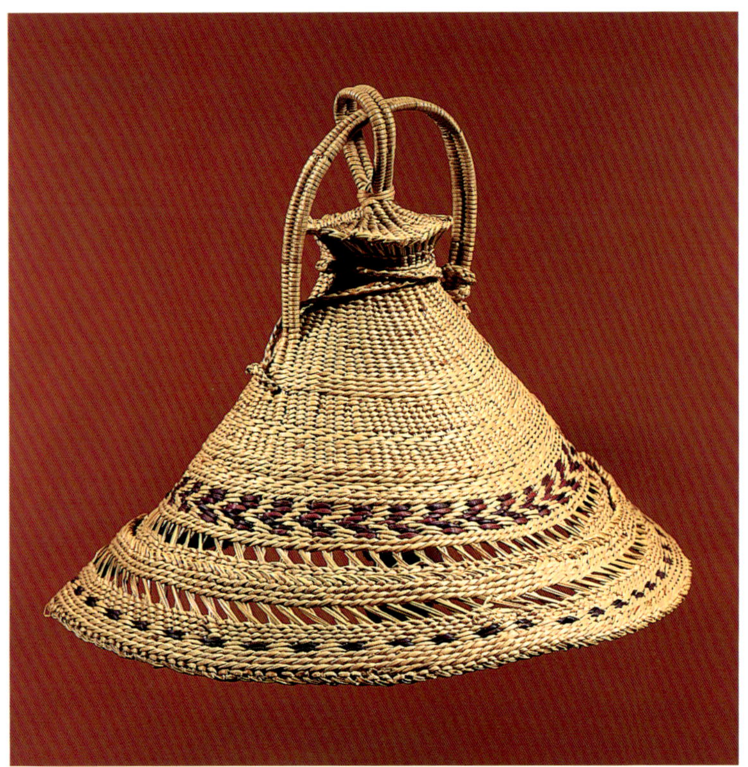

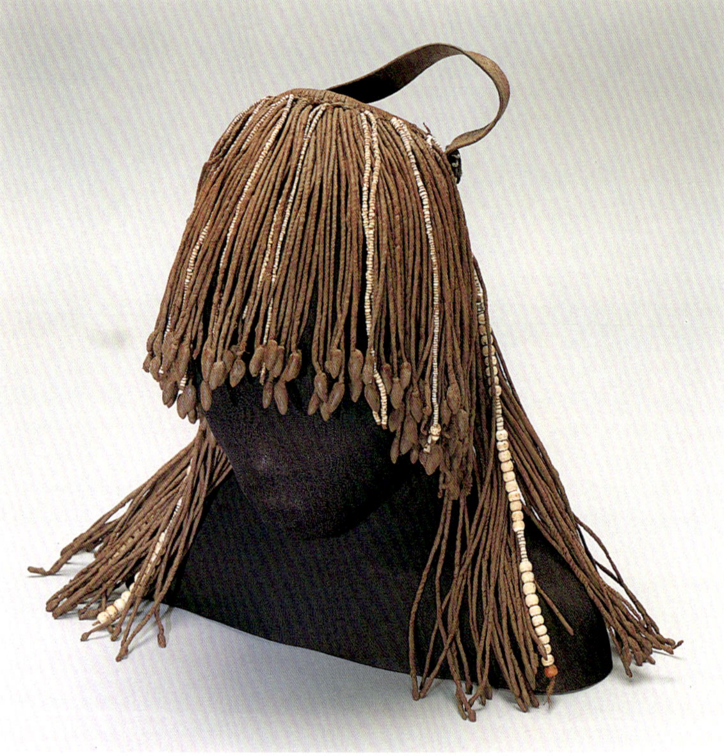

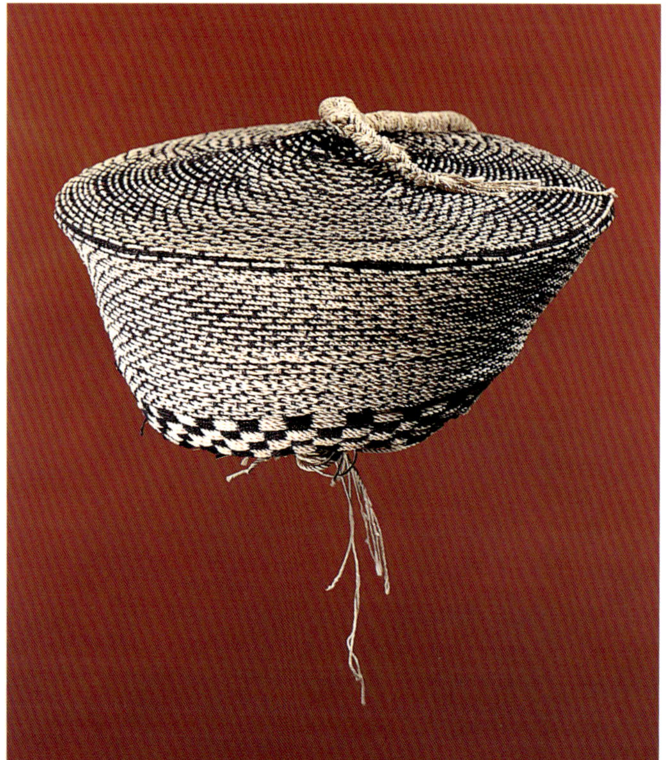

**Figure 4.12**, above left. Man's hat *(khaebana)*. Sotho, Lesotho. Reed. H. 25.0 cm. FMCH X68.2770. Museum purchase.

**Figure 4.13**, above. Girl's wig *(ehando)*. Himba, Namibia. Leather, fiber, clay, shell, iron. H. 48.0 cm. Department of Anthropology, Smithsonian Institution NMNH 407,572. Photograph by Diane Nordeck. This wig is made from twisted baobab fibers attached to a leather circle; when removed,the wig can be carried by the strap on top. The glass beads are European in origin and were traded into the area from Angola.

**Figure 4.14**, opposite. Himba girl wearing a fiber wig *(ehando)* with trade beads and buttons. Photograph by G. D. Gibson, Cunene District, Angola, 1973.

**Figure 4.15**, left. Woman's hat *(isicholo)*. Zulu, South Africa. String, cloth, basketry, fabric, straw. H. 40.0 cm. Gift of Mr. and Mrs. Richard B. Rogers and William Lloyd Davis.

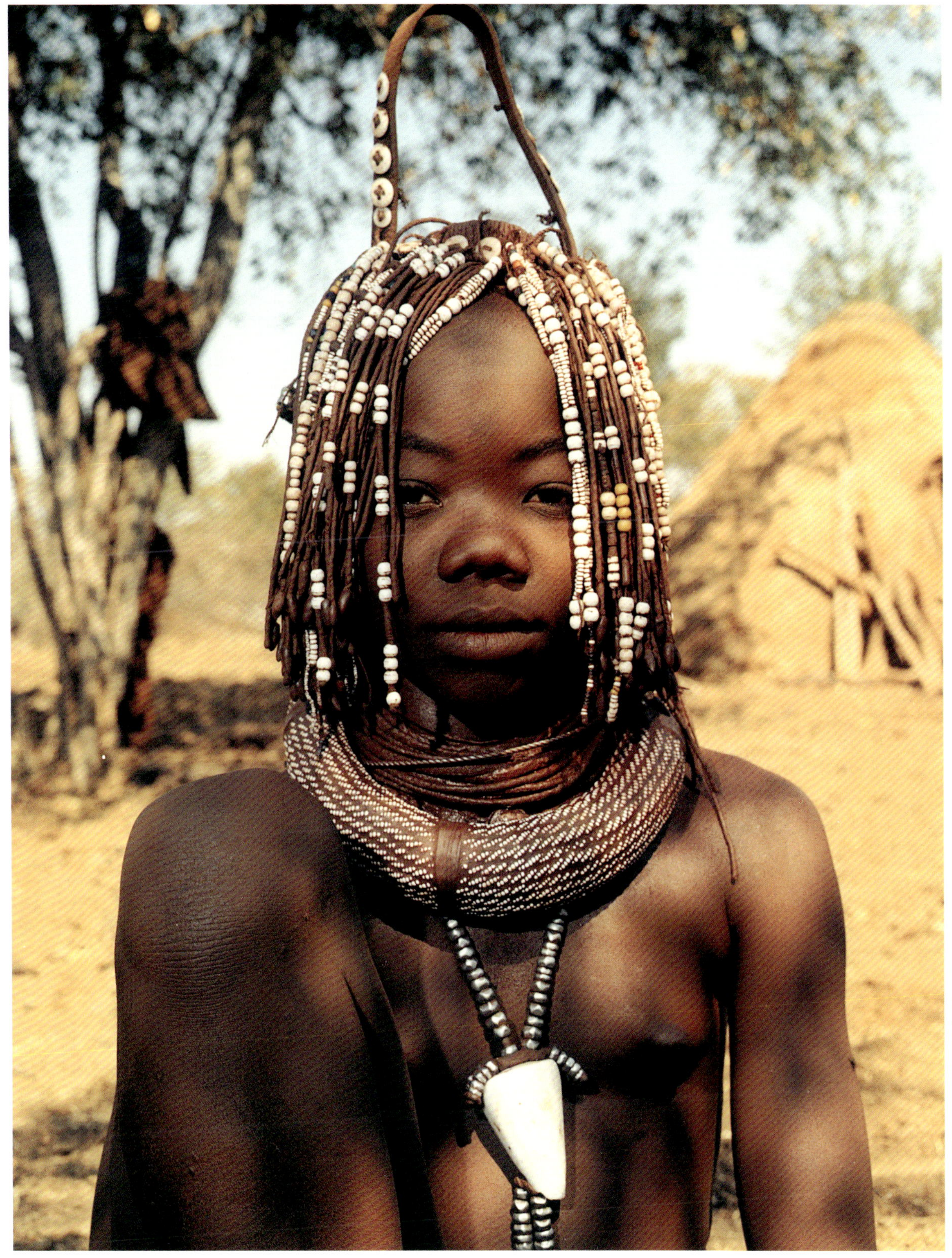

by many men and women throughout Zaire as part of daily dress and also as emblems of title. Whether this Nkutcu cap was an insignia of office or just the head-wear of a particularly well-dressed man is uncertain, but the elaborate high-relief designs suggest that it belonged to an individual of good taste, considerable means, and high status.

In addition to linear patterns woven in as part of the design, basketry hats can be embellished with a host of other materials. Depending on the extent of the embellishment, the basic materials and construction of the hat may remain open to view, or they may be completely covered over with decorative materials. Wide-brimmed basketry hats (Figs. 4.8) worn by the Fulani and others in the Sahelian region of West Africa are embellished with leather strips sewn to the brim and crown. Although the application of leather strips sewn along the rim serves to strengthen the most vulnerable part of any wide-brimmed hat, leather strips attached in various places on the brim and a leather topknot are mostly decorative. A leather strap with leather tassels secures the hat in place when it is worn. Although attributed to Fulani herdsmen, hats of this type are now made for sale by Fulani and others, and are worn as protective and fashionable headgear by men of many groups (Fig. 4.9).

Virtually the same hat is transformed through the application of decorative leather panels that completely cover the hat's basketry frame (Fig. 4.10). Attributed to the Lobi, this hat is actually a variation of the so-called Fulani herder's hat, a broad-brimmed variety that is worn by men from a number of groups in the Sahel. Although the hat was owned by a Lobi elder (Fig. 4.11), the decorative leather strips embellished with geometric and linear patterns in contrasting red and black are of a style produced by Gurensi and Kassena leatherworkers in the Bolgatanga and Navrongo regions of northern Ghana. Given the extent of this decorative embellishment, this hat may have been reserved for use on market days and for other social gatherings when being well-dressed for a public occasion demanded something beyond everyday wear.

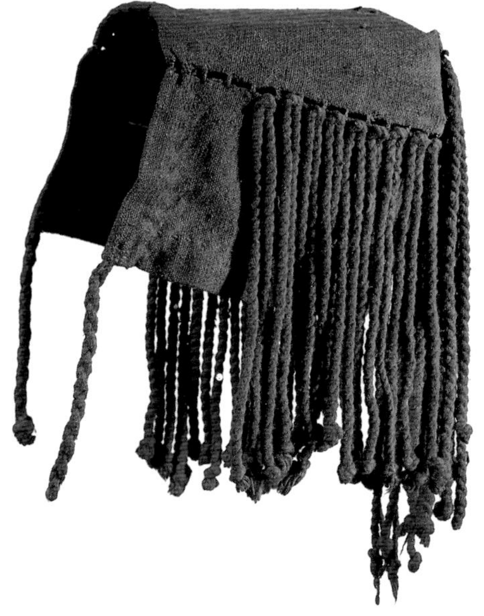

**Figure 4.16.** Man's headdress *(gorowije ine).* Dogon, Village de Bandiagara, Mali. Cotton, earth pigment. H. 33.0 cm. FMCH X88.784c. Collected by the National Museum of Mali and the UCLA Museum of Cultural History Joint Textile Documentation and Collecting Program.

Protection from the sun and rain is offered under the broad rims of basketry hats worn by Lesotho men (Fig. 4.12). Men make their own hats, for among the Lesotho, hatmaking is a skill "learned in boyhood days when herding cattle in the hills" (Tyrell and Jurgens 1983:168). Largely undecorated, the conical hat has a flared rib at about its midpoint and is embellished at the apex with a decorative looped basketry flourish. Apparently this style of hat (*khaebana;* Sechefo n.d.:2), a standard part of Lesotho male dress for generations, is made from the root fibers of Lesuoane grass which grows in marshy areas. Documented in the literature as practical headgear worn by Lesotho men to protect them against the rain, this style of hat has been appropriated as a vital symbol of Lesotho national identity. At the 1984 Olympic Games in Los Angeles, the Lesotho team wore these basketry hats as part of their national dress in the Parade of Athletes.

Although forms and, at times, materials may vary, headdresses, hats, caps, coiffures, veils, and head-scarves serve similar functions of practicality, propriety, status, fashion, and identity for women and men. The Himba girl's wig called *ehando* (Fig. 4.13) requires a high degree of expertise and hours of preparation. Once it is completed it offers a ready-made alternative that fulfills societal norms. This style of headdress serves to announce the unmarried status of a young girl (Fig. 4.14).

Beaded and basketry headdresses, as well as elaborate coiffures, have been a vital part of the social and ethnic identity of Zulu women for more than a century. A variation of the *isicholo* married woman's hair style and beaded hat is a black-and-white basketry hat of a broad flaring style popular today (Fig. 4.15). These hats were commonly available for sale in trade stores throughout the Zulu region in the 1970s and 1980s. Once purchased, the new hat was prepared for wear by its owner. This involved rubbing the hat with red ochre. Women regularly cover the hat with head-scarves for practicality and fashion. The basic shape of the hat is still clearly evident under the scarf, thus satisfying requirements of fashion and propriety in an economical, yet culturally appropriate, way.

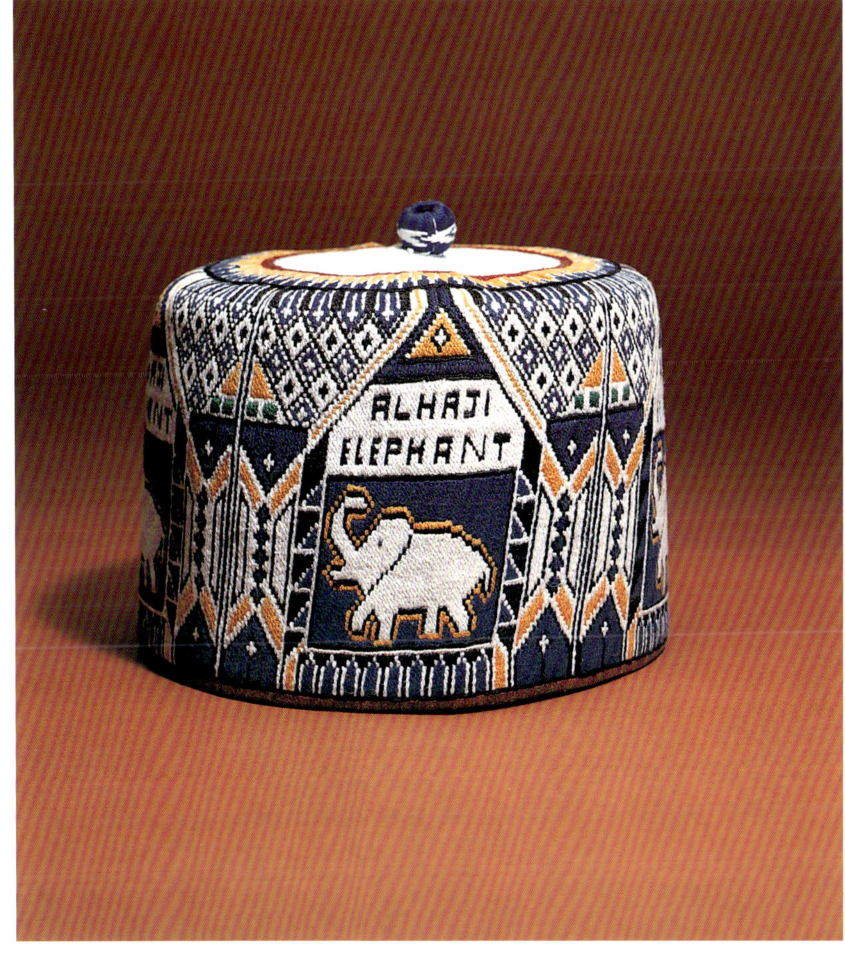


**Figure 4.17**. Man's hat *(fulan)*. Hausa, Nigeria. Cloth, thread. H. 14.5 cm. FMCH X92.54. Anonymous gift.

## WOVEN AND EMBROIDERED HEADWEAR

Locally woven and imported cloth is used in the fabrication of caps worn by men throughout Africa as part of daily dress. Once again, the choice to cover the head acknowledges locally held notions of propriety, yet also offers the opportunity to make individual statements about fashion, status, and prosperity. Close-fitting conical caps or bonnets *(gorowije ine)* worn by Dogon men are made from locally woven narrow-strip cloth (Fig. 4.16). Cotton cloth ties secure the hat to the wearer under the chin. Hats of this style may be dyed with natural earth-brown and indigo pigments, and they may be embellished with twisted cotton strands banded at the ends with thin strips of aluminum. This style of cap is an old one, in existence in the Bandiagara escarpment region of Mali even before the arrival of the Dogon. Indeed, Bedaux (1988:45) documents a similar cotton cap that dates to the eleventh or twelfth century worn by the Tellem people who inhabited the region prior to the

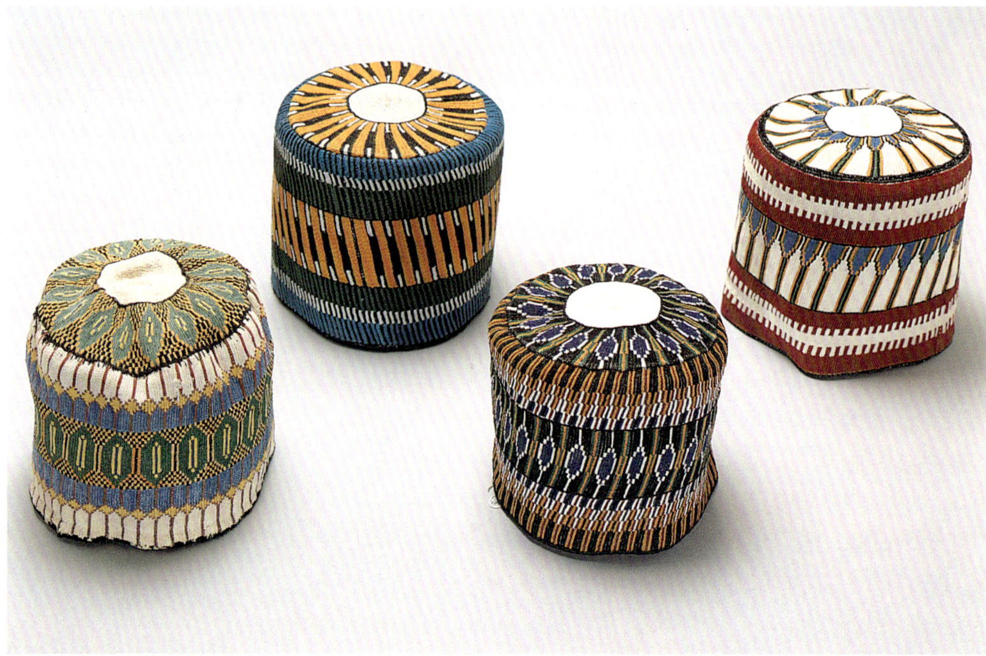

**Figure 4.18**. Men's hats *(fulan)*. Hausa, Niger. Cloth, thread. Department of Anthropology, Smithsonian Institution NMNH a. E425,349; b. E425,359; c. E425,352; d. E425,353. Height of tallest:, 16.5 cm. Photograph by Diane L. Nordeck.

Dogon. Today, this type of hat is commonly worn by Dogon men of all ages as part of daily dress. Brilliant white hats of the same style are used by Dogon men in funerary celebrations and other ritual occasions. Ezra (1988:24–25) illustrates a 1967 photograph of Dogon men in ritual dress, including the white cotton, conical-shaped cap, during the *Sigi* commemorative celebration that occurs every sixty years or so.

Hausa men's hats *(fulan)* are made of narrow-strip cloth that may be decorated with elaborate embroidery. The Hausa are credited with introducing this form to Nigeria and for its wide dissemination within West Africa. The embroidered patterns that ornament Hausa hats are commonly curvilinear in design and Islamic in inspiration. The writing on the hat "Alhaji Elephant" collected in Nigeria, links the honorific title of Alhaji, one who has made the pilgrimmage to Mecca, with the image and name of the elephant, a praise name for powerful and important men (Fig. 4.17). Other embroidery designs may refer directly to historical or topical events, and certain hat forms and designs have become associated with particular ethnic groups. Four Hausa-style hats that were popular in Niger in 1985 are a case in point (Fig. 4.18).

The hat *Allah ya ba damana da albarka* (May God grant us a good rainy season) was created following the famine of 1973 (Fig. 4.18a). It is a prayer for plentiful rains and an abundant harvest. The motifs represent the pile of millet stalks stacked in the center of a field after harvest, the green leaves of the second dry season garden crops surrounding the millet harvest, and the garden enclosure made of spiny branches to keep out cattle and small ruminants.

The hat design known as *fulan Tahoua* (hat of Tahoua) is one of several hats identified with the Tahoua region in Niger and it represents a particular historical incident. The central, horizontal band motif recalls the designs on the wall of the house of the warrior, Kaocen (Fig. 4.18c), an Izkazkazen Tuareg from Damergu who was active in local resistance to the French in the early part of the twentieth century. He participated in a rebellion in the Kanen area led by the Sanusiya warriors and he subsequently led a second Tuareg revolt against the French in 1917 in which his 600–800 warriors laid seige to the French garrison at Agadez. He was killed in 1919.

*Fulan Damagaram* (hat of Damagaram) celebrates the former glories of the chiefdom of Damagaram, whose capital city of the same name is the modern-day city of Zinder (Fig. 4.18d). Damagaram rose to prominence under the reign of Sarki Tanimune (1851–84) when the trans-Saharan trade routes shifted and began to pass through the city. The two horizontal motifs on the hat represent the wall surrounding the city of Kano in the latter part of the nineteenth century. The broken, disrupted area in the white wall motif in the bottom band is said to symbolize the sacking of Kano by the Damagaram cavalry. Damagaram warred with Kano, but never succeeded in subjugating the emirate nor in entering the city itself. They did, however, defeat the emirate of Hadejia, a vassal state of Kano and the design probably refers to this historical episode.

*Fulan Maiga* (hat of Maiga) is named after Seyni Maiga, a Zarma nobleman said to have been the first to have worn a hat of this particular design and fold (a single, longitudinal depression in the center; Fig. 4.18b). Hausa hatsellers in Niamey today say that this is still the type of hat most preferred by Zarma men.[1]

Yoruba men from Nigeria wear a variety of hats and caps. Hausa-inspired knitted and woven skull caps, for example, depart from their Islamic models through the use of bold, contrasting red, green, and black-and-white color blocks (Fig. 4.21). Taller, more cylindrical hats called *filà* are made from locally available strip cloth or commercially printed textiles, such as the popular cowrie shell design (Fig. 4.22). These hats are usually lined with cotton cloth and may be embellished with limited or allover embroidery patterns. Indeed, these more elaborate caps usually complement a matching ensemble, which consists of a flowing Hausa-style robe or an embroidered smock and trouser set. When lurex threads came on the market some decades back, they were incorporated as a design element in the narrow-strip weaving traditions throughout much of West Africa, adding a bit of glamour and sparkle to the clothing made from strip cloth.

Clearly recalling Muslim antecedents, the red fez is often an insignia of office that is worn as part of daily attire (Fig. 4.23). Although this particular fez was collected in northern Nigeria, identical hats (many manu-

**Figure 4.19.** A Hausa hat washer in Madaoua, Niger. Once the hats are embroidered and sewn together, they are washed and blocked on wooden hat forms. The hat in the man's hand is called *kuye* (sticks). The long vertical bands represent the traces of millet rows left in the soil after harvest. The orange and blue hats with embroidered perforations are imported from Nigeria. The blue and white hat on the table represents the mosque and is usually embroidered without the aid of pattern lines. The design on this hat is called *muhadu abanki* ("things that come close together and bump into each other") because this style was formerly so popular that men wearing the hat were literally bumping into one another in the marketplace. Photograph by Christine Conte, 1985.

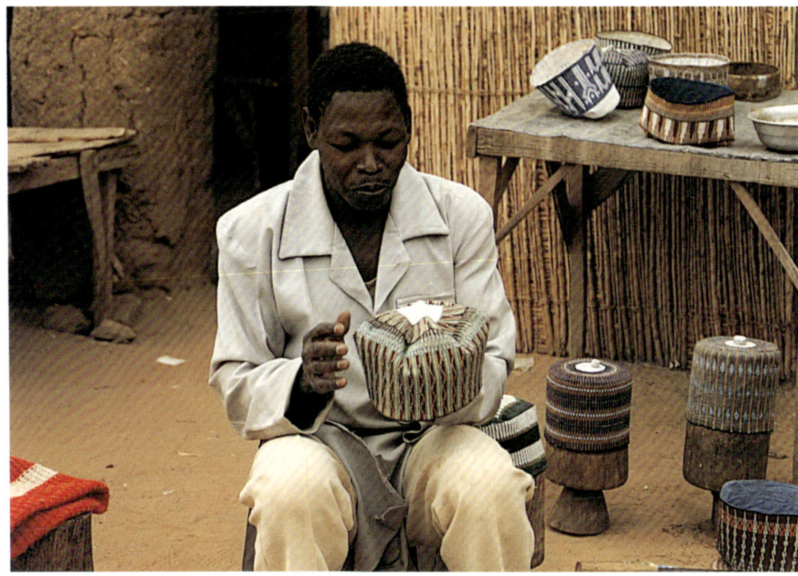

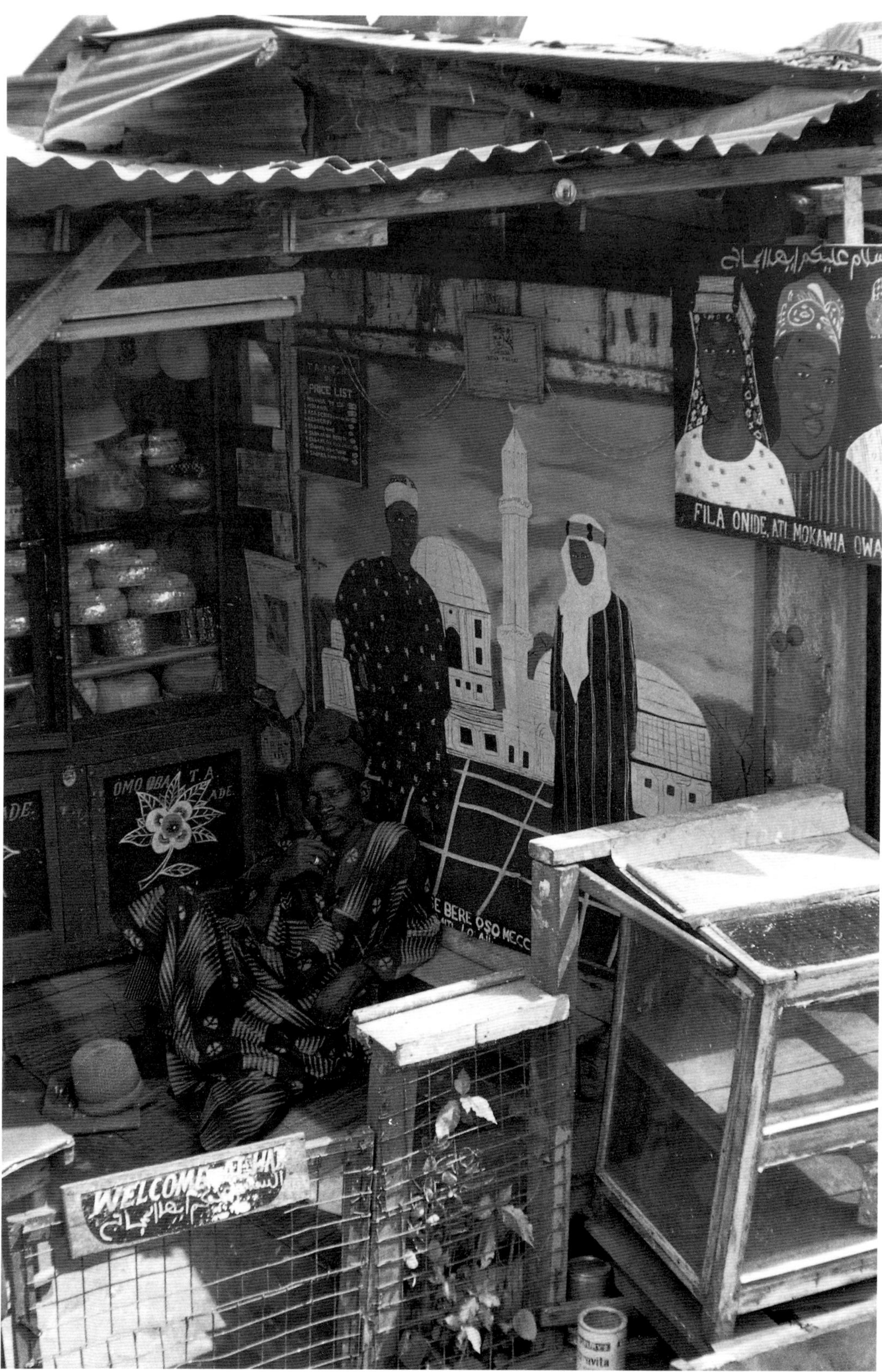


**Figure 4.20**. Hat shop in market. Ibadan, Nigeria. Photograph by Eliot Elisofon, 1970. Neg. no. VI-18, 7A. Eliot Elisofon Photographic Archives. National Museum of African Art.

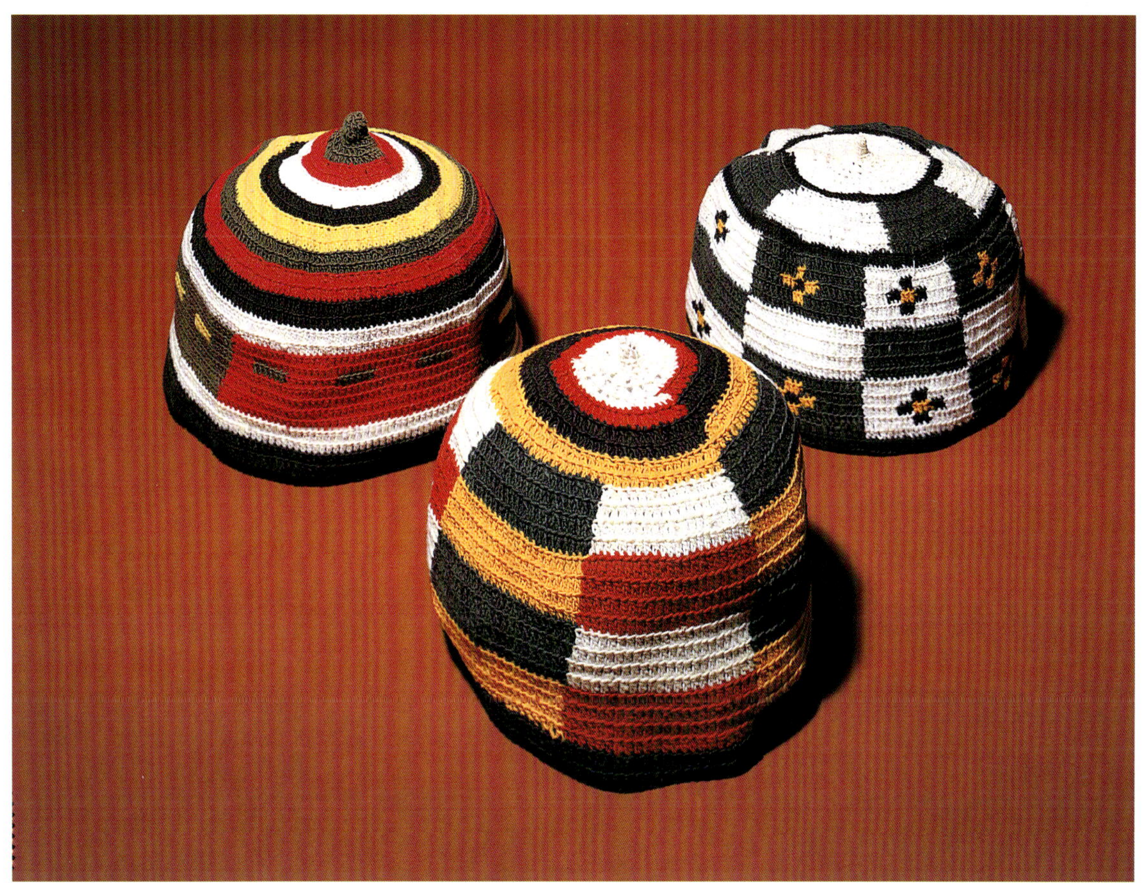

**Figure 4.21**, above. Men's hats. Hausa, Northeast Nigeria. Cotton. H. 12.0 cm. FMCH X86.4576, X86.4577, X86.4578. Gift of Arnold Rubin. Knit caps, found in markets throughout West Africa, are convenient and affordable alternatives for daily headwear. Although Islamic in design, the brightly colored knit patterns depart from the more common white, embroidered, Muslim-influenced models.

**Figure 4.22**, right. Men's hats *(filà).* Yoruba, Nigeria. Cloth. H. 23 cm. FMCH X89.120, X89.121, museum purchases; X86.457, gift of Arnold Rubin.

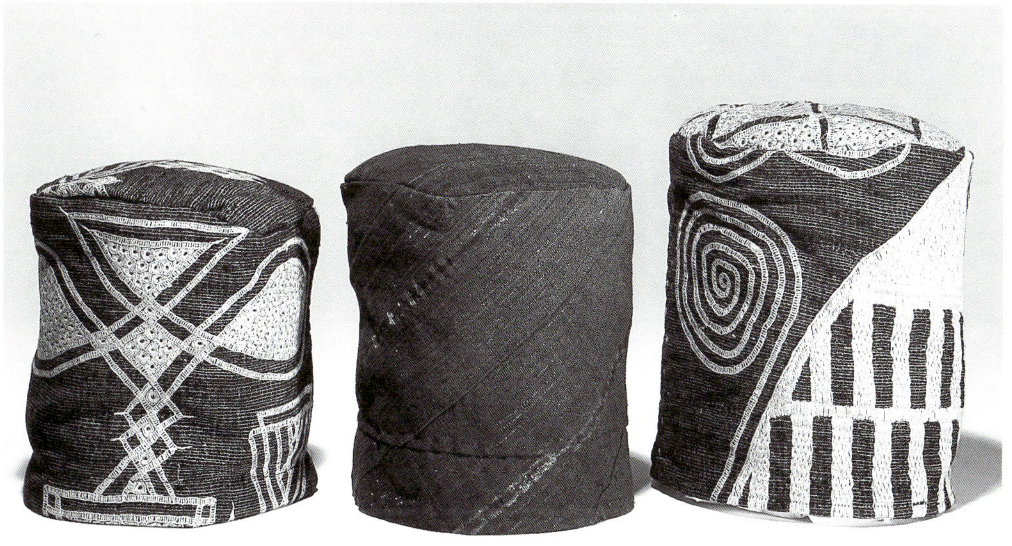

factured abroad) are worn throughout Africa by both Muslim and non-Muslim men (Fig. 4.24). Made of solid felt material of a deep red hue, the color alone may signal its use by ritual specialists. Among a number of related groups in northern Ghana, Togo, and southern Nigeria, for example, the red fez is reserved for shrine priests, custodians of the earth, and important village chiefs (Fig. 5.36). The Moba of northern Togo use the red fez in these same contexts; it is also worn by young men at the conclusion of their initiation rites during their symbolic reentry into the community.

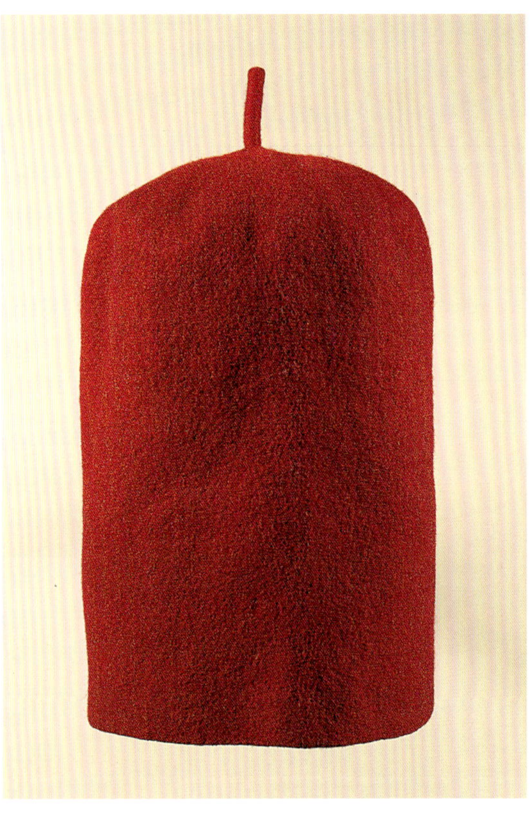

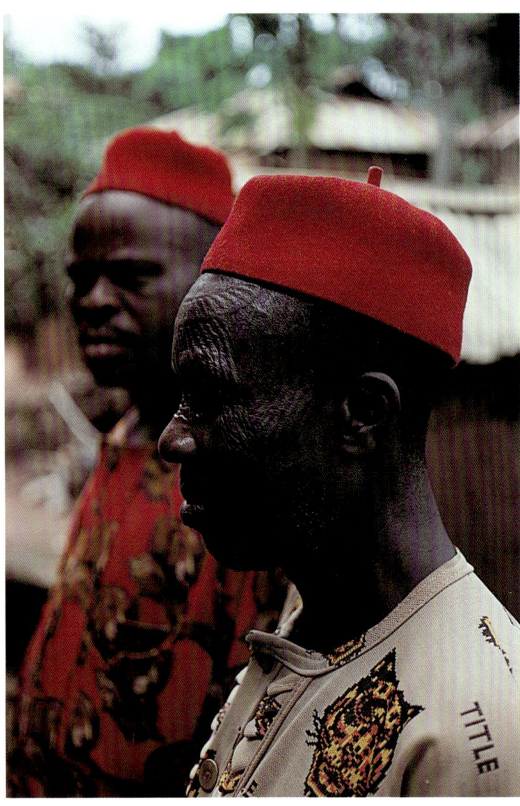


**Figure 4.23,** left. Fez. Undetermined group, Nigeria. Wool, felt. H. 29.0 cm. FMCH X83.843. Gift of Arnold Rubin. There is a very faint manufacturer's stamp on the inside of this fez similar to the markings found on French berets, which suggests that this hat was manufactured in Europe, the Middle East, or northern Africa and imported into Nigeria.

**Figure 4.24,** above. Two Igbo men wearing red fez hats as everyday headgear. Photograph by Herbert M. Cole, 1966.

Along the Swahili Coast of Kenya and Tanzania, men wear a variety of embroidered caps (Fig. 4.25) also of Islamic inspiration. These caps (*kofia ya kiua)* are characterized by an amazing variety of curvilinear and geometric embroidered designs. The caps are made by men who trace the embroidery patterns in pencil onto the fabric, but it is women who do the actual embroidery. Similarly, openwork crocheted caps are designed by men but women are responsible for the needlework. There are particular styles that identify caps as coming from Malindi, Mombasa, or Lamu along the coast of Kenya, or from the island of Zanzibar or mainland Tanzania (Figs. 4.26, 4.27).

Apart from the practical value that daily headwear affords, one cannot overlook the aesthetic dimensions of everyday hats and caps. Whether the intention is to offer protection from the elements, to conform to notions of social propriety, or to make individual fashion statements on less formal occasions, daily wear hats function as aesthetic enhancements to everyday, lived experience. The care with which everyday hats and caps are constructed, the manner in which they are worn, and the decorative embellishments that make an ordinary hat distinctive — all these factors contribute to the beauty of the hat and to the aesthetic experience of the wearer.

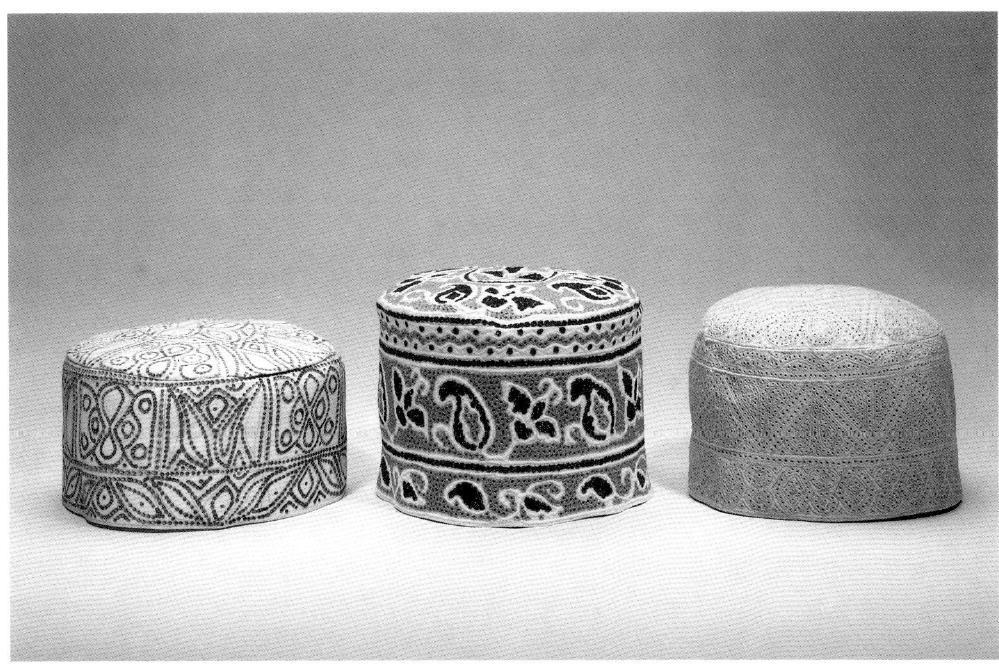

**Figure 4.25,** left. Men's hats *(kofia ya kiua).* Swahili, Lamu Kenya. Cotton. H. 21.0 cm. a. FMCH X94.26.7, b. X94.26.6, c. X94.26.4. Museum purchase. Three variations on the common Swahili hat called *kofia.* The hat designated "c " is embroidered in silk by hand and is the most expensive and prestigious of the three. Example "b" is hand-embroidered with cotton thread, and least notable is "a" with punched holes and no embroidery.

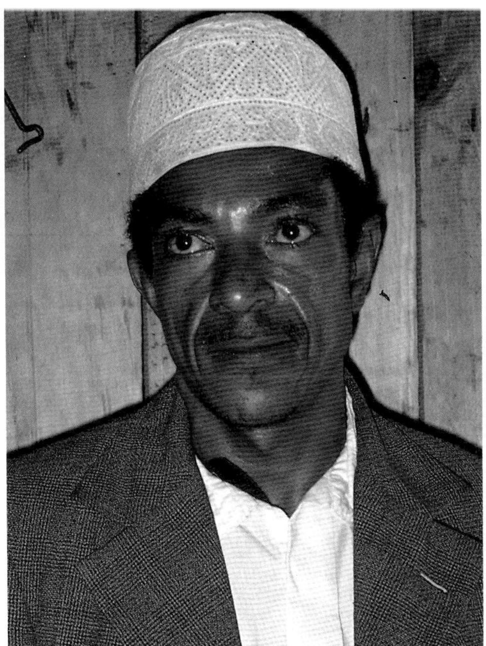

**Figure 4.26,** below left. Said Ahmed Kirume of Lamu wearing a hat (*kofia ya kiua)* embroidered in silk by his wife Sada Ahmed Salim. The primary motif of the hat is the heart *(kopa).* Swahili peoples, Kenya. Photograph by Christraud M. Geary, 1994.

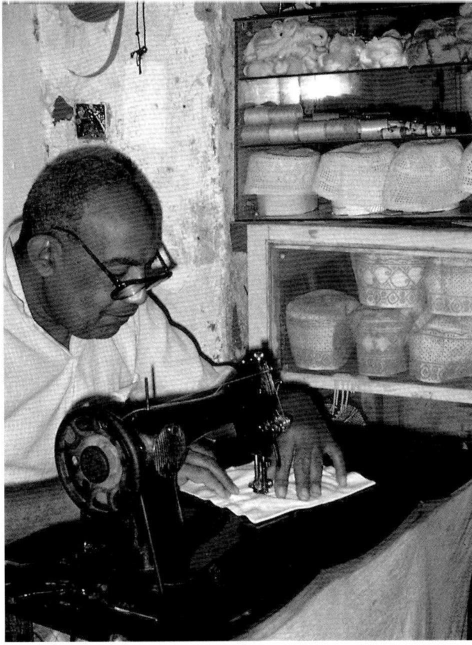

**Figure 4.27,** below right. Tailor preparing the patterns used to embroider a *kofia*-type hat. Lamu, Kenya. Photograph by Christraud M. Geary, 1994.

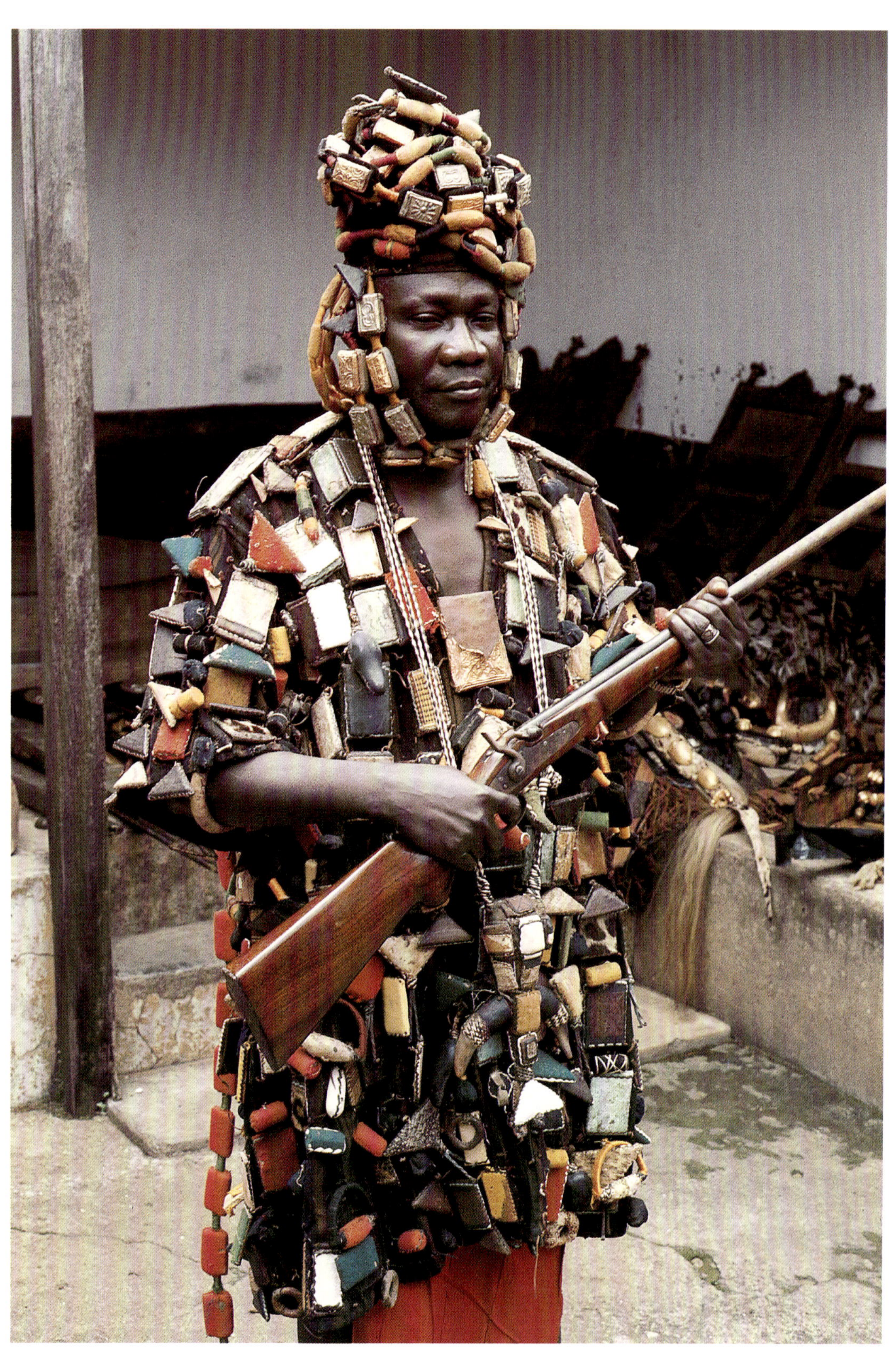

# 5 SPECTACULAR HATS FOR SPECIAL OCCASIONS

CHRISTINE MULLEN KREAMER

People everywhere in the world invest particular time and attention preparing themselves for public presentation at special occasions and ceremonial events. In addition to the psychological, emotional, and intellectual preparation that some may require in anticipation of a presentation of self in a more public and formalized setting, considerable thought is invested in decisions about clothing, hair style, cosmetics, and other aspects of body ornamentation that are required or appropriate for any given event.

Clothing — defined as apparel, garments, or body coverings — is distinguished from dress to some extent, and from costume to a considerable extent, in the manner in which it is worn and in the assumptions made (consciously or unconsciously) about the ways in which attire defines the occasion as either mundane or special. In English, the word "dress," while certainly suggesting apparel and the more practical aspect of covering one's body, connotes a measure of suitability for particular occasions, as in the phrases "casual dress," "formal dress," and the like. "Costume" similarly implies particular clothing for a specific kind of occasion and suggests that elements of costumed attire may well derive from or allude to particular regions, time periods, or professions, as well as to customs, traditions, and symbolic references. Further, in some instances, "costume" implies a sense of masquerade or a subsumption of one's everyday identity in favor of another, perhaps symbolic, identity. While meaningful distinctions between clothing, dress, and costume require cultural and historical specificity, acknowledging that differences in attire define the event as mundane or special — for wearer and viewer alike — is a useful entrée into an examination of headgear reserved for special and ceremonial occasions.

## OPPULENT DISPLAY OF PRESTIGE MATERIALS

### BEADED SPLENDOR

In Africa and throughout the world, dress for special occasions and ceremonial events often involves the use of particularly elaborate, precious, or exotic materials, a high degree of decorative embellishment, and/or forms that clearly depart from more mundane modes of attire. The special or ceremonial nature of the event is signalled by the adoption of dress and body ornamentation that is viewed as spectacular, either in the combination of forms, the choice of materials, or in the symbolic messages

**Opposite.** Ejisuhene Nana Diko Pim III wearing the "great" war shirt and hat. Ejisu, Ghana. Photograph by Doran H. Ross, 1976.

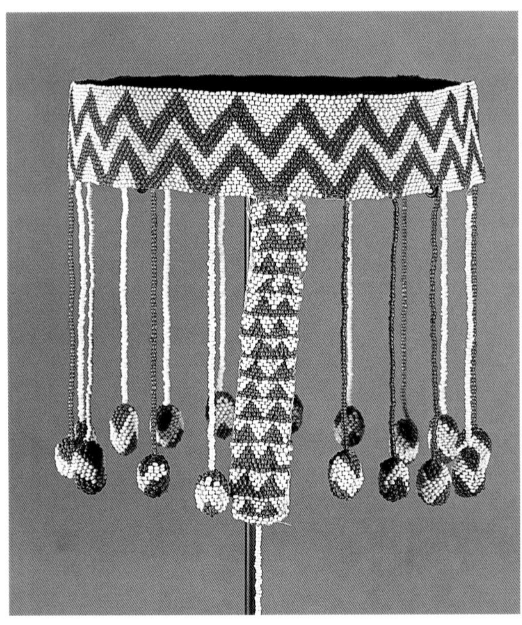

**Figure 5.1**. Royal headband. Tutsi, Rwanda and Burundi. Beads, wood, raffia, thread. H. 27.0 cm. Private collection.

conveyed through the form or context of special occasion dress.

Leadership attire is a particularly important case in point, for in much of Africa leadership dress and regalia serve as visual metaphors for the social, political, and, at times, religious powers of rulers. Thus, it is not uncommon for leadership dress and regalia to be particularly opulent in form and made of precious materials, to convey the wealth and prestige of the chief as well as the collective prosperity of the community.

Long viewed in Africa as valued items of trade and as signifiers of wealth and prestige, beads make powerful visual statements about social prominence, individual and collective prosperity, and power and authority. There are fine glass bead-making traditions in Bida, Nigeria. In Ghana, contemporary beadmakers use crushed soft drink and other bottles to make their wares. Nonetheless, although widely used throughout Africa as ornaments for the body — clothing, ritual dress, leadership regalia and the like — most extant glass beads in Africa were made outside Africa, "the products of Venetian, Czech, or Dutch glassworks, with an insignificant contemporary representation from Japan and India" (Liu 1984:42). The importance of beads as prestige materials derives in part from their prominence as valued, imported trade items. As part of the trade network, as well as a sign of wealth derived from participation in or control over that network, beads are a logical choice for personal adornment destined to convey statements about power, prestige, and social position. In addition to references of wealth and power that beads convey, particular colors of beads, and the beaded designs themselves, may hold culturally-specific symbolic meanings that convey messages critical to the use and interpretation of the beaded materials.

As a visual metaphor for political power and the wealth and prestige associated with leadership, beads form an important part of royal regalia. Our discussion earlier in this volume about Yoruba beaded crowns indicated the many ways in which beads convey aspects of the political, religious, and economic power of the Yoruba chief. This power derives, in part, from the chief's control over the ways in which beads may be used. The same is true for the Cameroon Grassfields, for the Fon (king) is said to control access to the use of beads as forms of personal adornment. Among the Tutsi of Rwanda and Burundi, elaborate beaded headwear is worn by Tutsi royalty. On ceremonial occasions women of royal and high status wear headbands with beaded fringe designs (Figs. 5.1, 5.2) or beaded bands that wrap around the head in complicated configurations.

An exuberance of beaded splendor is conveyed in the rather Baroque treatment of the bicorn chief's headdress made by the Pende of Zaire (Figs. 5.3, 5.4). The headdress shape conforms to Pende stylistic conventions: the bicorn headdress is said to allude to the strength and power of the buffalo in a reference to the associated powers of chieftaincy. Although all the stylistic elements are there — the appendages or

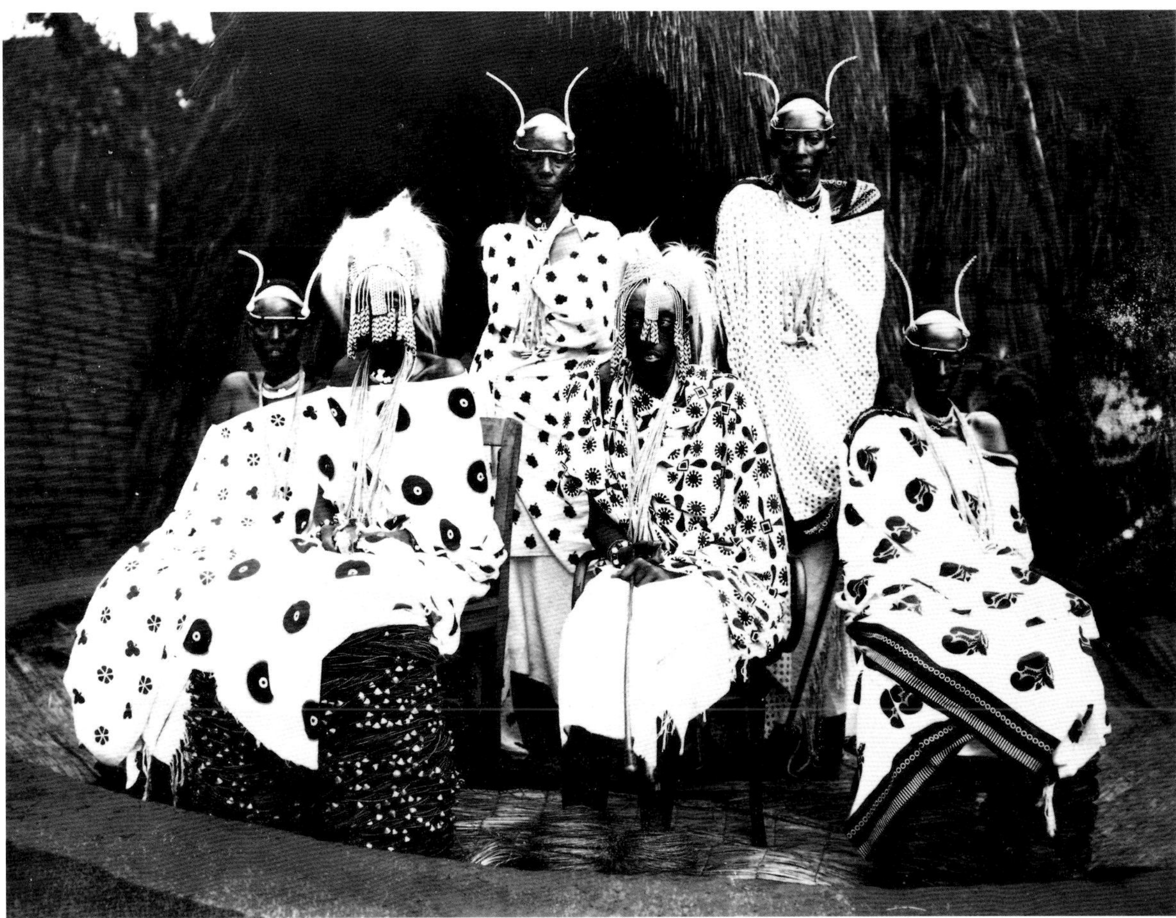

Figure 5.2. *Mwami* (king) of Rwanda with his family. The king and his family are shown wearing beaded diadems as part of their royal headwear. Photographer unknown, ca. 1910. White Father's Collection. Eliot Elisofon Photographic Archives. National Museum of African Art.

horns on each side, the central knoblike protuberance, a finial at the crown — these formal elements are almost subsumed to the dizzying effect of the multihued beaded patterns. While the range of colors departs from the norm, the arrangement of the beads in zigzag, lozenge, triangle, and circle designs is consistent with the more common, and sedate, black-and-white beaded headdresses. Among the Pende these headdresses are called *misango mapende*. The form is said to have originated in the Lunda chiefdom. According to Bourgeois, the headdresses are common not only to the Pende, but since the 1940s Yaka and Suku chiefs have purchased this type of beaded headdress from their Pende neighbors (1982:30). The knobbed form of the headdress is common in raffia fiber headwear throughout the region, as noted in the Mbala chief's hat called *mpu a nzim* (Fig. 5.5) that is ornamented with four clusters of *n'simbu* shell currency (Darteville 1953:167).

The symbolic significance of beaded patterns is demonstrated in an examination of the Tabwa diviner's headdress (Fig. 5.6). Composed of a fiber and beaded headband surmounted with feathers, the beaded headdress draws visual attention to the forehead, a place — for the Tabwa as well as many other peoples in Africa and

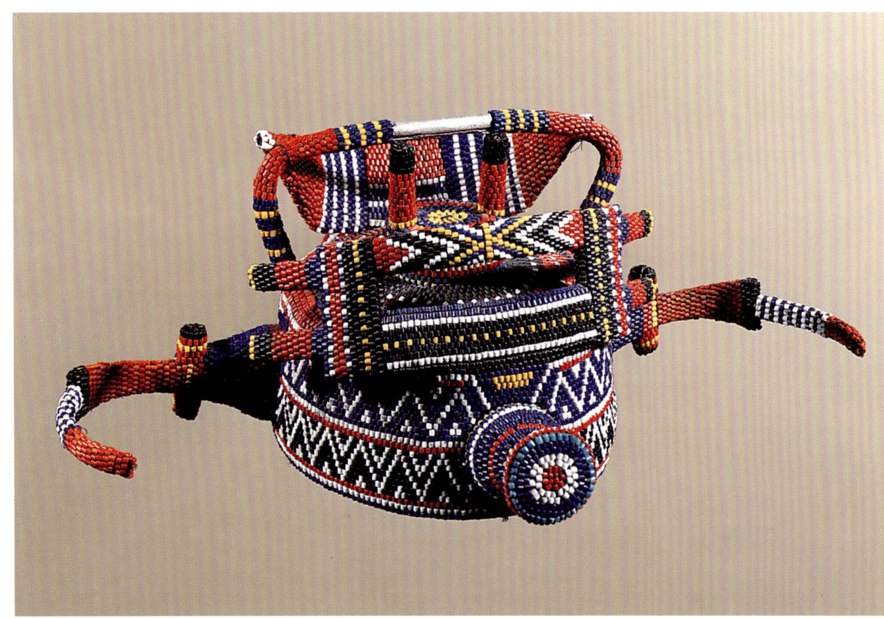

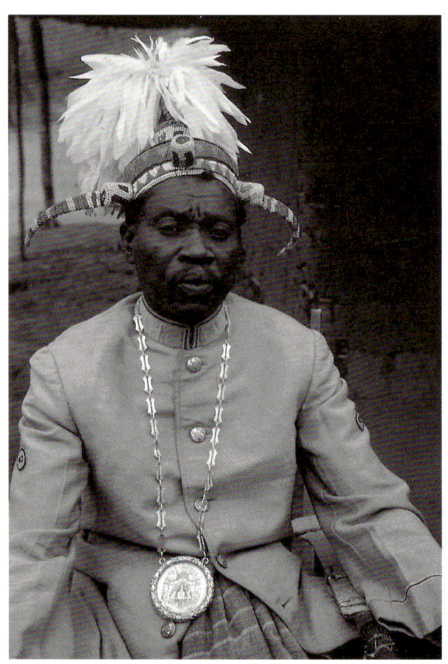

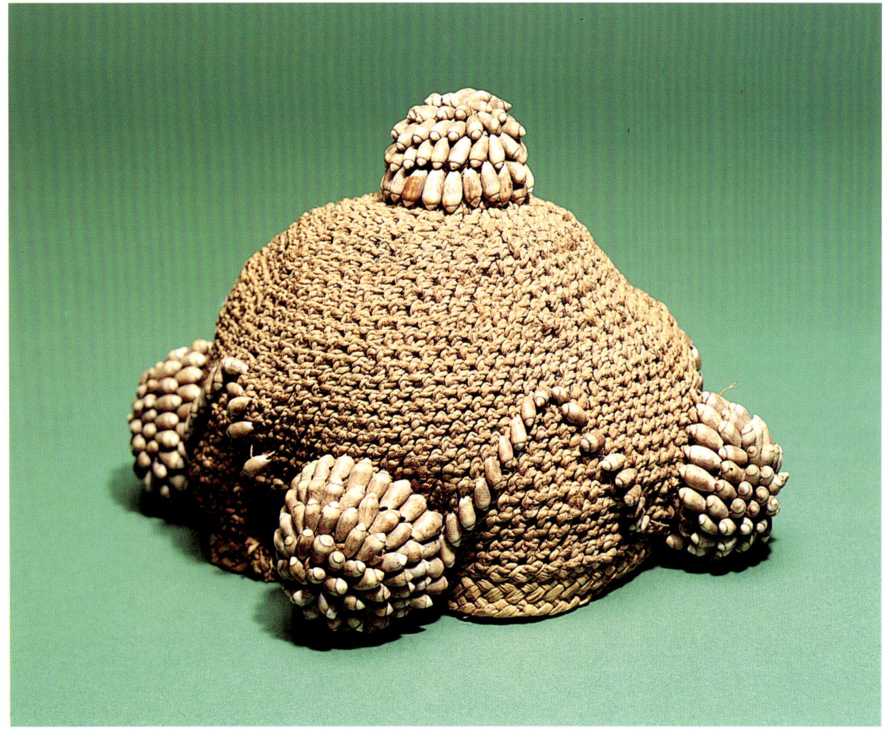

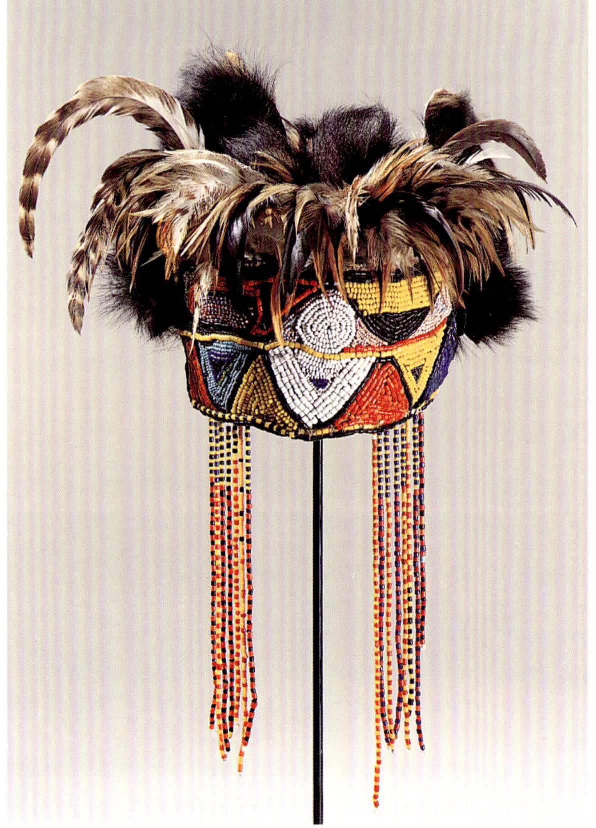

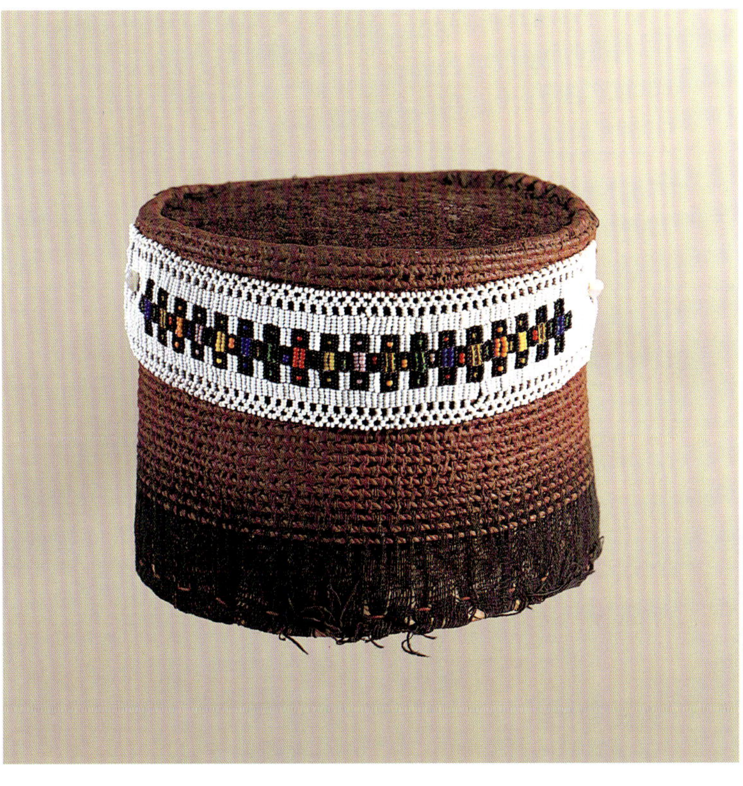

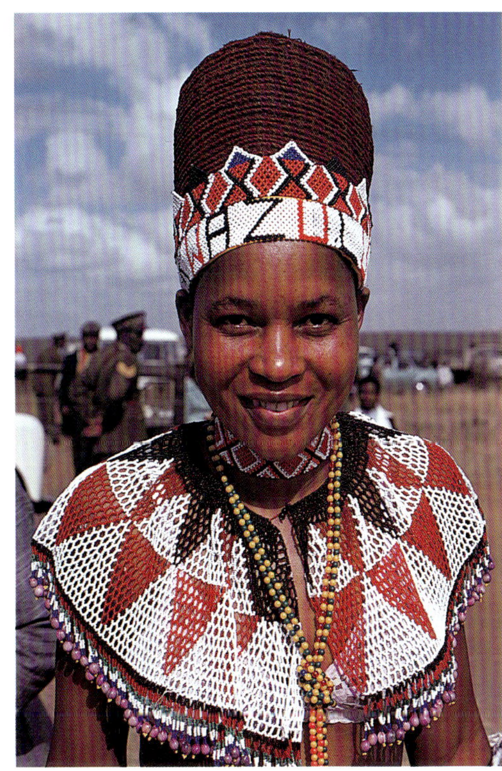

throughout the world — that refers to an individual's wisdom, perception, and second sight, as well as intelligence and creativity.

According to Allen Roberts, this particular type of headdress and Tabwa beaded patterns, the spirits themselves are represented in the geometric patterns of the beads. The opposing isosceles triangles are a pattern known generally as *balamwezi,* the rising of the new moon, which is found on virtually all categories of Tabwa arts, including sculpture and body decoration. However, beyond this more generalized meaning, the central triangle motif of the diviner's headband is a reference to the "eye of Kibawa" who controls the domain of the dead, and the juxtaposed triangles on either side of the center are "the wives of Kibawa" who, along with other spirits, possess Bulumbu cult adepts to help them divine and heal the afflictions of their clients (Roberts 1986:35). The geometric patterns clustered in such a way as to allude to the second sight, or perceptiveness, of the diviner, as well as to the realm of the ancestors, reinforces the powers of the diviner to see into both worlds — the world of the living and the world of the dead — as he attempts to resolve those problems and concerns that plague members of the Tabwa community.

In addition to the symbolic importance attributed to certain kinds of beaded patterns, the colors of beads may hold culturally-specific meaning. Among the Zulu, the color white refers to purity and love, and is particularly appropriate for headwear associated with marriage.[1] In some Zulu beaded headdresses, it is the shape rather

**Figure 5.3,** opposite top left. Chief's crown *(misango mapende).* Pende, Zaire. Beads, metal, fiber. H. 18.0 cm. Collection of Robert Alan Friedman.

**Figure 5.4,** opposite top right. Pende chief, Muela Buana village, near Gungu, Zaire. Photograph by Eliot Elisofon, 1951. Slide no. C PND 2 (2248). Eliot Elisofon Photographic Archives. National Museum of African Art.

**Figure 5.5,** opposite bottom left. Chief's hat *(mpu a nzim).* Mbala, southwestern Zaire. Raffia, shell. H. 15.0 cm. FMCH X65.5495. Gift of the Wellcome Trust.

**Figure 5.6,** opposite bottom right. Diviner's headdress *(nkaka).* Tabwa, Zaire. Beads, hide, feathers, cotton. H. 59.0 cm. Private collection.

**Figure 5.7,** above left. Married woman's hat *(isicholo).* Zulu, South Africa. Hair, fiber, beads, red ochre, thread. H. 14.0 cm. Collection of Robert Alan Friedman.

**Figure 5.8,** above right. Zulu woman wearing a columnar basketry hat with beaded embellishments. Photograph by Carolee Kennedy, 1977.

than the color that links them with married women, although Carolee Kennedy (personal communication 1994) feels that the predominantly white color scheme reflects a preference common from the 1930s to 1950s.

Fashions, like "traditions," are never static. Both are part of dynamic processes that are, by their very nature, in constant states of assessment, evaluation, modification, innovation, and transformation. The Zulu beaded hat (Fig. 5.7), called *isicholo*, is a case in point. This style of hat was originally inspired by the mud-smeared top-knot hair style identifying married Zulu women in the nineteenth century.[2] A beaded headband *(umnqwazi)* encircling the forehead at the base of the coiffure was "a sign of respect to the male members of her husband's family" (ibid.). By the late 1930s and 1940s, this hair style was modified to a broader cylindrical hairdo that tapered only slightly to a wider, flatter crown (Conner and Pelrine 1983:15, fig. 9).

The columnar-shaped beaded hat recalls this version of the married woman's hair style (Fig. 5.8). Worn high on the head, the beaded hat visually reinforces the sil-

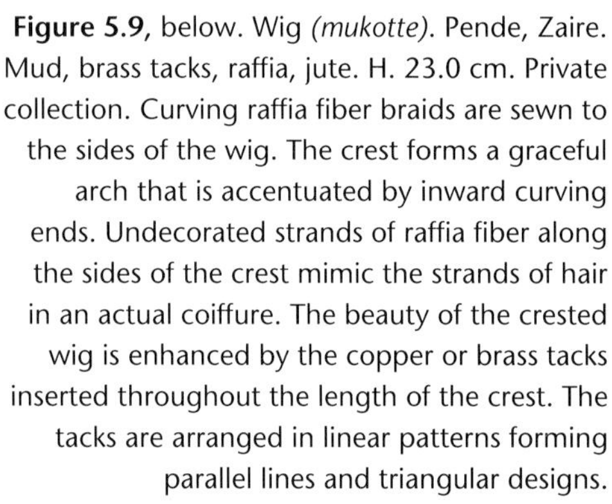

**Figure 5.9**, below. Wig *(mukotte)*. Pende, Zaire. Mud, brass tacks, raffia, jute. H. 23.0 cm. Private collection. Curving raffia fiber braids are sewn to the sides of the wig. The crest forms a graceful arch that is accentuated by inward curving ends. Undecorated strands of raffia fiber along the sides of the crest mimic the strands of hair in an actual coiffure. The beauty of the crested wig is enhanced by the copper or brass tacks inserted throughout the length of the crest. The tacks are arranged in linear patterns forming parallel lines and triangular designs.

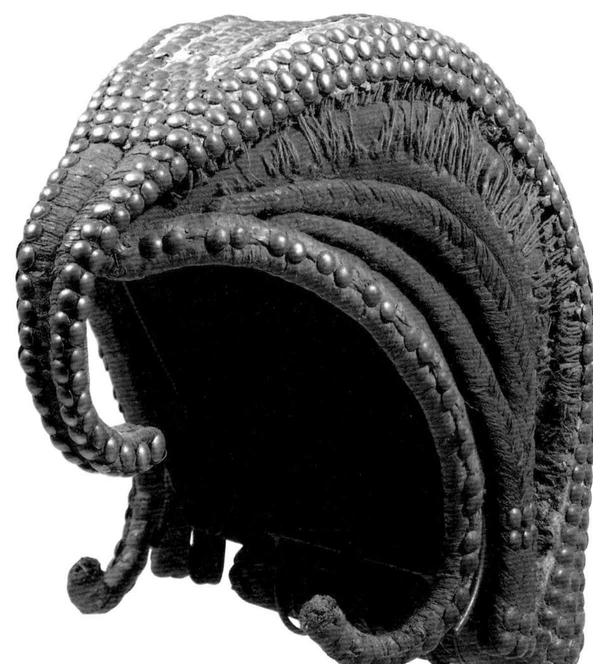

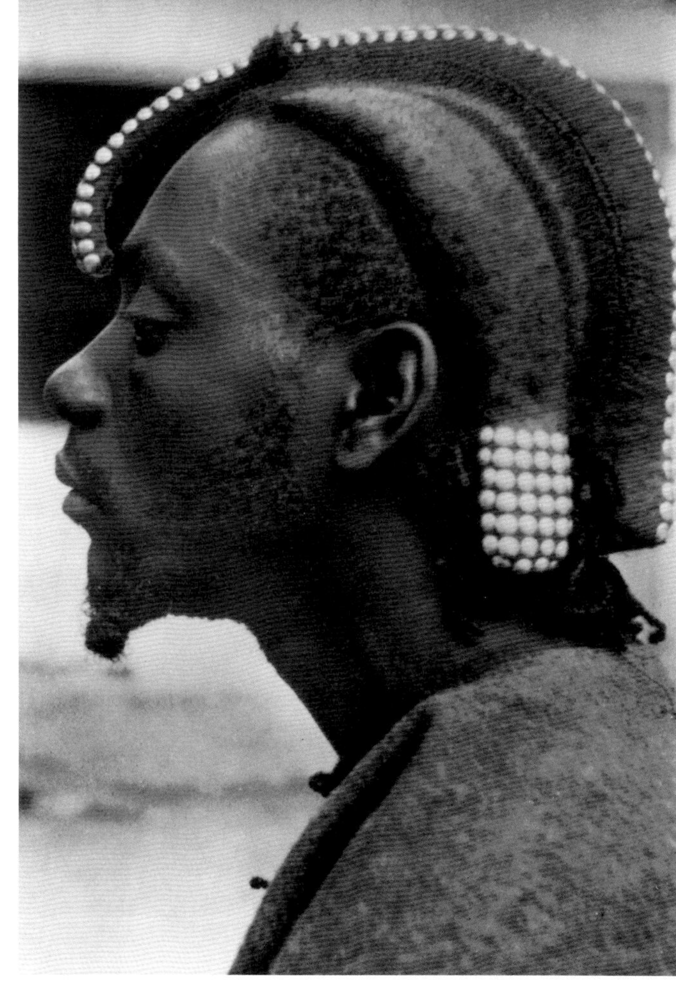

**Figure 5.10**, right. "Type Bapende" (Pende man), Zaire. Photograph by Casimir d'Ostoja Zagorski, 1926. "L'Afrique qui disparaît," Series 2, no. 60. Eliot Elisofon Photographic Archives. National Museum of African Art. This man is wearing the coiffure that inspired the wig in Figure 5.9.

houette of the older hair style, yet responds to the growing interest in beaded ornamentation among the Zulu. Its exclusive use as a married woman's hat satisfies Zulu norms of social propriety, and through the first half of the twentieth century at least, the hat was part of daily dress for Zulu women. During her research among the Zulu in the late 1970s, Carolee Kennedy saw few women wearing this type of beaded hat on a daily basis; it was worn only on special occasions, such as weddings and regional festivals (personal communication 1994).

Another example of an ornamented headdress influenced by a traditional coiffure is the Pende crested wig (Fig. 5.9), called *mukotte,* which "replaces a similarly shaped coiffure that is made with long hair, clay, oil, copper nails, cowrie shells, and/or beads" (Biebuyck and Van den Abbeele 1984:70). Apparently, there are several local and regional variations to both the coiffure and the wig. The coiffure may be worn by men or women (Fig. 5.10), although the literature seems to indicate that the fiber wig is preferred by men. The wig is made of a raffia fiber framework covered with a base of raffia cloth. The coiffure depicted in this wig is a popular hair style worn by a number of groups in the region, including the Mbala who adopted it from the Pende (ibid.). Although worn as part of ordinary dress, the crested wig (and one assumes the coiffure that it recalls) could be embellished with a crown of parrot feathers for special occasions (de Sousberghe 1958:pl. 284, cited in Biebuyck and Van den Abbeele 1984:70).

## EMBROIDERED ELEGANCE

Headdresses may convey power, wealth, status, and prestige through the use of any number of manufactured, imported, or found man-made materials, as well as by the amount of time and attention devoted to its manufacture and decoration. There are many factors that place a headdress into the category of special or ceremonial wear: particularly well-crafted items; the addition of decorative embellishments that signal the skill of the maker; the aesthetic appreciation of the work on the part of the wearer; and the rarity, preciousness, or sheer expense of the materials.

Elaborately stitched and embroidered hats, worn in many parts of Africa, fit into the category of special occasion headwear by virtue of their decorative elaboration which sets these hats apart from more mundane daily wear. The added time involved in the embroidery process, translated into enhanced value (and, no doubt, the actual production cost and resale price of the item) would, for practical reasons alone, suggest that such hats would be worn for special occasions. The occasion need not be a ritual event, however, as particularly exquisite examples of headwear are, throughout Africa, reserved for regularly scheduled social gatherings, such as market days. More than mere covering from the elements, such hats are worn in a public presentation of self, in which one generally seeks to make a fashion statement, or at the

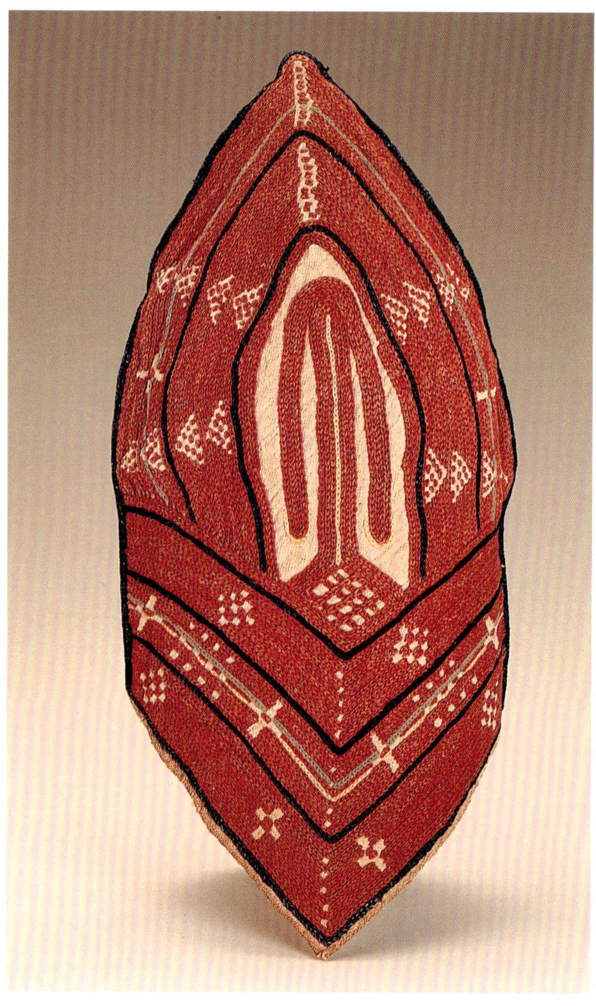

**Figure 5.11**. Man's hat. Guro, Wan, or Malinke, Côte d'Ivoire. Cotton, dyes. H. 41.0 cm. National Museum of African Art NMAFA 89-1-1. Anonymous gift. Photograph by Franko Khoury.

very least, to dress up in one's finer clothing. Notions of propriety fit in here, as well, for public presentation through dress acknowledges (even if it does so by dismissing) widely held norms of appropriate dress and public decorum. Thus, aspects of the practical nature of headwear — head covering, propriety, decorum — are combined with visual statements on one's social standing and prosperity (perceived or actualized) in the choice of headwear worn on public — and, therefore, special — occasions.

Special occasion headwear may contain threads of silk, gold, silver, and glittery synthetics embroidered by artists in delicate linear patterns. Spangles, beads, shells and other materials may also be included in the embroidery work. Well-dressed men throughout much of West Africa wear elaborately embroidered cotton caps that complement their smock and trouser ensembles.

Hats of the "mitre" style are made and worn in many parts of West Africa, including Mali, Liberia, and Sierra Leone, and as far east as Nigeria, northern Cameroon, and Chad (Lamb 1984:143). Among the Bamana of Mali, this hat is called *bama da* "crocodile mouth." The long tapered flaps leading up to the wide opening for the head recall the gaping maw of a crocodile. The Lambs (1984:143) note a similar name for the hats among a number of groups in Sierra Leone. Embroidered designs on these hats take the form of geometric and curvilinear patterns, and may also include stylized animal motifs and ideographs. The embroidered patterns separate hats of a more mundane nature from embellished decorative headgear that may be reserved for more special occasions, such as going to market or to festivals and community gatherings when one would want to be particularly well-dressed.

There is variation in the way these mitre-like hats are worn. The triangular shaped flaps may be positioned laterally near to or covering the ears, or one triangular flap may extend down the back of the head, while the front flap is flipped up to reveal the forehead. Although usually made of narrow-strip cloth, locally woven broad-loom cloth as well as imported cloth may also be used for these hats.

In many parts of West Africa, mitre-style hats that include elaborate embroidery designs are trade items originating from their center of manufacture in Guinea-Conakry (Lamb 1984:143). Thus, the precise ethnic identification of this hat is uncertain, given that the ethnic group of the weaver and hat maker may not be the ethnic group of the wearer. Nonetheless, it is of a style that is fairly commonly worn by Guro, Wan, and Malinke men in Côte d'Ivoire, where it was purchased (Fig. 5.11).

For men in the Cameroon Grassfields, covering the head is de rigeur as appropriate dress for daily, special, and ritual occasions. Gebauer (1979:82) notes that in the nineteenth- and early twentieth-century Grasslands societies, slaves were prohibited from covering their heads, while freemen were

> obliged to do so. To meet this demand, the commoners developed the plain, foldable, goblet-like cap of black, durable fiber. Men of rank favored more decorative headgear made of raffia fiber. Cotton fibers inspired artisans to loop beautiful geometric patterns into knitted caps.

Throughout the Cameroon Grassfields there are a wide variety of colorful knit and embroidered caps worn by men of varied social standing to conform to these dictates of fashion and propriety.

Gebauer (1979:111) reports that at the turn of the century Hausa traders introduced the hand-embroidered hat which is still popular in the Grassfields and throughout West Africa. Hausa styles greatly influenced Grassfields dress in the nineteenth and twentieth centuries, inspiring Grassfields tailors to produce flowing embroidered and applique gowns that, with modifications and innovations, borrowed from the Hausa model for their basic form (Gebauer:110).

Broad-crowned flexible hats called *ntamp* (Lamb and Lamb 1981:184) from the Cameroon Grassfields (Figs. 5.12, 5.13, 5.14) were probably worn as part of daily dress, defining a man of relatively high status and adequate means. The addition of the bird's feathers projecting out from the crown would indicate particularly high status or embellishment for a ceremonial occasion. In some instances, the permission of the Fon is required before an individual can wear certain feather ornaments.

The Grassfields is noted for a variety of collapsible cotton knit caps. The *ashetu* hat (Lamb and Lamb 1981:181) imitates a style of coiffure distinguished by projecting tufts of hair. Reproduced in this hat, the tufts of hair are rendered as projecting knit burls that ornament either side of the head. The burls are embellished with alternating bands of color. Vertical lines of color separate the right and left sides of the elaborate "coiffure." While the body of the cap is tightly knitted, the burls are knitted more loosely and then stiffened with tiny wooden inserts to make the burls project upward (Figs. 1.9, 1.10).

Although the bulk of hats in this section address the messages embedded in headgear worn by men, there is a wide variety of headwear worn by women to signal important events and special occasions. Elaborate coiffures, jewelry, and wrappers draw attention to the head and to the norms of social propriety and fashion that come into play in the choice of form and occasion for elaboration of the head. As with men's hats, elaborate embroidered designs often distinguish headwear reserved for special and ceremonial occasions.

**Figure 5.12**. Man's hat *(ntamp)*. Bamenda, Cameroon. Vegetable fiber, feathers. H. 14.0 cm. Collection of Robert Alan Freidman.

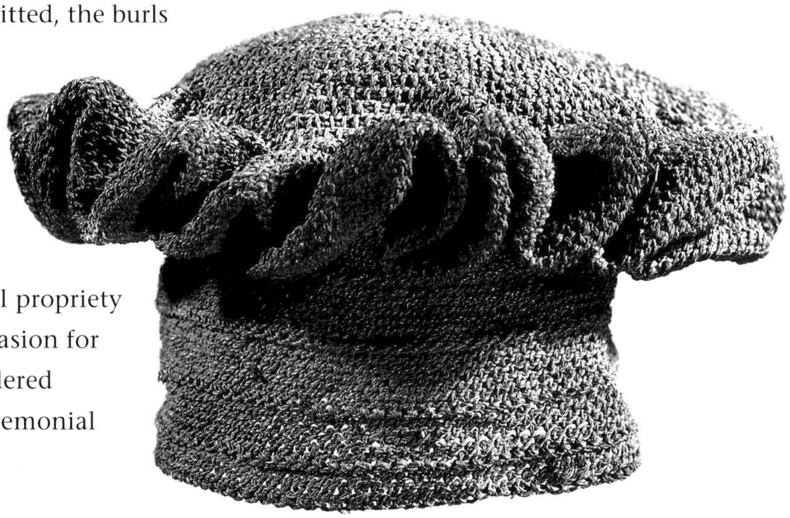

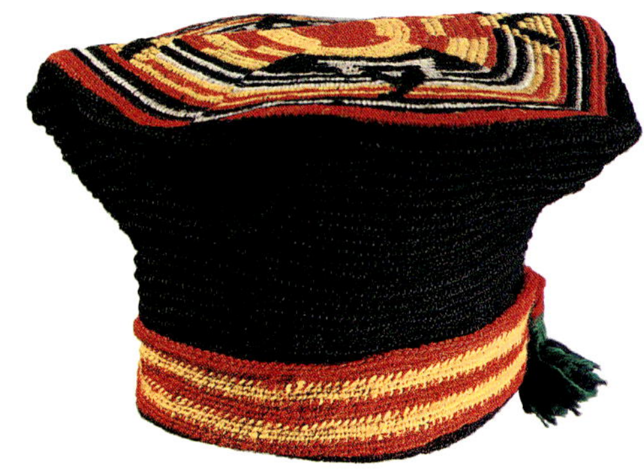

**Figure 5.13,** right. Man's hat *(ntamp).* Bamenda, Nigeria. Wool, fiber. H. 15.0 cm. FMCH X86.2628. Gift of Jim Pieper. This hat was collected in the Bamenda community in Gboko town, part of the Tiv area of northern Nigeria.

**Figure 5.14,** below. Fon (king) Abumbi II of Bafut, Cameroon, in a palace courtyard. These colorful yarn hats are worn daily by men throughout the Grassfields kingdoms of the Cameroon. In the Grassfields, it is considered improper for an adult man to appear in public without some form of hat or headcovering. Photograph by Christraud M. Geary, 1969. Eliot Elisofon Photographic Archives. National Museum of African Art.

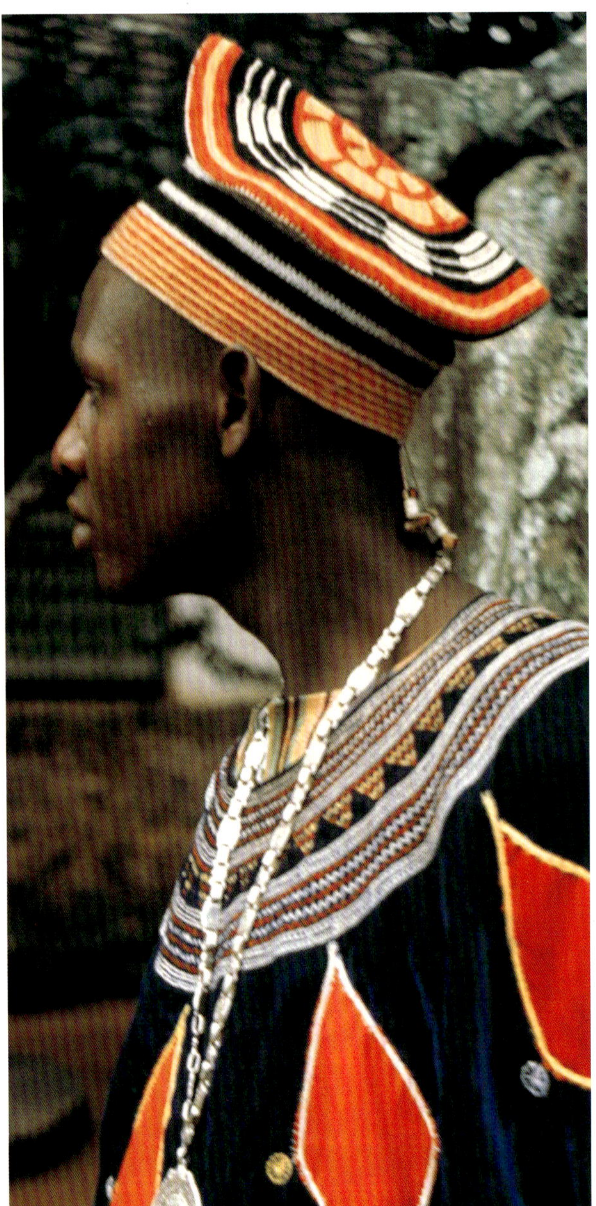

Often overlooked in an examination of women's body adornment are caps that cover the head as ceremonial dress or as part of daily wear. Caps with trains from Tunisia *(qoufiya*; Fig. 5.15) are worn by women at their marriages and for other festivals (Sugier 1968:61). In addition to their ceremonial context, the veils are superb examples of the artistry of African embroidery. In Tunisia and Morocco, embroidered clothing is obligatory for most women who may spend a considerable amount of money and time making embroidered clothes for their wedding day and trousseaux (Stone 1987:14). The elaborate nature of Tunisian marriage clothing is not without its practical application: the gold and silver thread traditionally used to create the elaborate embroidered patterns can be viewed as a woman's nest egg to be used when needed (Stone 1987:15).

One type is found in eastern Tunisia from Bizerte south to Sfax and Kerkena. Orange silk material is transformed into a shimmering statement of feminine beauty through elaborate embroidery of gold-colored metallic thread. The train is attached to a cap made of sturdy, locally woven cotton. The upper portion of the long train is embroidered in curvilinear patterns along the sides, leaving the orange silk material unadorned; the bottom third of the veil is fully embroidered. A colorful fringe of white, red, orange, and blue threads creates a particularly festive look.

Among the Galla (Borana) of southern Ethiopia, and northern Kenya, women wear a variety of leather skirts, wrappers, shawls, and trains. In photographs taken in the early 1950s, Adamson (1967:356–7) illustrates the leather dress of Borana women, including long leather skirts, cowrie-ornamented leather bands worn bandolier-style across the chest, and ornamental panels with leather and calabash fringe worn across the lower back and buttocks. The headdresses worn at marriage (Fig. 5.16) are composed of three sections — a broad central train that falls down the center of the back, flanked by thin panels on either side. The cap of the train is slightly rectangular and projects up from the head. Cowrie shells in linear, floral, and circular patterns are sewn to the leather. Copper or metal disks may also be attached to the headdress for further embellishment. This type of leather train (*ankerba*) is part of the leather attire worn by married women among the Borana (Galla people who moved from Ethiopia into Kenya) and neighboring groups (Biebuyck and Van den Abbeele 1984:114). In addition to being worn, there are suggestions that the headdress may have been suspended over the entrance of the newlyweds' house .

**Figure 5.15**, left. Woman's wedding train *(qoufiya)*. Tunisia. Silk, metallic thread, cotton, sequins, beads. H. 96.0 cm. FMCH X86.1753. Gift of Caroline and Howard West.

**Figure 5.16**, below. Woman's wedding train *(ankerba)*. Galla, Ethiopia. Leather, cowrie shells. H. 163.0 cm. Private collection.

## EXOTIC IMPORTS

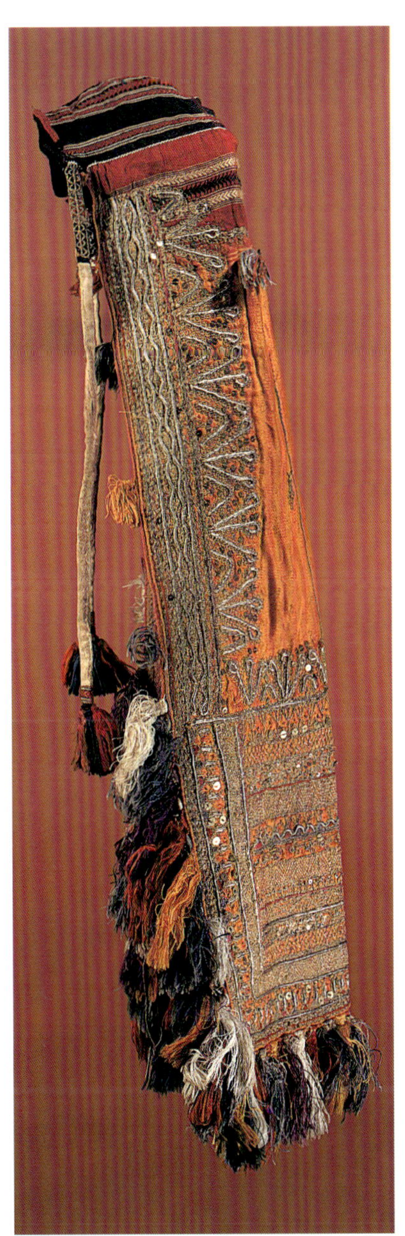

While the preciousness of a material — such as imported beads, gold, silver, or copper — or the degree of handiwork or decorative elaboration may signal that a headdress is reserved for special occasions, the adoption of forms, materials, and motifs of foreign inspiration in the creation of special occasion headwear may be yet another way to convey messages of prominence, prestige, wealth, or education.

Although fairly rare, full-size wooden hats inspired by French colonial headwear were carved by the Baule of Côte d'Ivoire prior to independence in the 1960s. These hats, as well as Baule figure sculptures that include details of clothing, show a keen sense of fashion — including dress inspired by the colonial presence and influences from various parts of Europe, most predominantly metropolitan France. Their appeal to the Baule lies not in their imitation of exotic foreign dress, but in the appropriation of dress that, linked to colonial authority in the Baule's history, carried with it associations of power, authority, and prestige.

Carved of wood, these hats are skeuomorphs of the regulation pith helmet and the *képi*, or French military cap (Figs. 5.17, 5.18) worn by officers in the French army.[3] While the pith helmet is largely undecorated on the outside — save for the concentric grooves that define that hat style — the interior rim of the helmet is painted with red pigment. Ravenhill stated that in the 1970s he saw a dozen or so pith helmets and military hats for sale in the cen-

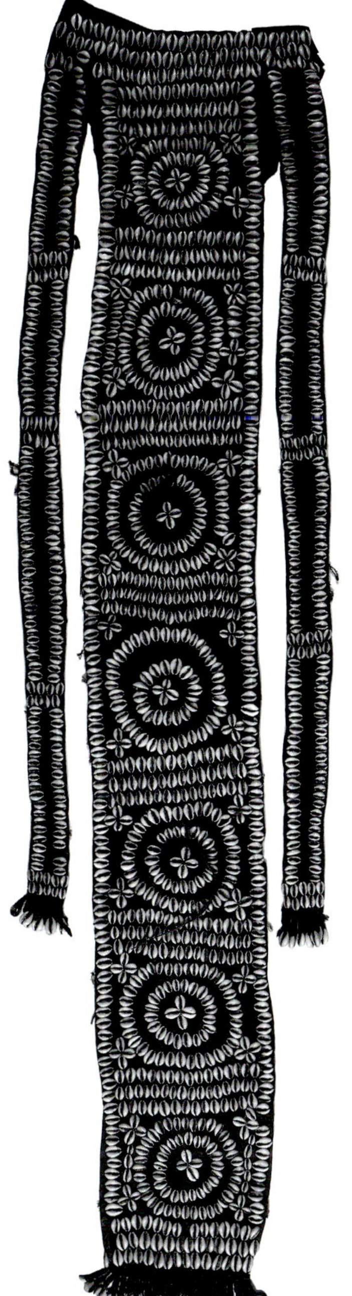

tral market in Bouaké. He notes that the interiors of some of the hats were lined with wallpaper and/or pigment (Philip Ravenhill, personal communication 1994). Both hats show signs of use. It may well be that these hats are related to the genre of Baule display art called *sika blawa* (Ravenhill, personal communication 1994), which are regalia and prestige objects covered in gold *(sika)* foil. Although these examples bear no evidence of having been ornamented with gold foil, they may fall under the category of gold-plated display objects, which includes royal regalia, figure sculpture, and other wooden objects. In their discussion of gold in West African art, Fisher and Himmelheber (1975:25) illustrate a 1934 photograph of the market stall of a gold-leaf specialist who is displaying his wares presumably for sale. Among the neatly arranged display of gold-leafed linguist staffs, state swords, and flywhisks with gilded hilts, is a life-sized pith helmet embellished with concentric incised ridges around the crown of the hat. Given its context, and the glossy sheen apparent in this black-and-white photograph, it may be that the hat illustrated was covered with gold leaf.[4] Vogel (1991:236) illustrates a full-size gold leaf pith helmet and notes its use as a display object in funeral contexts.

Among another Akan group, the Fante of south-central Ghana, western military regalia is said to have inspired

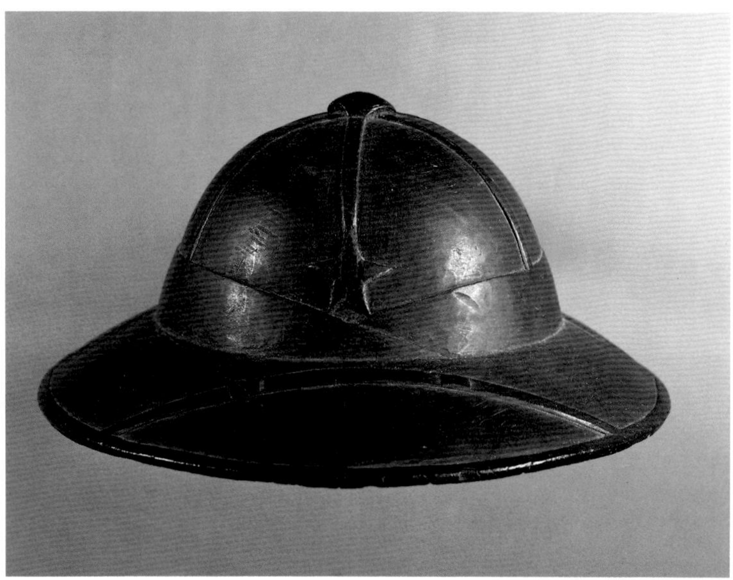

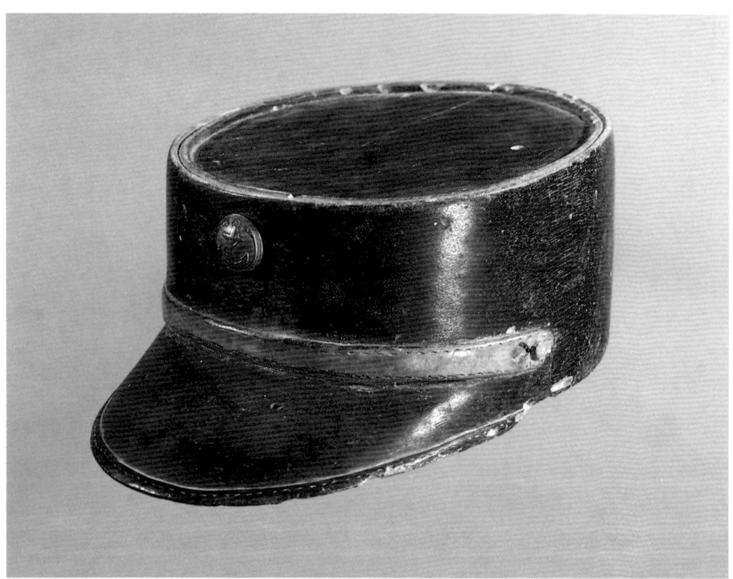

**Figure 5.17**, above left. Pith helmet. Baule, Côte d'Ivoire. Wood. H. 18.0 cm. Lent by Mort Dimondstein. The emphasis that the Baule place on elaborate coiffures in their figure sculptures as indicators of social propriety from a Baule perspective, is extended to include sculptural renditions of imported headgear. "The colonial pith helmet, one of the most important symbols of the colonial era, became one of the most common accoutrements represented in Baule art in this period" (Ravenhill 1984:114).

**Figure 5.18**, left. Gendarme hat *(képi)*. Baule, Côte d'Ivoire. Wood. H. 10.5 cm. Anonymous loan. A range of Baule carved figures wear hats that signal membership in the French colonial forces in Côte d'Ivoire: the fez-style hat indicating affiliation with the *Tirailleurs Sénégalais* colonial forces in Senegal, *gendarme* hats of the colonial police force, as well as a number of different styles of pith helmets from various periods of French administration. These imported elements are borrowed and used by the Baule, not merely in imitation of Western dress, but as statements to convey the status and success that such dress implied during the colonial period (Ravenhill 1980:10).

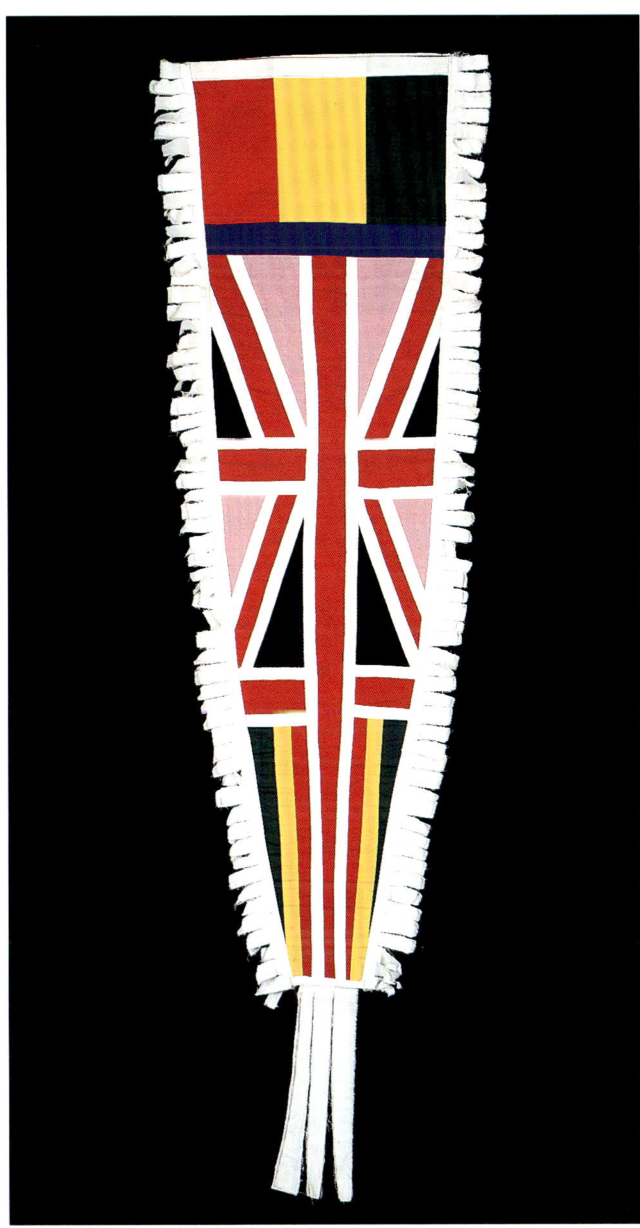

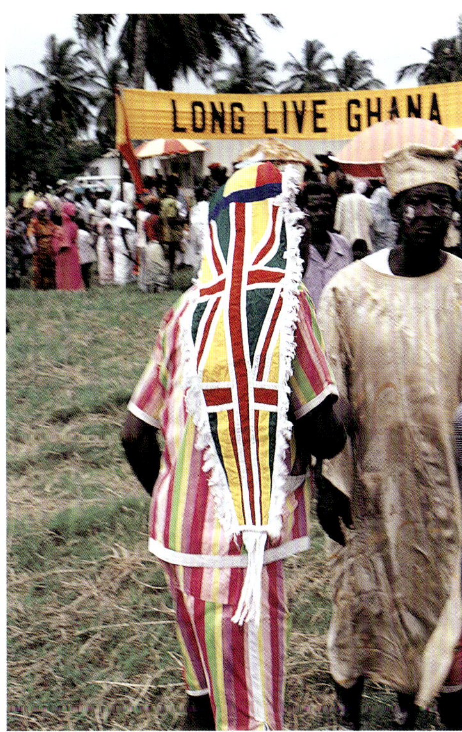


**Figure 5.19**, above. *Asafo* hat *(frankaa)*. Fante, Lowtown, Ghana. Fabric, cotton, thread. H. 115.0 cm. FMCH X81.1659. Gift of Mrs. W. Thomas Davis. The hats of traditional Fante warrior groups are called *frankaa*, the Fante word for flag. This hat combines the Union Jack with the Ghanaian tricolor — a lively merging of two power symbols.

**Figure 5.20**, above right. Member of a Fante *Asafo* company wearing a hat called *frankaa* at the annual Odambea festival dedicated to celebrating the harvest and to remembering the dead, Lowtown, Ghana. Photograph by Doran H. Ross, 1981.

the materials, forms, and motifs of the traditional military organization called *Asafo*. Fante history is marked by long and intensive contact with Europeans who came as merchants to the coast as early as the 1470s. Representatives of trading companies from Portugal, Holland, Sweden, Denmark, France, England, and other countries competed for trade in gold, various other commodities, and eventually slaves.

The *Asafo (sa,* war; and *fo*, people) are a common feature of most Fante towns. *Asafo* military companies are numbered and named and have their own emblems and company regalia. Even today, *Asafo* performs military, political, religious, and civic functions (Ross 1979:3). In addition to their role in state defense, *Asafo* organizations are the custodians of certain religious shrines and are active in public works projects that benefit the community. The history of *Asafo* suggests that European influence

> had a dramatic effect on both the organization of the companies and their patterns of military display...[including] the numbering of companies, marching in procession, musketry salutes, the use of distinctive flags, and the building of fort-like shrines based on European models (Ross 1979).

*Asafo* is noted for distinctive applique flags that are brought out for display on ceremonial occasions and for public festivals. The colors and patterns of the flags, as well as those for the company dress, are the exclusive right of each *Asafo* company. *Asafo* military dress is composed of a loose-fitting, short-sleeved, tailored cotton shirt, and a peaked or pennant-shaped cap (Figs. 5.19, 5.20). The cap is hand- or machine-sewn and may be embellished with applique designs and fringe in contrasting colors. The combination of European influences and Ghanaian innovation is clearly evident in this hat, which combines less-than-accurate renditions of the British Union Jack, balanced by the Ghanaian tricolors (red, green, and yellow) on either side. Like the flag itself the hat is called *fraanka.* A pouch or shoulder bag and a rifle usually complete the ensemble of the *Asafo* soldier. Female members of *Asafo* may wear similar garb or they may opt for an elaborate cloth-wrapper ensemble more evocative of royalty than the military. This military style of dress stands in marked contrast to the dress of the flag bearer, whose raffia fiber skirt and beaded bandoliers across his bare chest recall the dress of shrine priests, thus emphasizing the religious nature of *Asafo.*

## POWERS FROM THE WILDERNESS

In reviewing the literature on African headwear, it is clear that the choice of exotic, precious materials and elaborate forms is a critical way to signal the special nature of the wearer, the occasion, or both. Natural materials derived from the wilderness are a prominent feature in hats and headdresses used for special events, to signal special occupations, and to celebrate ceremonial occasions. It is not uncommon for chiefly headgear, hunter's hats, diviner's caps, and ritual and festival headdresses to incorporate the hides, beaks, feathers, horns, and crests of a range of wild animals to signal entrée to and mastery over the realm of the wilderness.

As Cole (1989:100) points out, the roles of political leaders are often linked with those of warriors and hunters in different parts of Africa. Thus, leadership dress that links the powers of rulers to those of successful warriors may include battle dress as well as actual or symbolic weapons to convey the warrior nature of a leader, prepared to go into battle to protect the community. These qualities may be further combined with allusions to hunters who, in many societies in Africa, hold a measure of power and prestige by virtue of the nature of their work which takes them into the physical and symbolic realms of the wilderness.

Leadership attire thus reinforces cultural and symbolic associations people have with particular kinds of objects and materials to ally chiefly powers with the strength, cunning, quickness, invincibility, and ferocity of wild animals. A quick review of African leadership arts show associations with the elephant, leopard, lion, bush cow, antelope, monkey, pangolin and a host of other wild animals that, through the use of actual or simulated skins and carved and cast representations in leadership regalia, make powerful visual statements that the chief's powers are not to be underestimated.

## FEATHERED FINERY

The use of feathers in the creation of headdresses and other forms of attire combine the opulence of highly valued decorative items with associations with the wilderness realm the birds inhabit. Feathers are a perfect design element for clothing and headwear, in part because of their many hues. However, their fragile nature and the rather tedious methods by which feathers are obtained and incorporated into attire prohibits their widespread use for daily wear. Feathered attire may allude to symbolic associations individuals and societies hold with particular kinds of birds, their habitats, and the qualities ascribed to them. They are beautiful decorative accents for a variety of headwear used by individuals as insignia of rank, emblems of authority and power, and spectacular and dramatic elements of performance attire.

Among the more striking examples of feather art are the headdresses from the Cameroon Grassfields. The Tikar feather headdress from the Grassfields is probably of a type worn by palace dancers in celebration and funerary contexts (Figs. 5.21, 5.22). These headdresses are fashioned from dyed feathers secured to a mesh cap (Gebauer 1979:111). The red tail feathers of the African gray parrot, as well as the feathers of other birds, go into making Grassfields headdresses. This type of headdress has its own built-in self-storage capacity, as the entire headdress can be turned inside out, with the feathers protected by the inverted fiber cap. When not in use, the hat can be stored in this manner, protecting all but the tips of the feathers from deterioration.

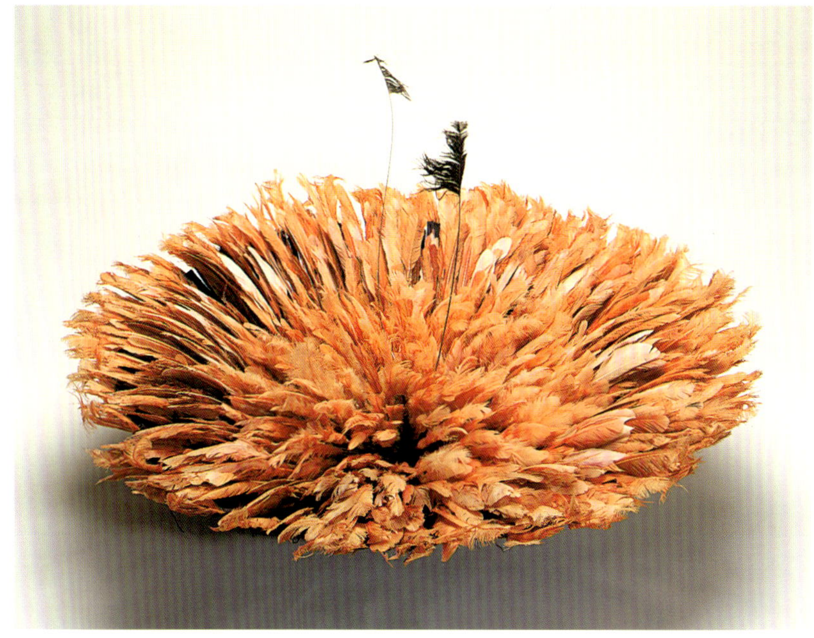

**Figure 5.21**. Headdress. Tikar, Cameroon. Feathers, vine, fiber, cotton cloth, string. H. 38.0 cm. FMCH X86.2477. Gift of Jerome L. Joss.

From beaded headbands and necklaces ornamented with aluminum, buttons, and beaded pendants, to elaborate headdresses and ruffs of wild animals now protected in national parks, the importance of jewelry and body ornamentation to define aspects of beauty, as well as social, economic, and political status is a defining feature among the Maasai of Kenya and Tanzania.

Among the more familiar animal headdresses are the lion mane headdresses and ostrich feather ruffs regarded as part of full dress regalia of Maasai warriors, known as *moran*. The ostrich feather ruff (Figs. 5.23, 5.24) dramatically extends the

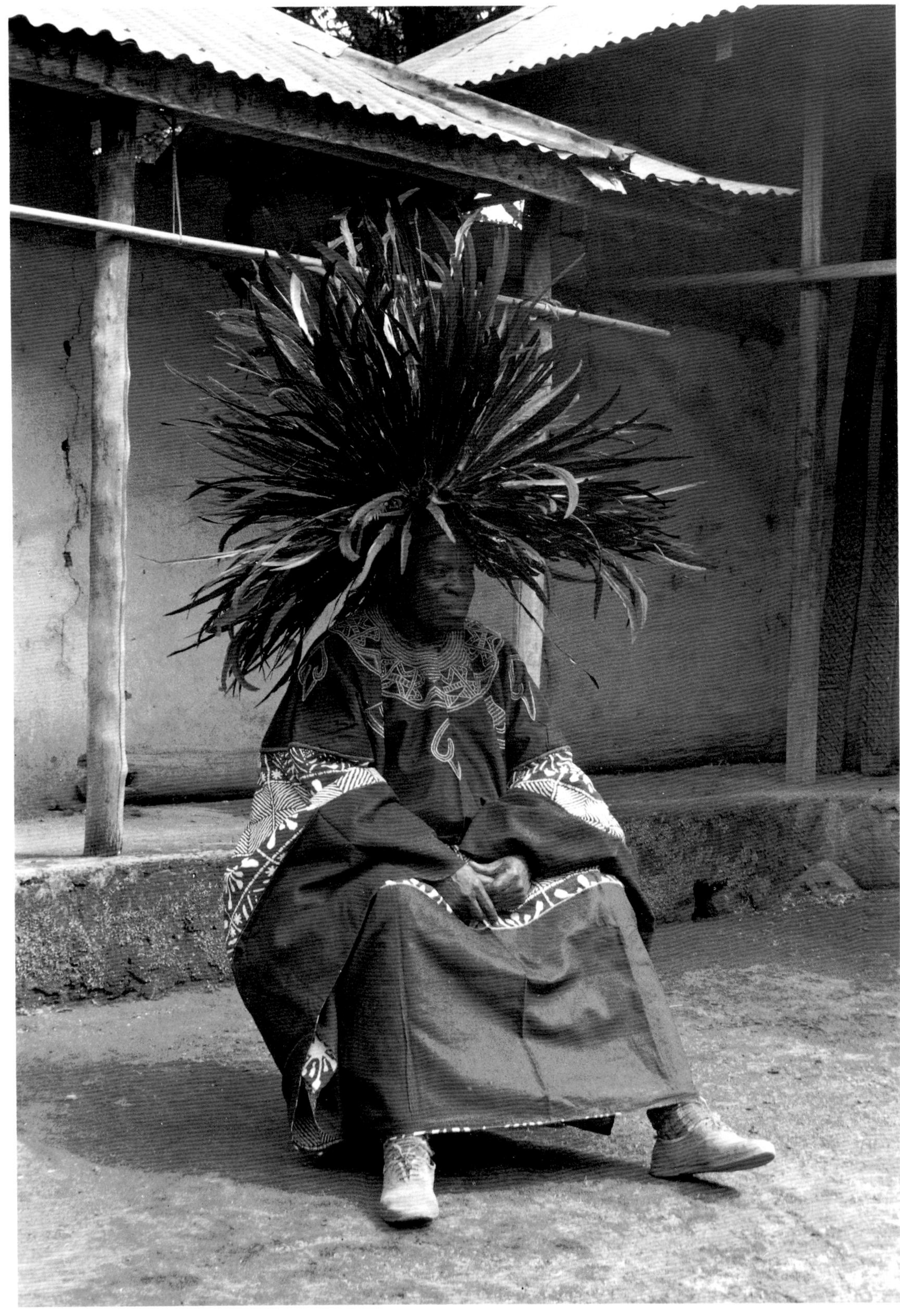

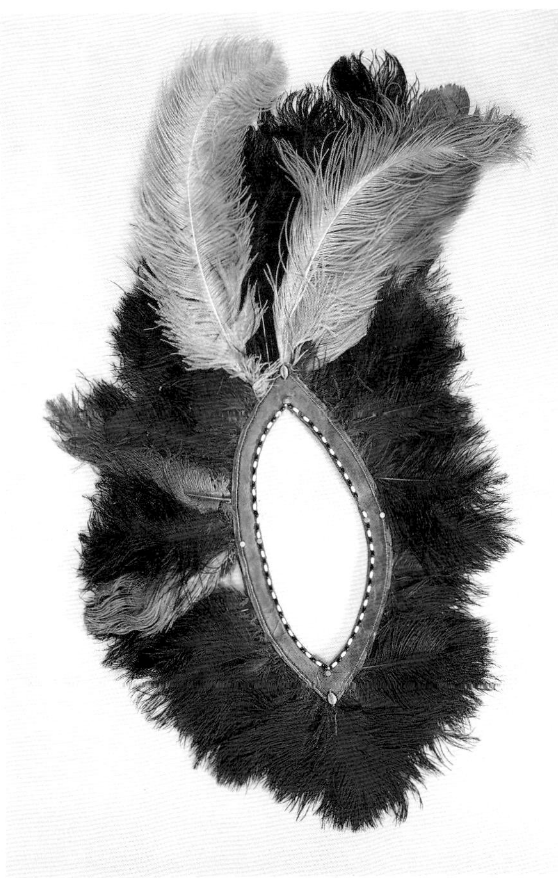

**Figure 5.23**, left. Warrior's face ruff *(enkuraru)*. Maasai, Kenya. Leather, ostrich feathers, beads, cowrie shells, wire, string. H. 38.0 cm. FMCH 398.51. Museum purchase. Most of the ostrich feathers were left in their dark natural color, but a few were dyed red. They are sewn to an oval leather band that frames the face. Strands of colored beads are sewn to the leather, drawing more attention to the face of the *moran.* The accession information on this Maasai ruff states that feathers from the female ostrich are affixed to the sides of the ruff, while feathers from the male are sewn on the top. This type of headdress is not restricted to the Maasai; it has long been used to connote warrior status among the Kikuyu and other groups of the region.

**Figure 5.22**, opposite. Fon (king) Vugha of Big Babanki, Cameroon. Photograph by Christraud M. Geary, 1969. Eliot Elisofon Photographic Archives. National Museum of African Art. Feather headdresses are also worn by certain other palace officials during non-Islamic festivals.

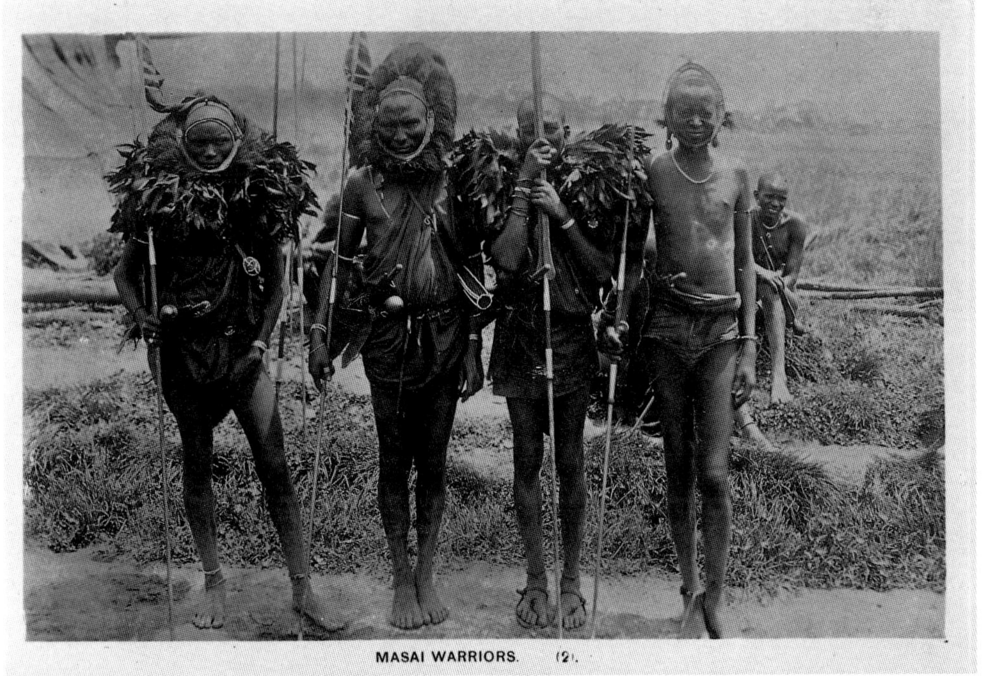


**Figure 5.24**, right. Warriors wearing face ruffs, Maasai, Kenya. Toned photographic postcard. Photographer undetermined. Real Photo Printers Lilywhite Ltd., Halifax, England. Printed in England, date undetermined. The Metropolitan Museum of Art, New York. Department of the Arts of Africa, Oceania, and the Americas. The Photograph Study Collection.

height and width of Maasai warriors, and accounts suggest that the very sight of Maasai warriors in their feather ruffs was enough to frighten off the enemy. The ostrich feather ruff called *enkuraru* is worn by warriors who have yet to kill a lion (Fisher 1984:22). The lion mane headdresses called *olawaru* are the prerogative of those warriors who have made a kill. While the lion mane headdress towers a foot and a half or more above the head, the ostrich feather ruff frames the face of the warrior. Today, these magnificent headdresses are worn mostly for ceremonies and entertainment dances.

## ANIMAL SKINS AND HIDES

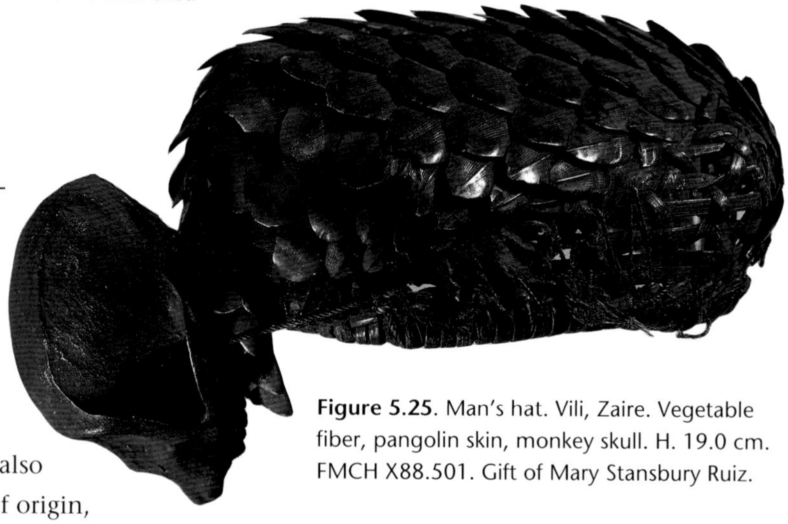

Worn by chiefs, elders, hunters, and members of men's associations, animal skin hats take a variety of forms. Other materials may be added to enhance further the impressive display of power these hats invoke. Monkey skulls, bird feathers, bird beaks, animal claws and teeth, civet and other wild cat skins, elephant hide and tails serve to reinforce visually the considerable powers wielded by the wearer. Seemingly more benign materials, such as cowrie shells and metal ornaments, also carry their own symbolic referents. Proverbs, sayings, myths of origin, and particular strengths and powers associated with specific animals are alluded to in headdresses that combine materials drawn from the natural world, particularly the wilderness.

**Figure 5.25.** Man's hat. Vili, Zaire. Vegetable fiber, pangolin skin, monkey skull. H. 19.0 cm. FMCH X88.501. Gift of Mary Stansbury Ruiz.

An amazing variety of pangolin hats are found among a number of groups in northeastern Zaire, including the Lega, Gombe, and Vili. The unique qualities of the pangolin — a mammal with fishlike scales on an armorlike hide that serve as protection from predators when coiled into a ball — make it an ideal symbol for the powers of chieftaincy or men's age-grade or titled associations. Its protective hide is the perfect metaphor for the impenetrable powers and defensive abilities of chieftaincy. The pangolin skin itself defines the wearer as one who goes beyond the boundaries of settled village life into the realm of the wilderness. Thus, whether used in actual form, as in the case of the pangolin hats from central Africa, or alluded to, in the case of Benin chiefly dress that imitates in cloth the scales of the pangolin, the pangolin is an animal associated with power and authority.

The *bwami* association of the Lega of Zaire places a great deal of attention on hats *(kikumbi)* to signal movement from one level of the association to the other. The giant pangolin, for example, is connected to the highest grade within *bwami,* the *lutumbo lwa kindi.* Biebuyck notes that the

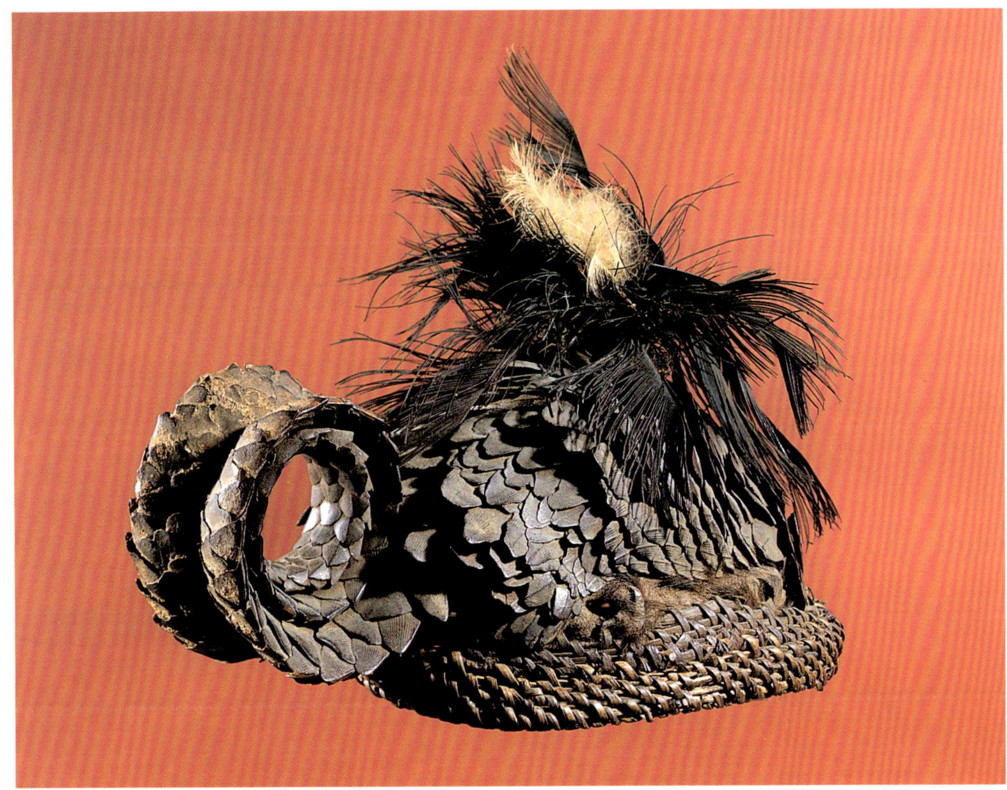

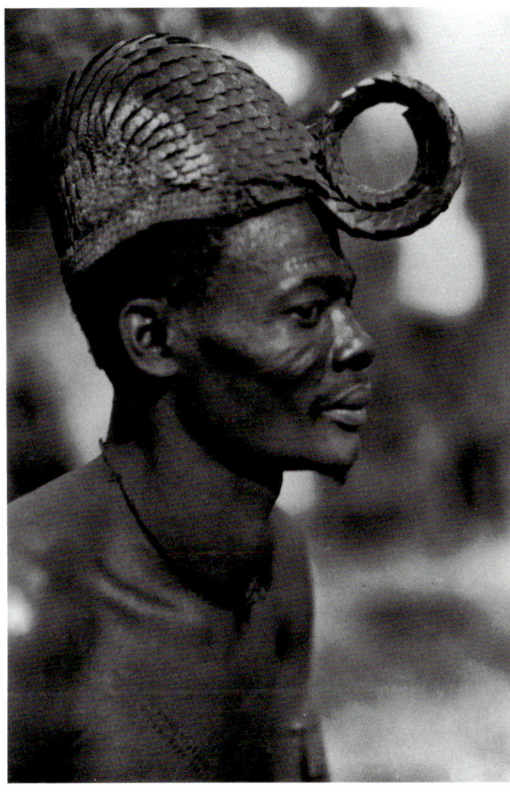

**Figure 5.26**, left. Man's hat. Gombe, Zaire. Pangolin skin, feathers, bamboo. H. 26.0 cm. Private collection.

**Figure 5.27**, right. "Type Gombe" (Gombe man), Zaire. Photograph by Casimir d'Ostoja Zagorski, 1926. "L'Afrique qui disparaît,"Series 2, no. 12. Eliot Elisofon Photographic Archives. National Museum of African Art.

> pangolin *(ikaga)* is a culture hero who is said to have taught people the technique for covering house roofs [phrynium leaves are arranged on the roof like the scales on the pangolin's body]. It is a sacred animal whose accidental death creates ritual disequilibrium, which must be expiated by appropriate rituals and distributions (Biebuyck 1973:pl. 91 text).

The pangolin claw is part of *bwami* cult paraphernalia and may be used as a warning signal; the scales or skin of the pangolin are seen as symbols of piety and respect (ibid.:189–190; Fig. 8.20). In *bwami* rituals, a row of pangolin skins or scales signifies that the path of initiation is long (ibid.:208).

In spite of their importance in *bwami,* and perhaps because of the prohibition of intentional killing of pangolins by *bwami* association members, pangolin hats are not common among the Lega and they are not part of required *bwami* attire. Rather, Biebuyck (1982:61) places pangolin hats — and other hats made of unusual materials such as colobus monkey hide, iguana skin, elephant ear, and the throat piece of the forest crocodile — within a category of additional hats that may reflect the "individual preferences and fantasies" of the owners who are high initiates in *bwami* (Fig. 8.21).

Both the Vili pangolin skin hat (Fig. 5.25) and the Gombe hat (Fig. 5.26) draw

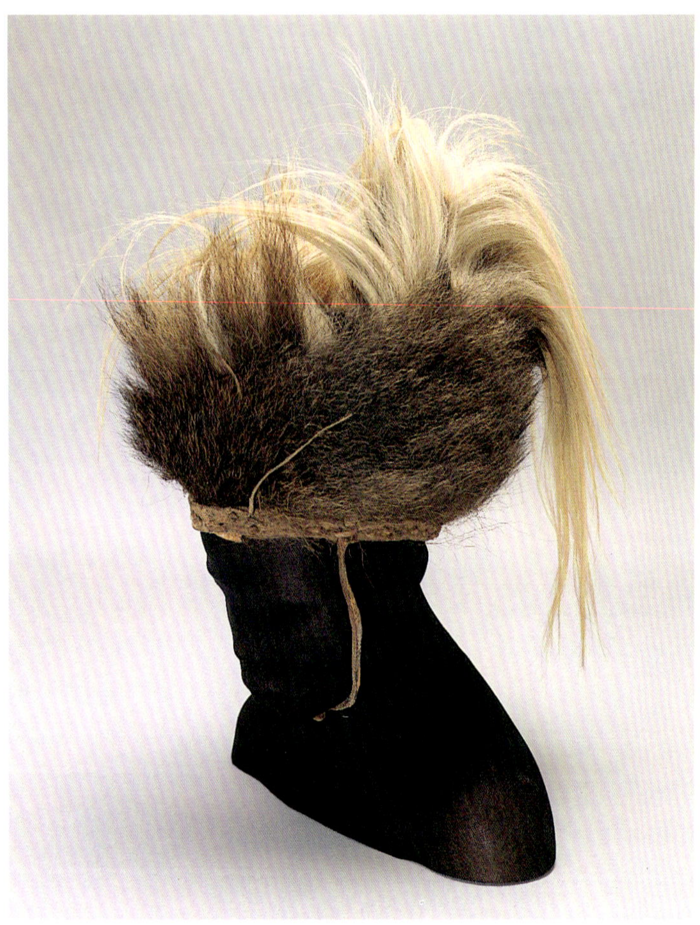

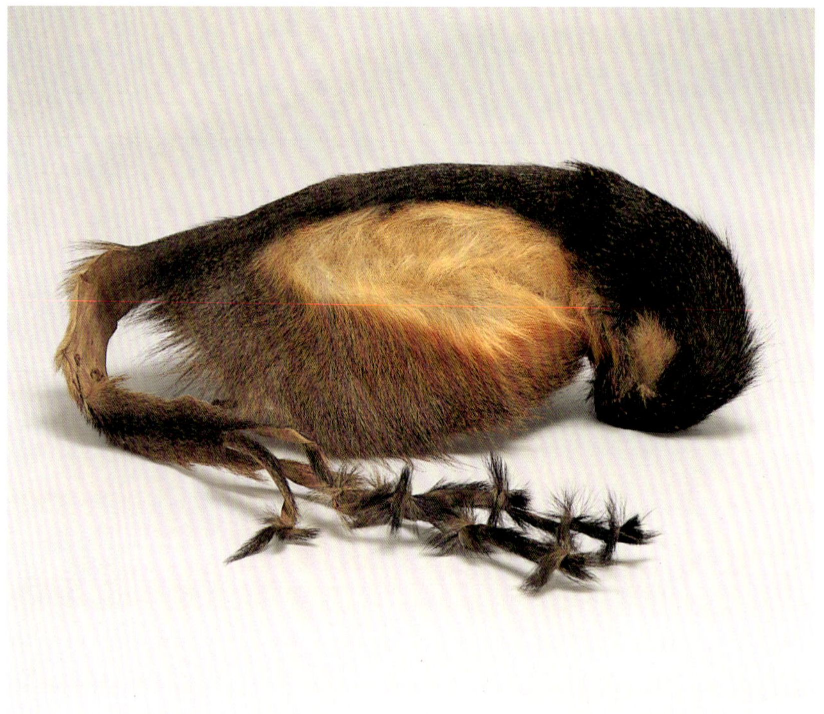

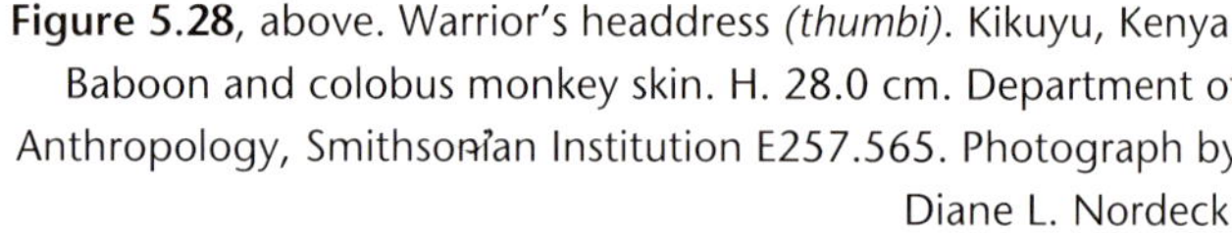

**Figure 5.28**, above. Warrior's headdress *(thumbi)*. Kikuyu, Kenya. Baboon and colobus monkey skin. H. 28.0 cm. Department of Anthropology, Smithsonian Institution E257.565. Photograph by Diane L. Nordeck.

**Figure 5.29**, above right. Man's hat. Upper Zaire River region, Zaire. White-nose monkey skin H. 18.0 cm. Department of Anthropology, Smithsonian Institution E169.203. Photograph by Diane L. Nordeck. A curious feature of this hat is that the legs of the monkey have been sewn to the body to make the sides of the cap. The person who created this hat made excellent use of the natural patterns of the skin. The tail of the monkey has been split into strands that hang down the back of the hat.

**Figure 5.30**, right. Headdress. Lega, Shabunda, Lualaba River, East Zaire. Skin, fur, textile, buttons, string, cord. H. 20.5 cm. FMCH 378.381. Museum purchase.

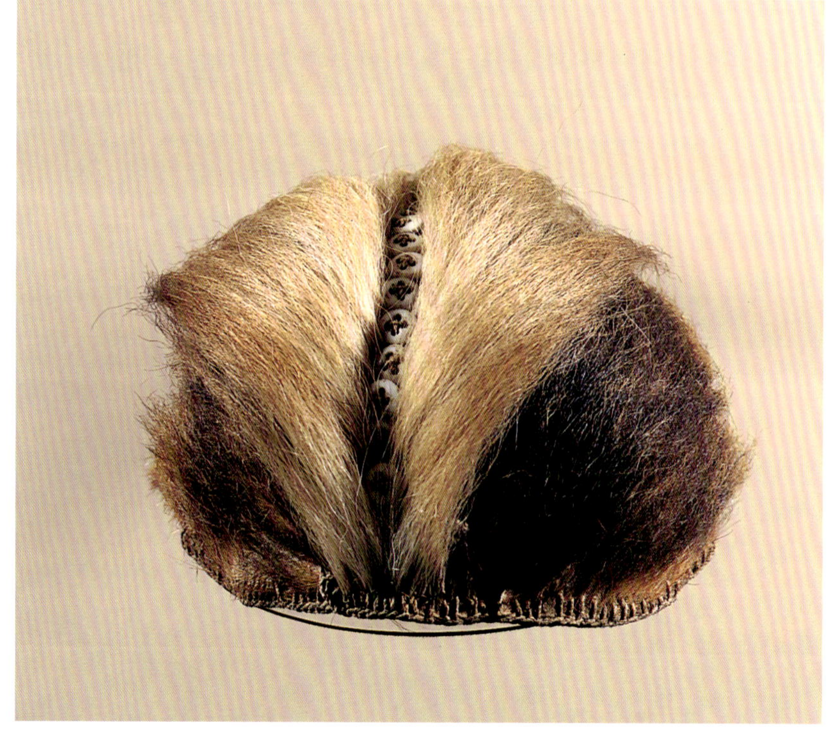

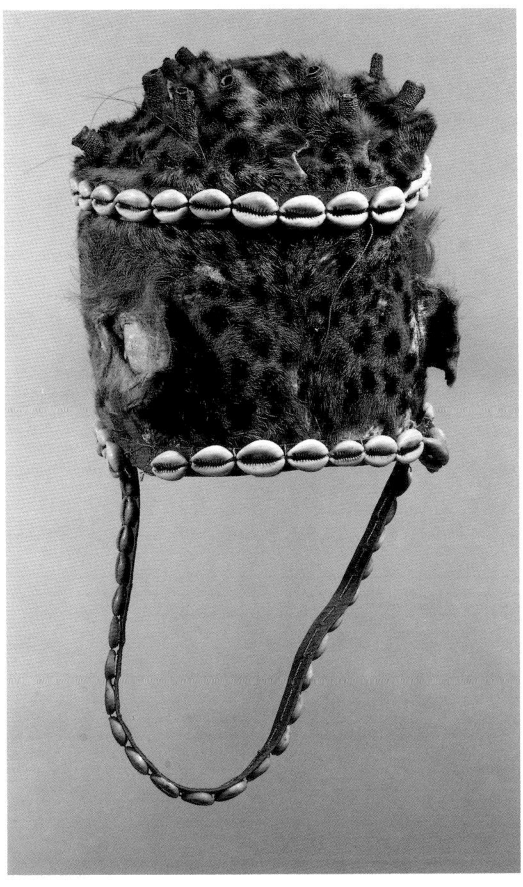

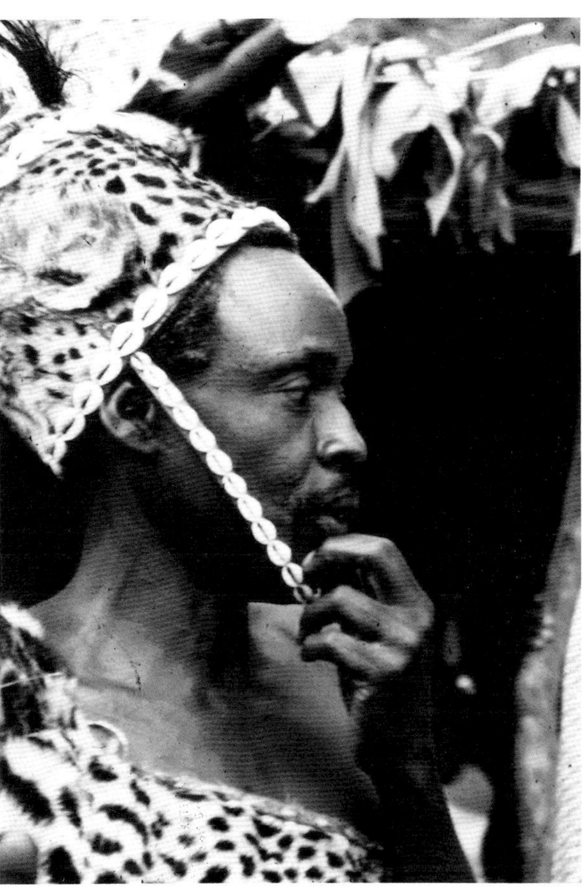

on the cultural associations ascribed to this animal. In the Gombe version, the pangolin tail is curled up upon itself and worn in the front (Fig. 5.27). The Vili hat embellishes on the visual metaphor of power by attaching a small monkey or chimpanzee skull to the hat. Given the symbolic significance of these materials in other parts of central Africa, and the fact that monkey skulls are often associated with healing and divination activities and, in some instances, serve as symbolic links to the world of the ancestors, it is likely that the hat was worn as an insignia of authority by an individual of considerable power and social prominence, either a chief, a diviner/healer, or a hunter.[5]

**Figure 5.31**, above left. Chief's hat. Sebei, Uganda, and Zaire. Leopard skin, cowrie shell, twine, leather, plant fiber. H. 38.0 cm. FMCH X85.1081. Gift of Walter Goldschmidt.

**Figure 5.32**, above right. The grandson of the Sebei prophet Matui at the ceremony for the exhumation of the prophet's bones. Photograph by Walter Goldschmidt, 1962.

Animal skin headdresses are found among many of Kenya's peoples, particularly those living in the northern and western parts of the country — the Maasai, Kikuyu, Luo, Samburu and others. A range of animal skins are and were used to define specific age-grades, warrior status, religious office (such as healers and diviners), and ceremonial and festival attire. Monkey and other skin headdresses from eastern and central Africa are shared across ethnic boundaries. Although accession information lists the monkey skin hat in Figure 5.28 as belonging to the Kikuyu, this style of headdress *(thumbi)* is a type shared by a number of neighboring groups

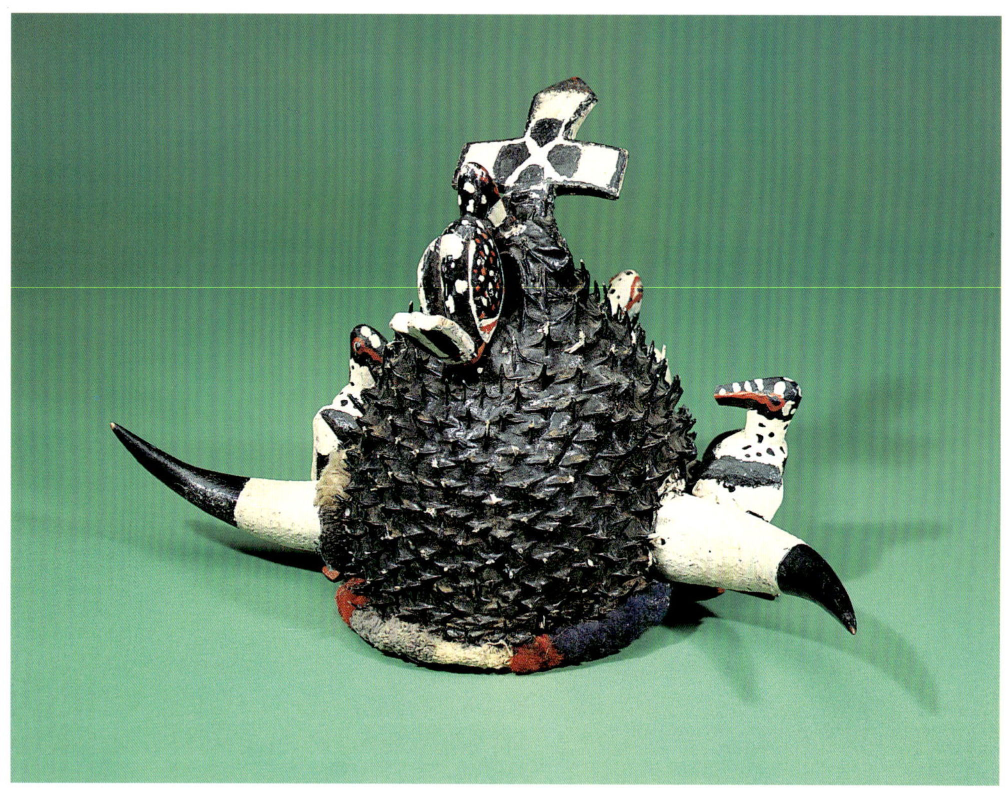

**Figure 5.33**. Initiate's hat *(iassaca)*. Bidjogo, Guinea Bissau. Blowfish skin, wood, horn, yarn, plastic, rubber, string, metal. H. 27.0 cm. FMCH X82.1111. Gift of Helen and Robert Kuhn.

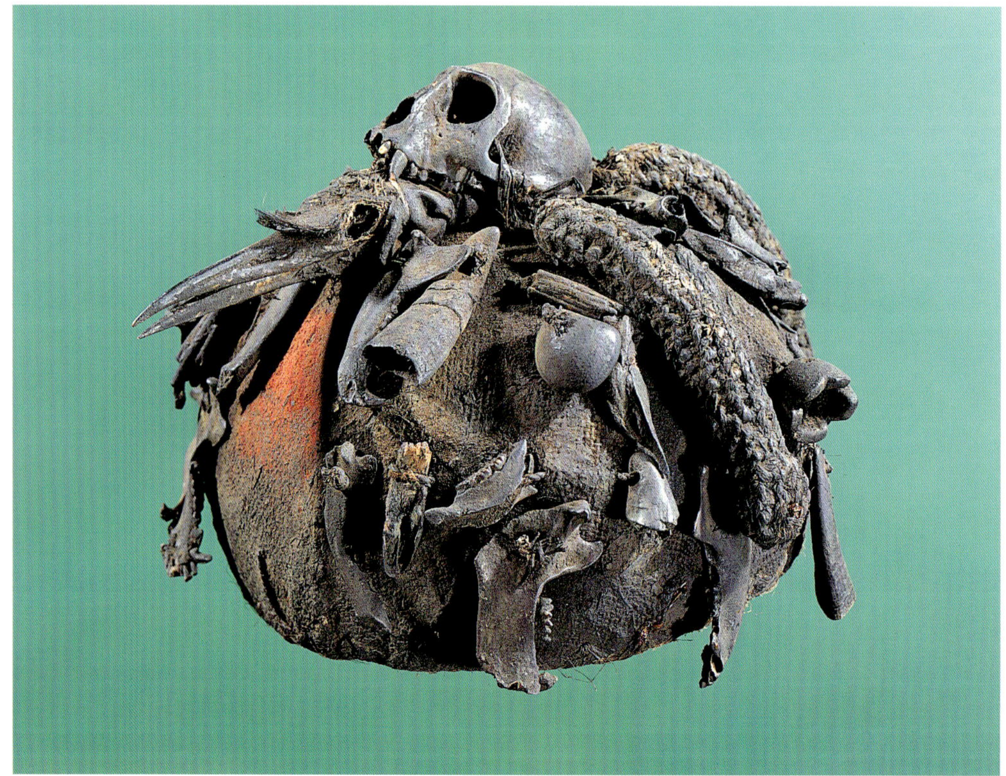

**Figure 5.34**. Man's hat. Bamileke, Cameroon. Monkey skull, crow's beak, duiker horns, lower jaws of unidentified rodents, seed pod, red ochre, fiber, hide. H. 25.0 cm. Private collection.

including the Luo, Samburu, and others. Adamson (1967:162), for example, illustrates a photograph of a Luo man wearing an almost identical headdress, identifying it as funeral dress. In the Adamson photograph, the complete ensemble appears to be composed of a number of hide cloaks and wrappers, a flywhisk, a large circular cowrie shell wristlet, and ornaments of shell, tusk, and bone around the neck. Judging from this and other photos in the text, the Luo had a wide variety of headwear derived from wilderness animals, including impala horns, ostrich feathers, monkey skins, and boar's tusks.[6]

Given the nature of the material, skins used in headwear and other items of clothing result in similar products. A case in point is this monkey skin hat from the Upper Congo River region of Zaire (Fig. 5.29). This hat maintains the integrity of the monkey form while making it an effective and impressive hat. The skin was identified by Smithsonian scientists as that of a white-nosed monkey. As with the Kikuyu example, the choice of where to place the light-colored portions of the skin suggests an appreciation for the natural beauty of these monkeys — a beauty translated into an object of personal ornamentation.

In fabricating animal-skin headdresses, modifications to the raw material may be relatively minimal in examples made from fairly unadulterated animal skins. Lega and Vili pangolin hats, for example, convey the size, texture, and shape of the giant forest pangolin. In viewing these spectacular headdresses, one is able to visualize, without too much difficulty, the wild animals from which the skins were taken. In contrast, other headdresses significantly alter the natural materials, either through extensive tailoring, the application of colorings and dyes, or in the combination and addition of other materials creating composite forms. In the Maasai ostrich feather ruff (Figs. 5.23, 5.24), the oval presentation of ostrich feathers, some of them embellished with red ochre coloring, recalls the beauty, but not the form, of the birds from which the feathers were taken. The same could be said for the Tikar red feather headdress (Fig. 5.21) from the Cameroon Grassfields.

Although the powers of the leopard are clearly alluded to in the Sebei headdress from Uganda (Figs. 5.31, 5.32), the tailored hat adorned with cowrie shells and other materials emphasizes the manmade nature of this headdress. However, combined with the leopard-skin robe that completes the ensemble, the message of power is dramatically reinforced and serves as an important reminder that the headdress is but one part of an ensemble. In addition to the power of the combined ensemble, the contexts in which the attire is worn enhance the dramatic impact and meaning of the attire. This particular leopard skin headdress and robe were worn by a chief and ritual specialist in a ceremony to exhume the bones of a deceased Sebei prophet (Goldschmidt 1976: 56 ff).

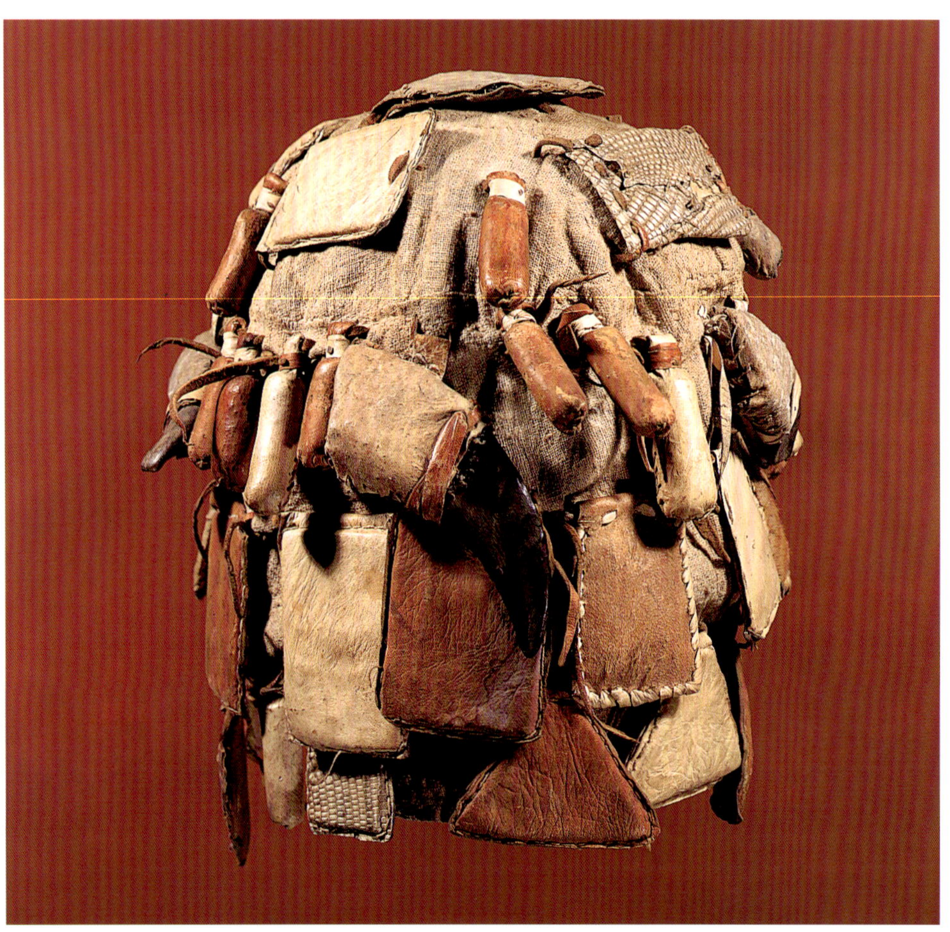

**Figure 5.35**. Hunter's hat. Hausa, Nigeria. Leather, reptile skin, horn, cotton, fur. H. 25.5 cm. FMCH X65.8231. Gift of the Wellcome Trust.

## COMPOSITES

There is considerable potential for extraordinary expressive power through the combination of diverse materials and/or images in the creation of composite headdress forms. Among the Bidjogo of Guinea Bissau, for example, the combination of seemingly disparate and unconnected marine and bovine creatures are combined effectively in men's association initiation headdresses (Fig. 5.33). The result is a fantastic and symbolically charged composite creature whose symbolic attributes may well surpass the literal associations made with any one individual element comprising the headdress.

The Bidjogo practice of combining bovine and marine elements into the ceremonial headwear of the male age-grade association has met with some fascinating results, as illustrated in this blowfish and cow horn hat *(iassaca)* that is ornamented with carved wood sculptures of birds. These elaborate headdresses are worn in initiation rites and public festivals by age-grade members. This less fierce combination — the benign blowfish embellished with nonthreatening upturned cow horns — is worn by the *canhoca* adolescent who, "leaving childhood and beginning to direct himself to the community, is identified with a domesticated or harmless animal" (Duquette 1979:31). The headdresses of older, uninitiated young men *(cabaro)* evoke a more ferocious and wild appearance by alluding to wilderness animals, such as the bull and the hippopotamus, and dangerous fish, such as the sawfish. The behavior of young boys and men in each of these grades captures some of the qualities attributed to the animals depicted in their headdresses.

In certain circumstances, such headdresses may also be worn by women who are associated with maintaining the shrine of "the Great Spirit," *Orebuko-Okoto* and the descendant spirits. They are also worn by young women (*defunto* or *orebuk)* who participate in a ritual period (*fanado)* during which they serve as surrogates for young men who have died before completing their coming-of-age ceremonies. In this way, the deceased man is able to enter the world of the ancestors. A woman who participates in this type of initiation ritual is able to acquire the ritual paraphernalia and takes on the status of the age-grade called *cassukai,* that of mature men (Duquette 1979:34).[7]

A variety of protective medicines and amulets are combined in hunter's hats among the Bamelike and the Hausa (Fig. 5.35). These caps are a visual summary of the powers attributed to the hunter, a specialist whose work takes him beyond the settled existence of village life into the dangerous wilderness realm. Successful hunting requires not only specific knowledge of the animals and plants of the surrounding environment, but also a fair measure of spiritual prowess to enable the hunter to negotiate the mystical dangers believed to reside in the bush. The dress of hunters, then, conveys mastery over the realm of the wilderness through the use of wilderness materials and allusions to medicines controlled by the hunter that protect him from the dangers of the bush, yet ensure his success in catching his prey.

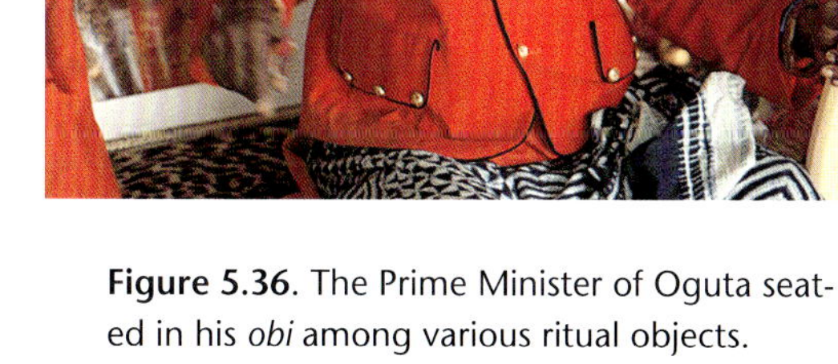

**Figure 5.36.** The Prime Minister of Oguta seated in his *obi* among various ritual objects. Photograph by Herbert M. Cole, 1983.

Hats that are used in daily wear can be objects of elaboration to create ceremonial and ritual headwear. For example, among the Igbo, a non-Islamic group in southeastern Nigeria, an Igbo priest adds feathers to a standard red fez to create part of his costume (Fig. 5.36). Among the Kuba, the small raffia hats worn daily by an initiated man may be the subject of further elaboration with the addition of feathers and hat pins as individuals take higher titles in Kuba society (see "Headdresses and Titleholding Among the Kuba" in this volume). Karamojong, Turkana, and Pokot men often add long ostrich feathers to their mudpack hairdos when participating in ceremonial events (see Figs. 2.21, 3.11). These embellishments redefine daily wear to objects intended for contexts of spectacular display.

## CONCLUSION

Although this chapter has been organized by materials and techniques into categories that define special occasion headwear, it could have been organized by the functional categories in which such headwear is worn. Indeed, particular categories of social experience seem to lend themselves to the wearing of special, even spectacular, attire.

It is no coincidence that in Africa and elsewhere in the world some of life's defining transitions — the change from youth to adulthood, marriage, assuming titles of leadership and authority, even death — are marked with elaborate ritual performances and special attire worn by participants and spectators alike. Initiation dress often combines exotic materials and composite forms to signal the powers of the initiation complex as well as the very real and symbolic separation of the initiate from the ordinary, everyday world while he or she is engaged in training. The symbolic nature of rites of passage for young girls and boys preparing to join the world of adults is signalled in a variety of highly ritualized, often spectacular dress that provides both literal and figurative references to the practical and esoteric knowledge, as well as to the secrets, challenges, and powers that are revealed during initiation training and acquired as one makes the transition from childhood to the status of young adult.

Special attire reserved for marriage offers an opportunity for the bride as well as her family and supporters, to reflect on the change of status and the acquisition of new social relations that occur at marriage. As an event that joins together two families and anticipates bringing children into the world, the marriage rite is a time of celebration. However, the importance of marriage goes beyond the ritual. The event itself creates a new state of social being, with a new and more complex set of social relationships. Thus, the significance of being married (as opposed to the rituals leading up to and culminating in marriage) is also a focus for specific attire that identifies one's marital status as part of a broader social system. That special and precious materials, elaborate techniques, and symbolic elements are incorporated into the attire of married women suggests the enormous importance attached to the institution of marriage itself and to the place of women in society.

As the dress of married women illustrates, identification of one's place in the social system is one potential outcome of specific kinds of dress. Indeed, particular forms of attire may designate one's occupation (such as a hunter, diviner, or priest) or one's place in society (such as an elder, senior wife, or titled person). In headwear that serves to define specific occupations, it is not uncommon to use materials that directly link with or allude to the work itself. Animal skulls, beaks, teeth and claws, bird feathers, as well as protective medicines and amulets from the wilderness are all appropriate materials not only to the work of hunters, but at various levels to the work of healers, diviners, and political leaders. In the case of leadership regalia and attire, opulent materials, time-consuming techniques, and elaborate forms unite into a coherent metaphorical statement about the power, authority, prestige, and wealth associated with leadership.

As many examples in this volume attest, considerable time and attention to form and the inventive use and combination of spectacular materials go in to the making of a variety of headwear. All these things provide important visual cues about the social position of the wearer and/or the contexts of use. These same factors figure into choices of attire that acknowledge norms of social propriety and express individual preferences and personal fashion statements. Therefore, one must be cognizant of the multiple usages, functions, and meanings of any one headdress — as part of an ensemble — depending on the wearer and the context.

It is the nature of special occasions to demand special attire. The spectacular headwear discussed in this chapter fulfills a multitude of social and religious functions. By and large, special occasion headdresses are spectacular works of art both within and outside the societies in which they are made and used, for their very composition and choice of materials suggest a conscious intent to astonish and impress insiders and outsiders alike with their opulence, their fantasy, and their beauty. The predominantly public occasions in which such headwear is worn acknowledges that the aesthetic experience is meant to be enjoyed by all — the wearer, the participants, and the audience. Even the outside spectator, with little or no cultural information with which to interpret the symbolism of meaning of such headwear, is bound to be affected by the powerful visual presence of such spectacular, special dress.

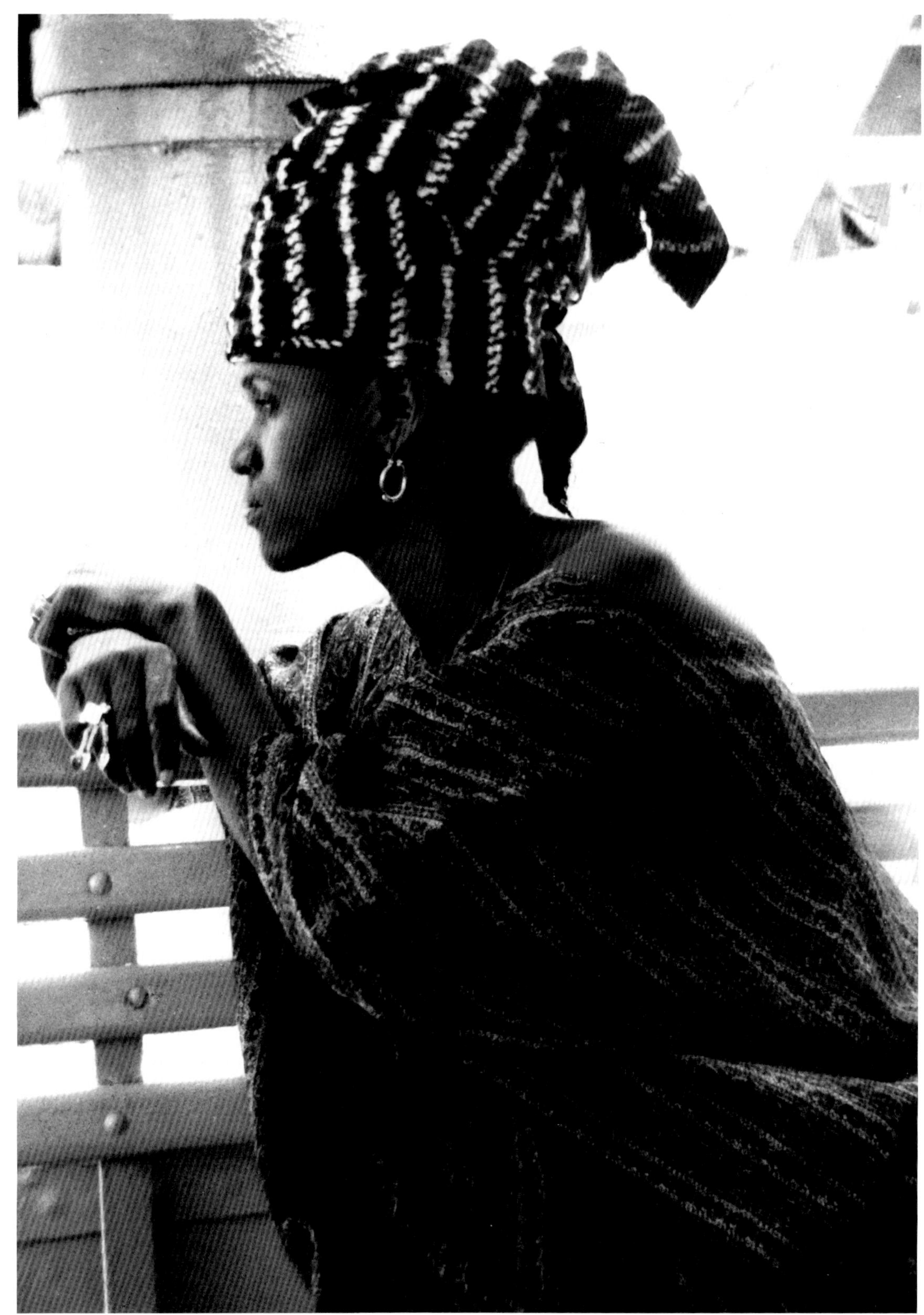

# 6 WRAPPING THE HEAD

## MARY JO ARNOLDI

The custom of wrapping the head with cloth is widespread on the African continent. Men's turbans are usually associated with an Islamic identity, and in some areas they are specifically associated with political authority. In most African Islamic societies from Morocco to Egypt, from Somalia to Madagascar, and from Senegal to Cameroon, men wear turbans to emulate and honor the Prophet, for it is said that Mohammed himself wore a turban. Among the Tuareg, men's distinctive turbans and face veils and women's headscarves express not only their Islamic identity, but symbolize more fundamental notions of Tuareg social relationships.

In West Africa, women's headties are not directly associated with Islamic practice and identity. Among the Wolof and Mande peoples of West Africa, women's headties express fundamental notions of propriety and are often indicators of a women's married status (Fig. 6.1). These notions have certainly been influenced by Islam which has a long history in this area. However, in southern Nigeria, among the Yoruba, where women's headties are considered a key element in formal dress ensembles, the practice of wrapping and decorating the head relates to critical Yoruba beliefs about the sacredness of the head and its role in defining aspects of personhood. In day-to-day practice, however, fashion dictates to a large extent the various styles and forms of headties that Yoruba women adopt.

### MEN'S TURBANS IN NORTHERN NIGERIA

In West Africa as early as the eleventh century, al Bakri noted that even in the nominally Muslim court of Ghana the king wore a tall hat decorated with gold that was wrapped in a turban of white cloth as part of his official prestige dress (Levtzion and Hopkins 1981:80). By the early nineteenth century, in northern Nigeria turbans and embroidered tailored robes (called *riga* in Hausa) were being worn regularly by an Islamic aristocracy which owed political allegiance to the powerful Sokoto Caliphate. Adopting Islamic dress was both a statement of religious piety and a prudent step in that it clearly identified the wearer with the interests of the new state (Fig. 6.2).

The Sokoto Caliphate was the dominant regional political authority in northern Nigeria throughout most of the nineteenth century. As a result of a *jihad,* an Islamic holy war, which began in 1804, the autonomous Hausa states — Nupe, Ilorin, Adamawa, and even parts of Bornu — were brought under the control of Sokoto and governed by the emissaries of Sheikh Usman dan Fodio. All the emirs, except one,

**Figure 6.1**, opposite. Woman on ferry to Goree Island, Senegal. Photograph by Eliot Elisofon, 1970. Neg. no. V-21, 32. Eliot Elisofon Photographic Archives. National Museum of African Art.

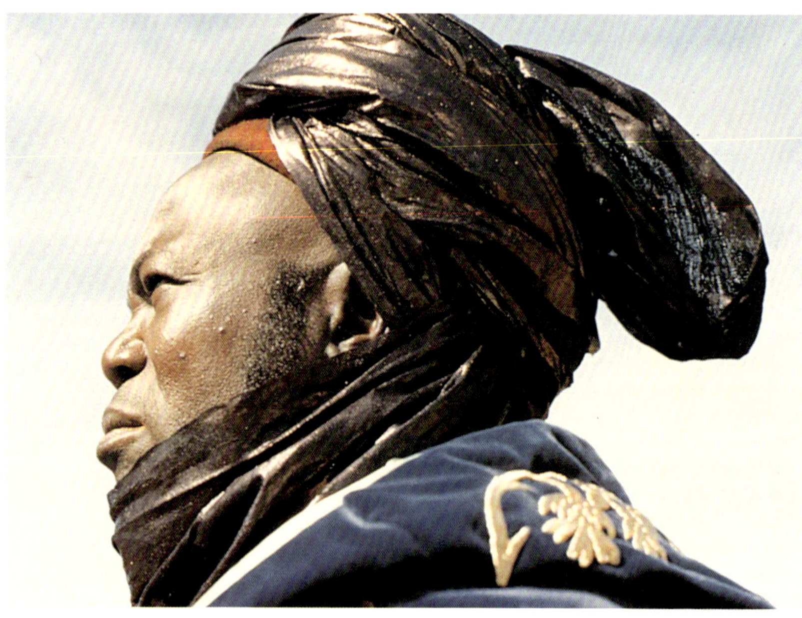

were from Sheikh Usman's own family or other important Fulani families (Hogben and Kirk-Greene 1966:381–383). By 1820, there were seven major emirates that comprised the Sokoto Caliphate with ten others in the process of formation (Last 1988:562). In the new Caliphate, the role of king was replaced by the emir. In some emirates, prior to the reform movement and the establishment of the Sokoto Caliphate, the person of the king was considered sacred and he personified the state. In the new Caliphate, the Sultan of Sokoto was given the title of Sarkin Musulmi, leader of all Muslims, and it was Allah who was the source of all state authority (Last 1988:563). The territory under the authority of Sokoto was extensive, and it was estimated that it took four months to journey from east to west and two months to journey from north to south. The emirates paid tribute to the Sokoto Caliphate, and it was Sokoto who sanctioned the appointment of emirs and resolved any disputes over succession (Last 1988:566–567).

**Figure 6.2**, above. Alhaji Bir Ahmadu Bello, the Sardauna of Sokoto, Premier of Northern Nigeria. Hausa peoples, Nigeria. Photograph by Eliot Elisofon, 1959. Slide No. C HSA 3.4 (1289). Eliot Elisofon Photographic Archives. National Museum of African Art.

There were two broad divisions within Sokoto society. The first was comprised of office-holders including titleholders, their kinsmen, scholars, clients, and their household slaves. The second consisted of those occupied with farming, trading, and craft occupations, and their slaves. Movement across these divisions was somewhat fluid, and scholars and slaves could be associated with either division (Last 1988:576).

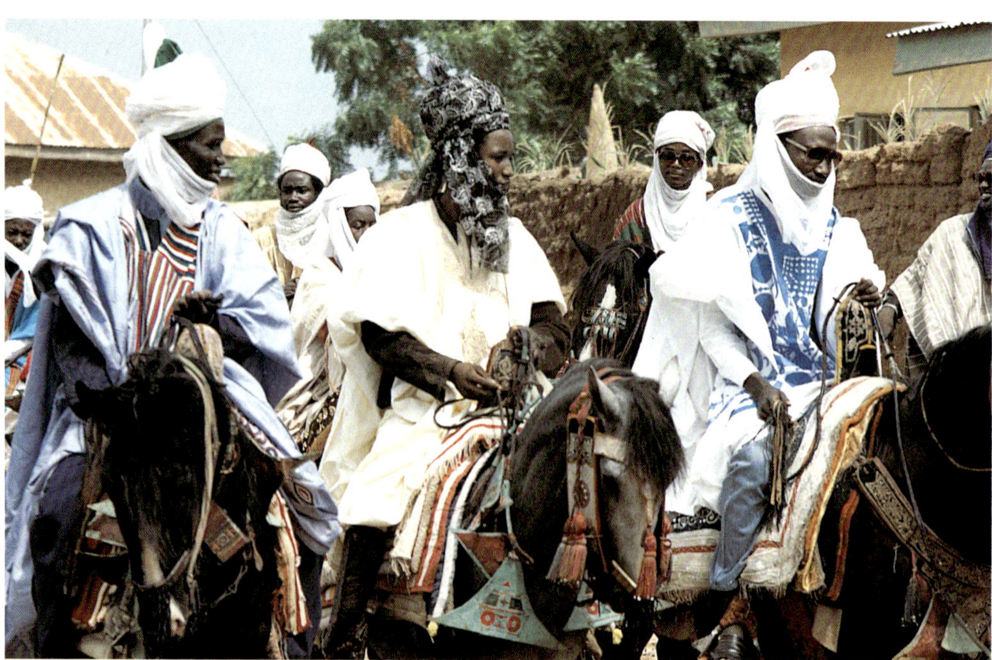

**Figure 6.3**, below. Nigerian nobles on horseback at Ramadan celebration. Gombe, Nigeria. Photograph by Herbert M. Cole, 1982.

Until the mid-twentieth century commoners normally did not wear hats and caps. The wearing of turbans among the aristocracy, court officials, and retainers associated a man with Islam and, when worn with the *riga giwa* (a Hausa term meaning "elephant robe" for the voluminous tailored robes worn by the aristocracy), marked him as a member of the administrative division of the Caliphate. Turbans and *riga giwa* were worn by the elite regardless of their ethnic affiliation, and they were indicators of high status and prestige (Kriger 1988:52). Photographs taken between 1908 and 1930 by Reverend Thomas Titcombe and Reverend Banfield in northern Nigeria document the widespread use of the turban and "robes of honor" in the Caliphate (Cannizzo 1989:57, 59; Kriger 1988:pls. 1, 2). Further afield, the turban and the northern Nigerian-style embroidered gowns were also adopted as prestige dress by other Islamic leaders including King Njoya of Fumbam, who was regularly shown wearing this ensemble in official portraits taken between 1908 and 1912. In various photographs, King Njoya is shown wearing either a white turban or a turban made from indigo cloth imported from the northern emirates and, in one photograph, a turban made with a combination of white and indigo cloth twisted together (Geary 1988:Figs. 1, 6, 10–12, 19–21, 23–26).

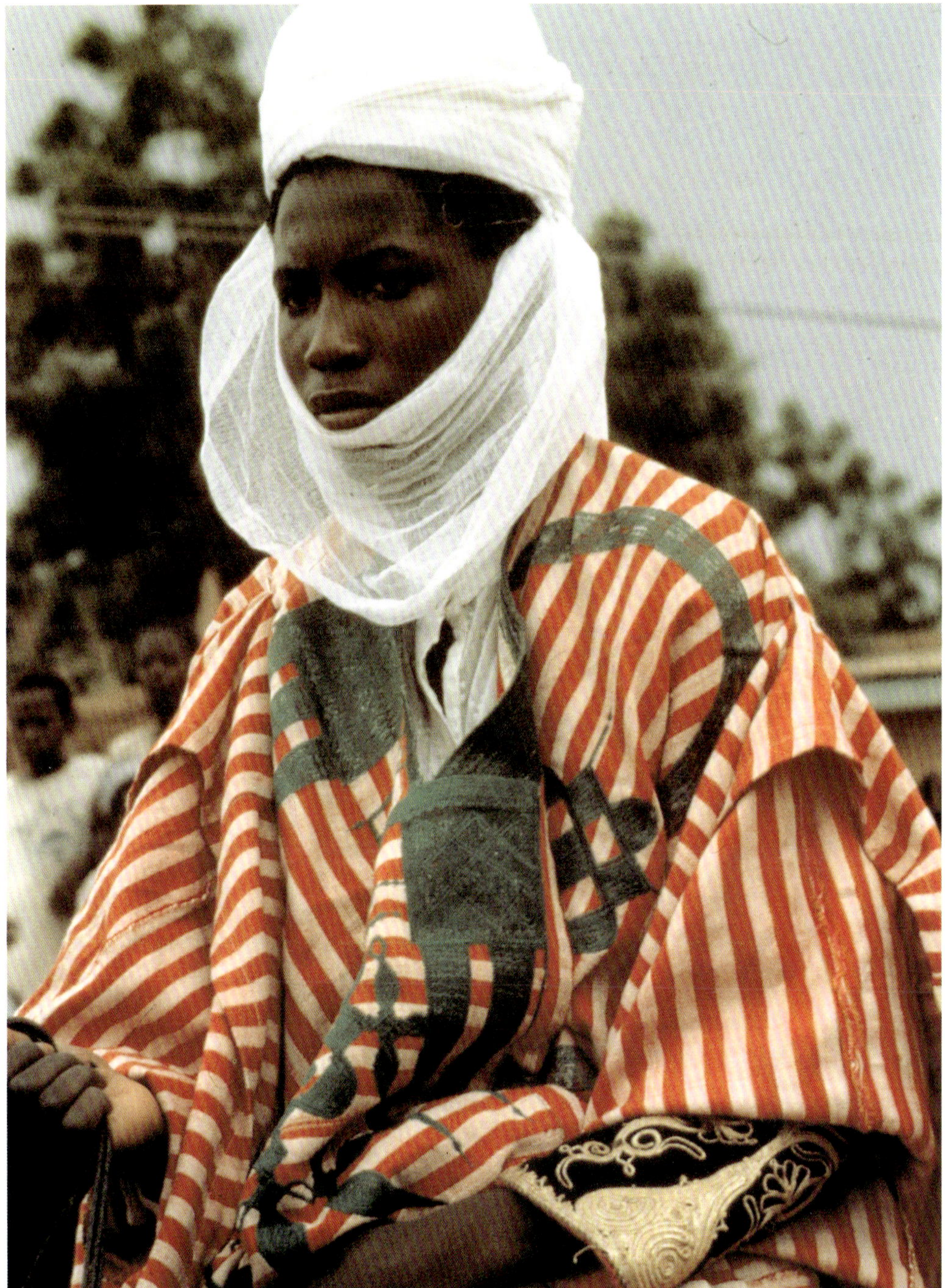

**Figure 6.4.** Hausa man in smock (riga) and turban. Northern Nigeria. Photograph by Herbert M. Cole, 1982.

Throughout the twentieth century and continuing into the present, this same turban and gown ensemble survives as the official dress for northern

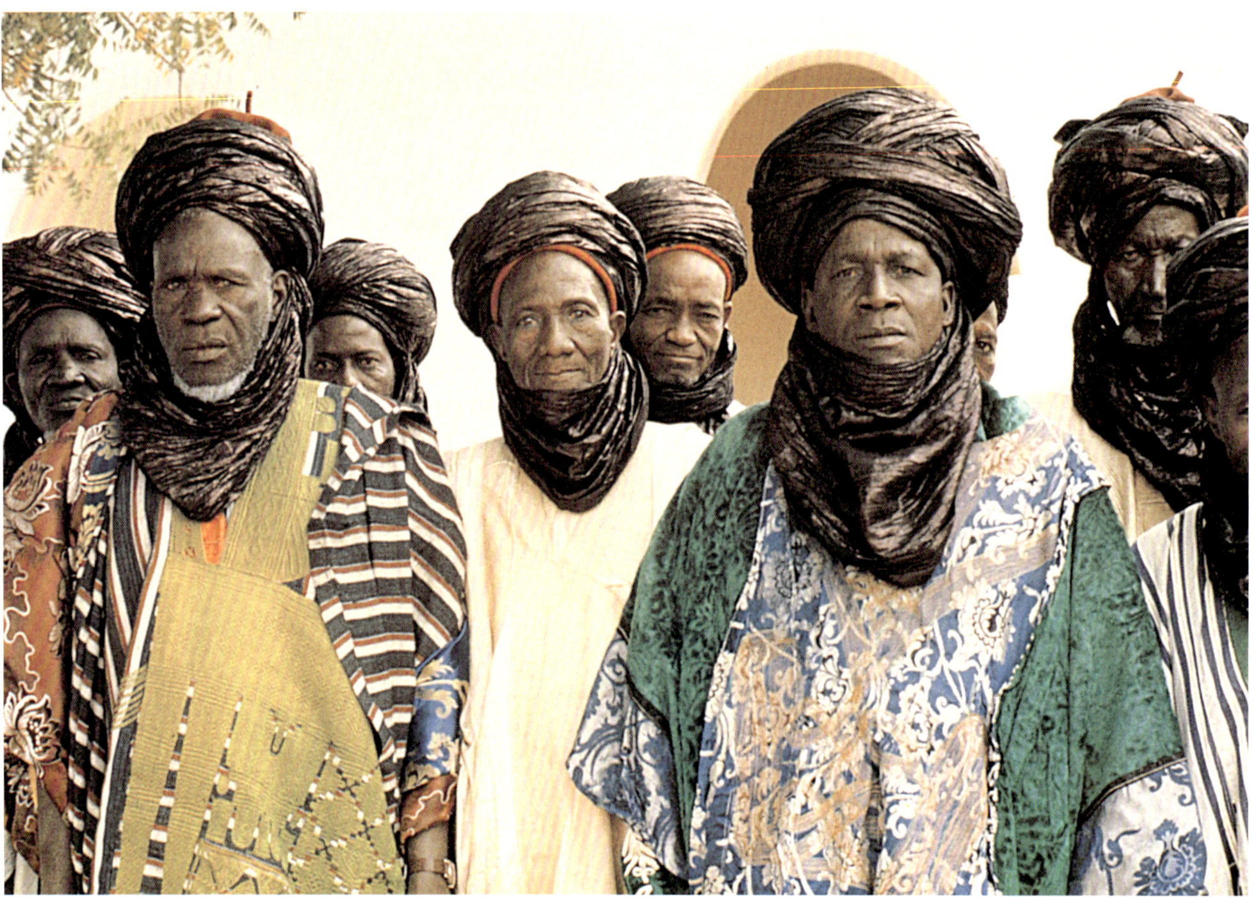

**Figure 6.5.** The Emir of Katsina's elite bodyguard at the morning greeting ceremony. Hausa peoples, Nigeria. Photograph by Eliot Elisofon, 1959. Slide No. C HSA 11.23 (1401). Eliot Elisofon Photographic Archives. National Museum of African Art.

Nigerian emirs and other elites (Hogben and Kirk-Greene 1966:frontispiece; Perani and Wolff 1992:pls.1, 2, 8, 13, 20). When an emir or other nobleman, wearing his voluminous turban and richly embroidered gown, moves through the crowd mounted on his horse with its heavily decorated saddle and trappings and surrounded by his retainers, he communicates to all his wealth, noble status, religious piety, and political authority (Fig. 6.4).

The most common turban style worn by the northern Nigerian nobility, religious leaders, messengers, and royal bodyguards consists of a strip of cloth several meters in length wrapped several times around the head over a cap, increasing its volume; it is generally positioned under the chin leaving the wearer's face fully exposed. In photographs taken in Nupe by Reverend Banfield, a Nupe *malam* (a religious official) has his lower face partially veiled, while in another photograph of the chief of Pategi and his retinue, none of the men have veiled faces (Kriger 1988:pls. 1, 2). In contemporary photographs of the Sultan of Sokoto and of the Emir of Kano, both men wear a separate face veil of semitransparent imported lacelike material when leading processions during major religious festivals (Perani and Wolff 1992:pl. 20). Face veiling does not seem to be essential when these leaders attend secular events.

Particular styles of turbans or particular textiles or colors may be reserved for specific occasions or for different segments of the aristocracy or their retainers. For example, in Kano and elsewhere many nobles wear white turbans when attending religious events. White is associated with piety throughout the Islamic world, and emirs generally wear white turbans and white gowns throughout northern Nigeria on religious occasions. The Emir of Kano and the members of his family wear a distinctive style of turban called the *harsa*. The *harsa* turban is worn when the Emir or a member of the royal family leads Friday prayers at a mosque or when they officiate at religious festivals. This turban style is peculiar to the Kano emirate and the royal family; it was first worn by Emir Ibrahim Babo (1814–1816). The *harsa* is fashioned from a white cloth several meters in length and is wound around the head and tied with two loops that project upwards from the back and top of the head. The cloth ends are then allowed to flow down the back. The two upward projections and the flowing ends are said to replicate the Arabic script for "Allah." Formerly, the *harsa* turban was constructed from multiple strips of undyed *turkudi,* which is a locally woven cotton cloth. Today, finely woven imported gauzy cotton cloths from Cairo, the Middle East, and elsewhere are often used for the turban (Perani and Wolff 1992:76).

In the northern emirates, the turban is a central symbol of political authority. In Kano, the installation of an emir is called "turbanning" (Perani and Wolff 1992:76). For secular political events, emirs and other elites prefer dark indigo-blue turbans; for example, when receiving official visitors, attending installation ceremonies and for *durbars* (equestrian displays).

In Kano this indigo turban is called *dan kura* after Kura, the village near Kano that produces this distinctive cloth.[1] In Kura undyed *turkudi* cloth is immersed several times in an indigo bath until it is a deep, almost black, color (Fig. 6.5). The dyers then beat indigo powder into the cloth giving it its characteristic lustrous glaze. These indigo-dyed cloths are expensive and are a favorite of the Nupe people to the south and highly prized by the Tuareg to the north, who regularly use the cloth for men's turbans and face veils and for women's headscarves. Today, besides indigo cloth, elites throughout northern Nigeria also buy expensive imported luxury cloths including brightly colored laces and brocades to fashion turbans.

**Figure 6.6.** Tuareg man and his wife at the *cure salee* celebration in Ingall, Niger. The man wears a turban and face veil and his wife wears an elaborate folded headscarf. This annual gathering of all nomadic peoples includes Tuareg, Bororo Fulani and others from Algeria, Niger, and Mali. During this period, baptisms and weddings are also celebrated. Photograph by Kristyne Loughran Bini, 1990.

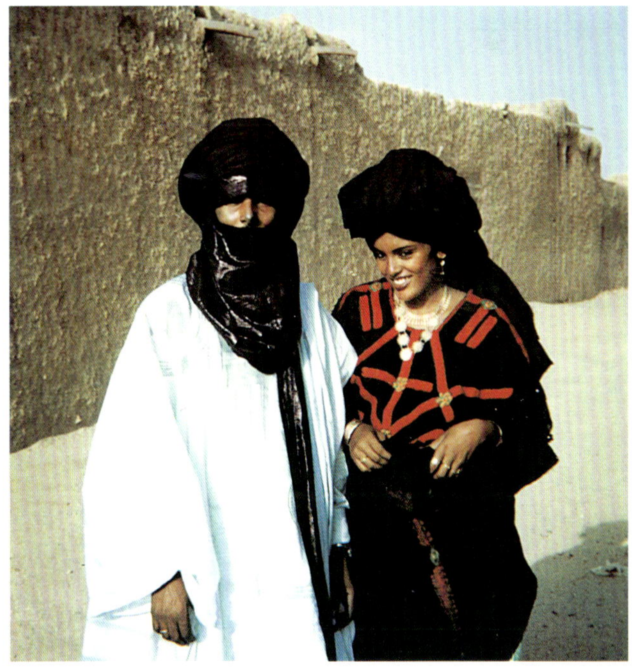

## PEOPLE OF THE VEIL—TUAREG MEN'S TURBANS AND FACE VEILS AND WOMEN'S HEADSCARVES

Tuareg men's turbans and face veils *(tagelmust)* have always held a particular fascination for outsiders. This headwear is referred to by writers, like al Bakri in the eleventh century, up to the present. Women's headscarves *(afar)*, which are less visually distinct, have by contrast gone relatively

**Figure 6.7.** Man and riding camel. Tenth anniversary of independence celebration. Tuareg peoples, Niamey, Niger. Photograph by Eliot Elisofon, 1970. Neg. no VII-7, 35. Eliot Elisofon Photographic Archives. National Museum of African Art.

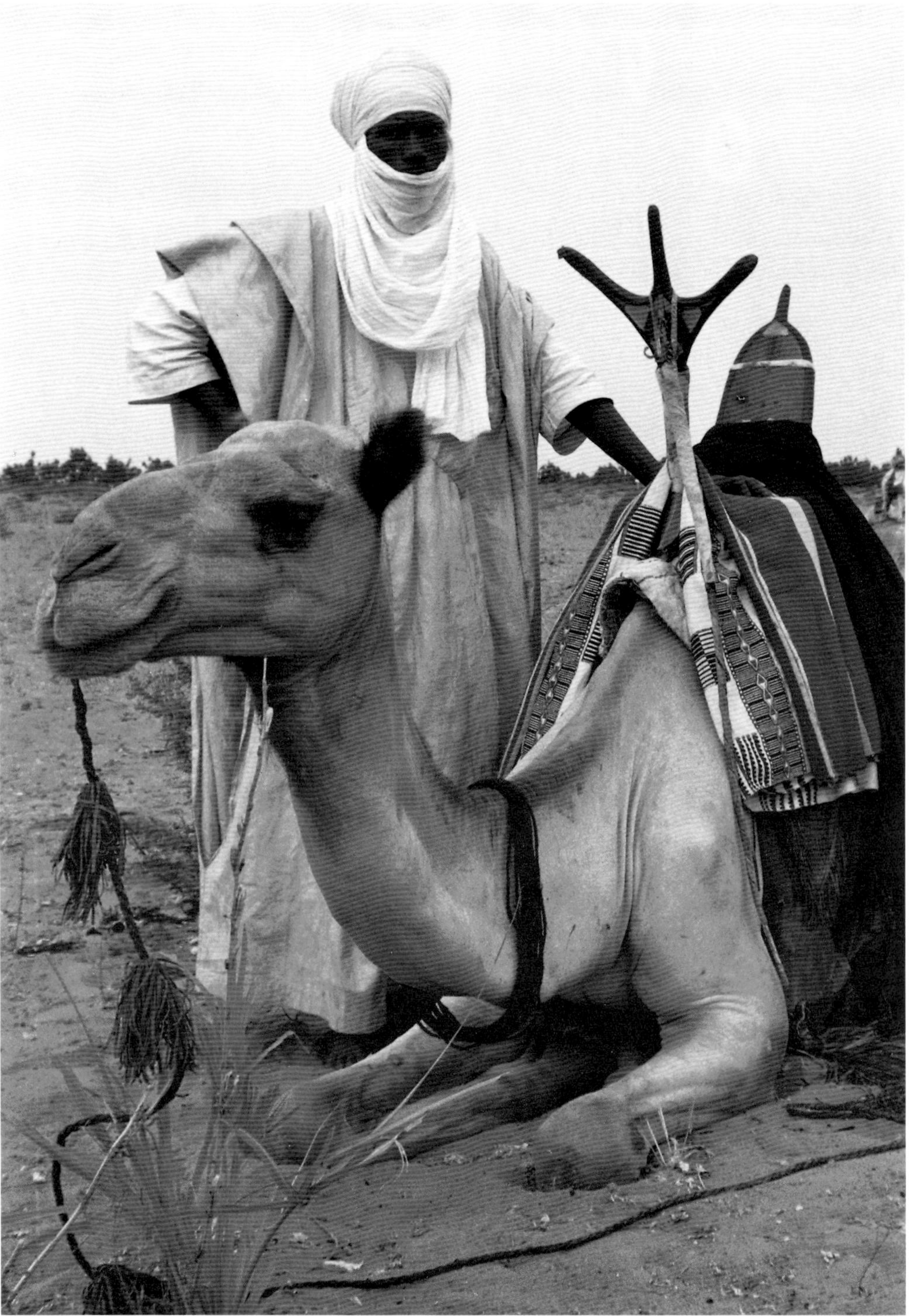

unnoticed in the literature. Yet, as Rasmussen (1991a) has recently argued, a Tuareg man's turban and face veil and a woman's headscarf are both symbolic extensions of the head and hair that express, although differently, shifting gender roles, sexuality, ageing, and transition.

While men's face veiling and women's headscarves fulfill Islamic requirements of modesty, they are also symbols of the Tuareg cultural value of reserve. These headdresses are directly linked to concepts of the person and to changes in an individual's status throughout his or her life (Rasmussen 1992:101). Among the Tuareg, the headdress is a potent symbol of adult responsibilities, accountability for actions, vulnerabilities, and self-worth. The wearing of headdresses is an important social practice in the noble class's observation of shame *(tekeraki)* and respect *(isimrarak*; Murphy 1964:1267; Fig. 6.6).

The Tuareg are nomadic and seminomadic peoples, who currently live in southern Algeria and southern Libya and in the northern regions of Niger and Mali. They practice pastoralism, sedentary gardening, and caravaning. Historically, the Tuareg were divided into several political confederations that functioned primarily in time of war. Each confederation consisted of several tribes that were territory-holding units under the authority of a chief. These tribes were further divided into clans. Tribes and clans are conceived of as descent groups whose members acknowledge a common ancestry. The fundamental unit of Tuareg society, however, is the *iriwan,* or house, which consists of from fifty to several hundred people who reside around a well and hold rights to the well and to the adjacent pasture land (Murphy 1964:1261). While there is no single unified Tuareg entity, they all speak dialects of Tamacheq, they are Muslims, and they share certain social and cultural institutions, beliefs, and practices. Tuareg society is highly stratified and includes several classes: the noble clans, vassal clans, blacksmiths, and former slaves. The term Tuareg is rarely used internally by the people themselves; it is an Arab appellation for their group. Rather, group identification finds expression in federation or clan identities such as Kel Ewey, "People of the Ewey," or in such terms as "People of Tamacheq," a reference to their language, "People of the Tent Posts," a reference to their traditional pastoral nomadism, or "People of the Veil," a reference to the distinctive turban and face veil worn by adult men in Tuareg society (Decalo 1979:227–228; Rasmussen 1992:352).

The head *(eghef)* is the seat of intelligence. Orifices are considered zones of pollution and it is therefore disrespectful to expose them before others. The mouth *(imi)*, which also means door, is a major point of vulnerability. Antisocial sentiments such as gossip and jealousy affect the victim by means of the mouth. The eye *(shet)* is also associated with misfortune and sorcery. Victims of gossip or evil mouth and evil eye often display head maladies (Rasmussen 1991a:106). *Goumaten,* spirits, also enter the body through the head, and spirit possession often begins with a headache

(Rasmussen 1994:86). Children, because they have no social status, are often described as having no head (Rasmussen 1991b:760), as are the very elderly, the insane, smiths, and ex-slaves, who neglect or drop the face veil and headscarf altogether (Rasmussen 1991a:106).

## MEN'S TURBANS AND FACE VEILS

Men's turbans and face veils are a dominant symbol of Tuareg male identity. The Tamacheq verb, *anagad,* to wrap the veil, is also the word for male honor (Claudot-Hawad 1993:34). In wrapping the head, a man winds several meters of cloth around his head to form a low turban so that the top of the veil usually rests on the bridge of the nose, and the bottom falls across the face to the upper part of the chest. The turban sits low on the head and completely covers the forehead, so that when the face veil is pulled high and tight over the nose there is only a narrow slit revealing the eyes. When the face veil is lowered and loosened it may fall just above the mouth, or at its lowest level may expose the entire face (Fig. 6.7).

The most expensive and aesthetically preferred turban cloth is *shegga,* an indigo-dyed cotton cloth made in the northern emirates of Nigeria. Kura, a village near Kano, is often associated with the production of this cloth. The length of the head cloth can be anywhere between two and one half meters to fifteen meters and made be made of seventeen or more narrow bands. In the 1950s, turbans were fashioned from twenty or thirty narrow bands (Nicolas 1950). In 1991 in Niger, Kristyne Loughran Bini observed that the most elegant and expensive turbans were made from nearly 100 narrow bands (personal communication 1994).

A young man begins wearing the turban and veil in his late teens and continues to wear this headdress throughout his active adult life with various degrees of covering and minor stylistic adjustments according to his social stratum, situation, and age. The young man's first wearing of the veil is a family ritual and marks his initiation from adolescent to adult status. This first veiling is followed by a week of seclusion similar to the seclusion of a married couple. The newly veiled man is transformed and is called *amawad.* His new social status grants him the right to court a woman, to carry a sword, to go to war, and to attend political meetings (Rasmussen 1991a:106). An adult man wears the turban and veil when at home or traveling, during the day and night, and when eating, smoking and even sleeping.

Adult men from noble clans follow the most strict protocols and their rigorous adherence to this practice signals their class identity and their rank within their clan. Nobles are also the class that is most heavily invested in maintaining reserve and respect in social relationships. Men from lesser clans and blacksmiths and former slaves are generally more lax with their veils, unless they are attempting to improve their social status.

The face veil introduces a form of social distancing between self and others, and this distancing involves an internal and external dialogue. It effectively hides the wearer's emotions and sentiments from others, while simultaneously maintaining and projecting his self-image as an honorable and respectful man (Murphy 1964:1268). The face veil underlines noble men's need to observe reserve and to protect themselves from its absence, which is called *awal,* gossip or literally evil mouth, the source of misfortune (Casajus 1987:317, Rasmussen 1991b:756). While the turban and face veil are associated with power, vulnerability, and danger, they are not always treated with reverence and in certain social situations there are aesthetic and playful aspects associated with veiling.

Throughout the day a man continually adjusts his veil pulling it higher and tighter, relaxing and lowering it in response to the mood and intentions of shifting social situations. A man is scrupulous in maintaining full veiling when he is in the presence of a chief, of older men, when engaged in formal courting or after his marriage, and when he is in the presence of his affines, especially his father- and mother-in-law. This full veiling demonstrates his respect for those others in social interactions. He may, however, assume a more relaxed veiling when he is in the company of his peers and trusted friends, or when flirting with women during social gatherings or festivals. During weddings there is a game called *ekesen taqubut* when any unmarried woman may try to snatch off any married man's face veil when he is inside her tent. If she is successful the man must offer her a small prize such as perfume (Rasmussen 1991a:108).

**Figure 6.8.** Tuareg women singing in their encampment outside Timbucktu, Mali. Photograph by Eliot Elisofon, 1959. Slide No. F TRG 4 (4601). Eliot Elisofon Photographic Archives. National Museum of African Art. The women are wearing the typical headscarf *(afar),* a simple veil placed over the head, wrapped at the neck and thrown over the shoulder.

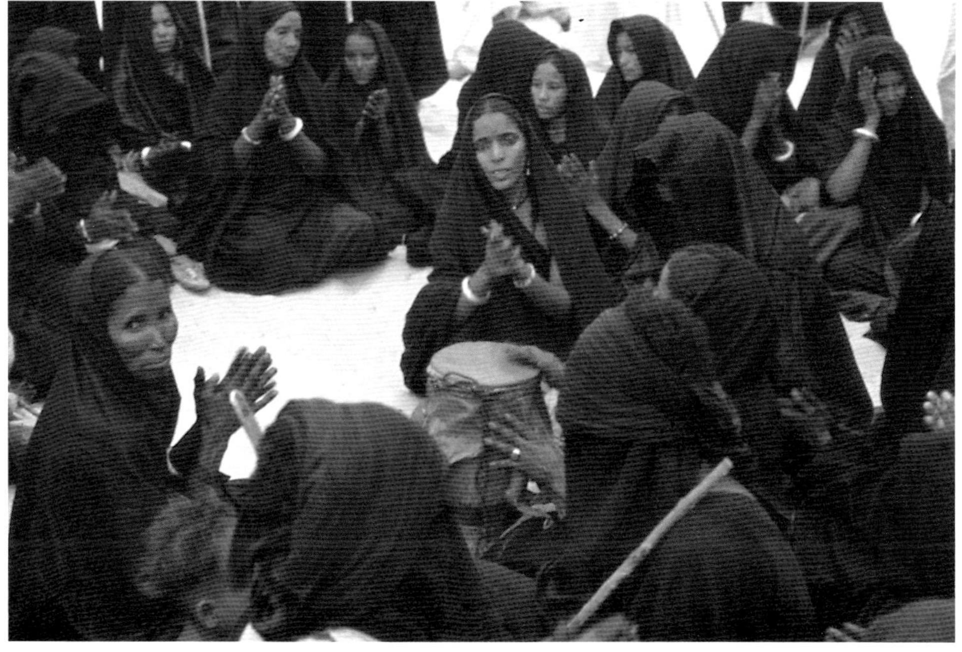

An older man may lower his veil slightly when in the presence of junior men, who owe him respect. Murphy notes that an older man who has made the pilgrimage to Mecca may choose to abandon the face veil altogether, for it is believed that he embodies sacredness in his very person and no longer needs to show shame or respect since his very status is adequate to guarantee the necessary social distance (1964:1268).

## WOMEN'S HEADSCARVES

The few references to women's headscarves treat them as casual and mechanical headdresses and assume that they differ entirely from the men's practice of face veiling. Rasmussen (1991a) persuasively argues that

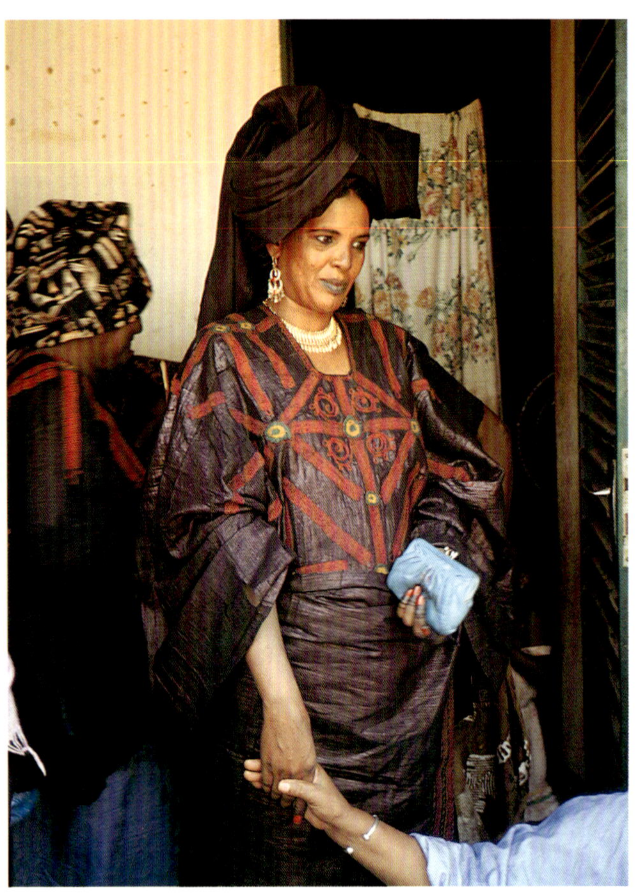

**Figure 6.9.** Tuareg woman at a baptism celebration. On this occasion she wears an elaborate folded headscarf of indigo-dyed cloth. Ingall, Niger. Photograph by Kristyne Loughran Bini, 1990.

although the two forms of headdress differ, they relate to each other in essential ways.

Women take up headscarves when they begin to be available to suitors because they regard them as elegant attire. Unlike with men, there is no formal ritual associated with taking up this practice. While the link between women's headscarves and marriage is less explicit, a woman does receive headcloths from her husband upon marriage, which suggests that a married women should cover her head. A married woman also owns her own tent and property including previously inherited herds of animals. By wearing headscarves, married women acknowledge their jural and property rights as owners of tents. While there is no female equivalent to the verb *anagad,* to wrap the veil as it refers to the male practice of face-veiling, Rasmussen suggests that the phrase *tamtot n ammas* (woman inside the tent) is also a potent image of a married woman inside the headscarf and alludes to her rights and status in marriage (1991a:114).

A married women is expected to partially cover her hair in public to fulfill the requirements of modesty, but she does not generally need to veil her face. In the course of everyday activities, a woman wears a simple headscarf that is wrapped at the neck and thrown over the shoulder (Fig. 6.8). Decorative silver weights, whose origins were keys for locks on leather bags, are often tied to the corner of the scarf that is thrown over the shoulder and their weight holds the scarf in place on the head.

On more ceremonial occasions and at festivals women wear an elaborate headscarf (Fig. 6.9). A large rectangular cloth is centered on the head and the two ends are brought across each other at the nape of the neck. The ends are then pulled forward crossing each other at front of the head and then the ends are folded and rolled into an elaborate configuration with the ends hanging down over the shoulders in back.

While women's faces are not regularly veiled there are occasions when reserve, shame, and respect require that the lower portion of the face, especially the mouth, be covered. Married women observe the same degree of respect and reserve as do men in interactions with their senior affines. When a woman finds herself in such a social situation, she will pull her headscarf over her mouth. If a woman partially covers her face with her headscarf when entering a tent, it is not because she is a woman or because she is timid, but because some of the men present might be her affines (Rasmussen 1991a:109). During certain ceremonies and rituals, key women participants veil their faces. For example, in conducting marriages, the mothers of the bride and groom keep their mouths covered by their headscarves, "like men who wear the veil" (Rasmussen 1991a:114). When women undergo the ritual cure for spirit possession they don men's turbans and full face veils. However, at other public events, a young women's adjusting and reworking of her headscarf is interpreted as a coquettish gesture, and at music festivals and other mixed-sex gatherings, a woman's headscarf may be the focal point of a game. At these events a suitor may race his camel by a woman and snatch off her headscarf. A scramble then ensues among the young men, and one of them retrieves the headscarf and returns it to the young woman (Rasmussen 1991a:108).

Many interpretations have been put forth for the Tuareg practice of headcovering and face veiling. Its purposes have been described in hygienic, magical, religious, and social terms. In any particular context one or more of these interpretations may indeed be valid. Head and head imagery is central in Tuareg beliefs about character and different states of being. Men's and women's headdresses lend a fluidity to social life because their use in particular social situations both marks and blurs behaviors and social boundaries. Decorating the head among Tuareg men and women is not a static practice, but changes over an individual's lifetime as a Tuareg man or woman ages and takes up new social positions. For both men and women the intended effect of covering the head is to hide personal sentiments and to remind the wearer of the need for caution and self-control in social relationships with others.

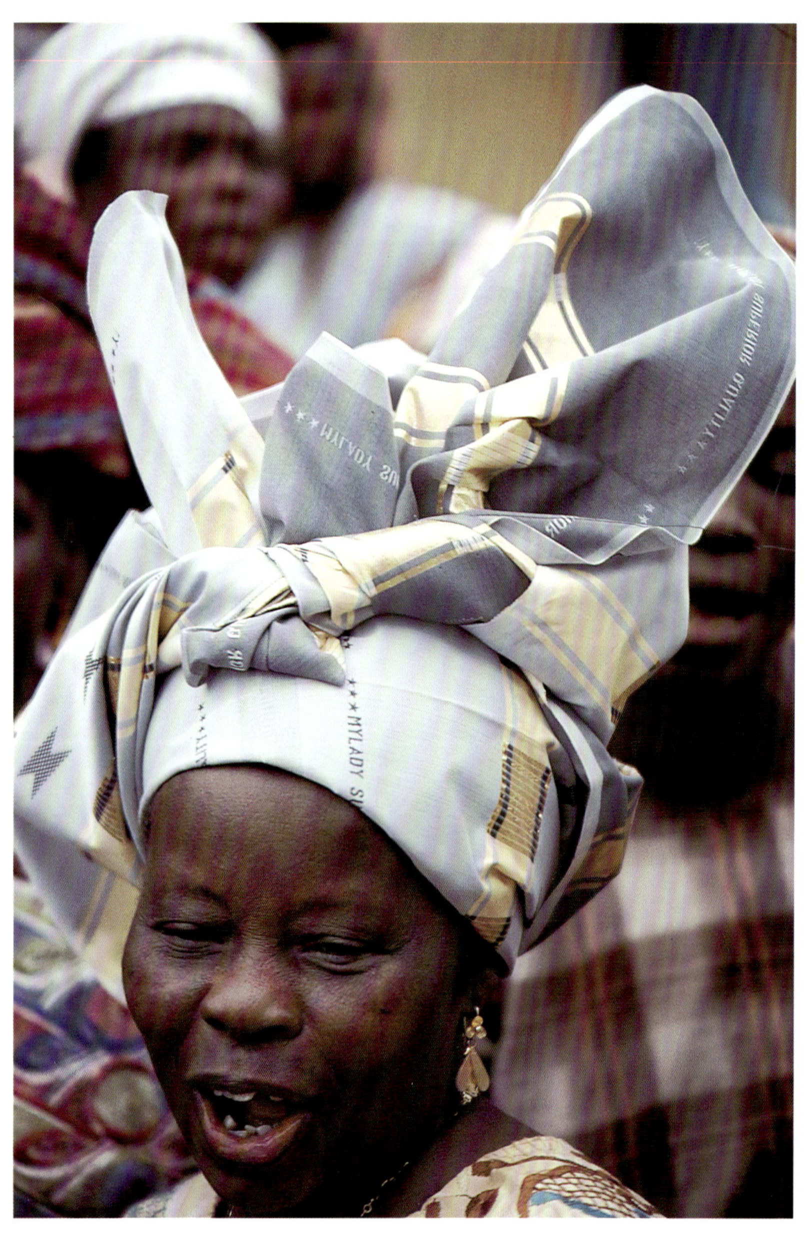

# 7 YORUBA HEADTIES

## MICHAEL OLÁDÈJO AFOLÁYAN AND BETTY WASS

The Yoruba are recognized throughout West Africa and the Yoruba diaspora for their sartorial splendor which is especially evident in the elegant headties *(gèlè)* worn by women. The creativity and skill in executing the tying of the Yoruba headtie is admired with awe. Beginning with a flat piece of fabric 1 1/2 to 2 1/2 meters long, a woman deftly wraps, tucks, pinches, folds, pleats, or spreads the material into an original creation that is called the *gèlè*. Combined with other appropriate items of Yoruba dress, the headtie is the crowning element that is essential to the outfit known as "Yoruba complete" (Figs. 7.1, 7.2). The headtie, more than any other item in the Yoruba ensemble, shows artistry and individuality. Yoruba women will identify and praise certain of their peers who excel in aesthetic sensitivity and who have the skill required to create a headdress with sculptural qualities. "*Ó lọ́wọ́ọ gèlè*" is often said meaning, "She has mastery of headdress styling." A woman may spend as much as an hour arranging her *gèlè* for a special occasion.

Almost any type of fabric may be fashioned into a headtie. Fabrics that are stiff but lightweight, such as damask, can be manipulated into luxurious poufs, while narrow strips of handwoven cotton can be sewn together to produce a fabric that has firmness and body contributing to a dramatic soaring effect. Velvet, lace, brocade, or machine-woven cotton are other popular fabrics for headties. A woman may choose to stuff the interior of the headtie with crinkled paper or she may add a wig as a base with her own hair to achieve the volume that is characteristic of these Yoruba creations. At the turn of this century, the Yoruba historian Samuel Johnson stated that

> female headgear consists of a band, of about 6 to 10 inches wide and 5 feet long (more or less). This is wound twice round the head and tucked on one side. It may be of plain cloth or costly, as she can afford. Well-to-do ladies use velvet cloths (1921:112).

At that time, Johnson described a wide variety of styles available in men's dress, but only a small range of items for women. No doubt the types of fabrics available increased along with stylistic options for women during the twentieth century. Different fabrics could be manipulated in headdresses to produce different effects, which, by the 1940s, Yoruba women were demonstrating as fully as they do today.

Although the *gèlè* worn with an upper body covering *(bùbá)* and one or two

**Opposite.** Yoruba woman wearing headtie of her own creation. Photograph by Herbert M. Cole, 1982.

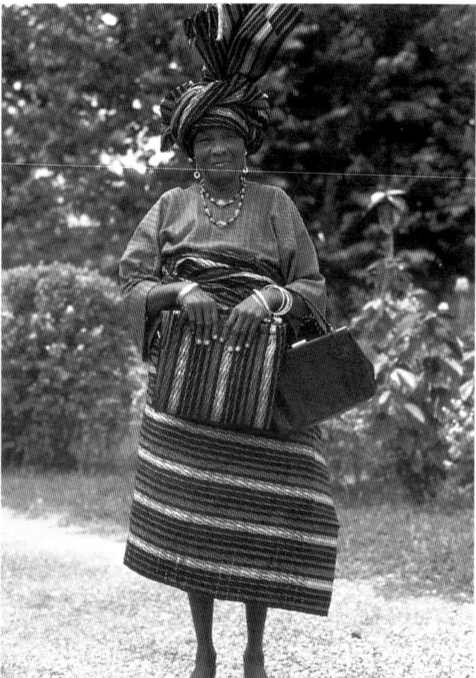

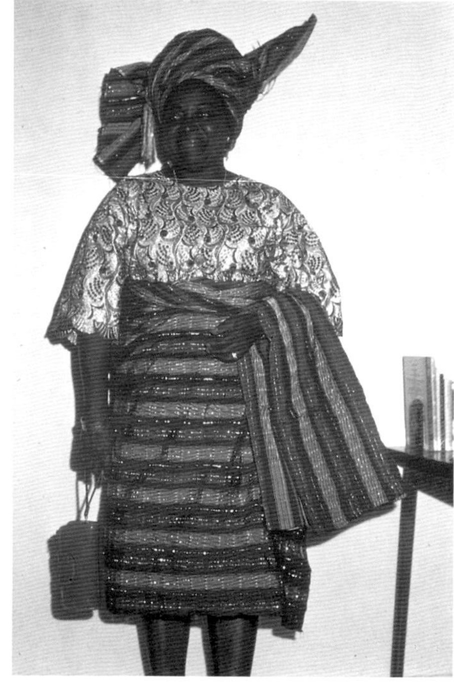

**Figures 7.1** right, **7.2** far right. Ensembles known as Yoruba "complete," with headties, wrappers, and stoles made of handwoven fabric. The fabric, mainly cotton, is woven in strips about four inches wide. Sewn together, the result is a material with firmness and volume that lends itself to stately arrangements such as those shown in the headties. Float yarns that appear on the surface of the fabric are characteristic of Yoruba handweaving.

wrappers *(iró)* are recognized consistently as traditional dress, they are readily subject to fashion change. As an example, the basic form of the *bùbá* and *iró* remain the same, but the shape of the neckline changes from time to time. The preferred width and length for the sleeves changes periodically, and at times it has been fashionable to enhance the *bùbá* with lace, ruching, or embroidery. The wrappers may maintain lengths comparable to skirts being worn in the western world. When skirts in Europe and America were worn short during the 1960s, the wrapper was simply folded to make it shorter. The most frequent fashion variation over time has probably occurred in fabrics. In a twelve-month period in 1949, anthropologist Justine Cordwell observed three major fashion changes in imported cloths in general, three changes in *bùbá* cloth patterns, and one major change in the fabrics used for headties (1952:276). She remarked that "Costume selection and composition affords the personal and immediate means of aesthetic expression to the average Yoruba individual" (1952:265).

Such creative satisfaction is exemplified in the manipulation of the *gèlè*. The headtie is rearranged each time it is worn (Figs. 7.3–7.6). While the arranging is known as "tying," it is not actually tied, but is shaped and tucked into the desired result. Women who were asked why they did not tie the *gèlè* into one permanent shape responded that they enjoyed making the variations. Rearranging the headtie for each wearing allows a woman to demonstrate her personal skill, it allows her to keep up with fashion as popular arrangements in headties change frequently, and it allows her to arrange her attire appropriately for different occasions (Fig. 7.7). The

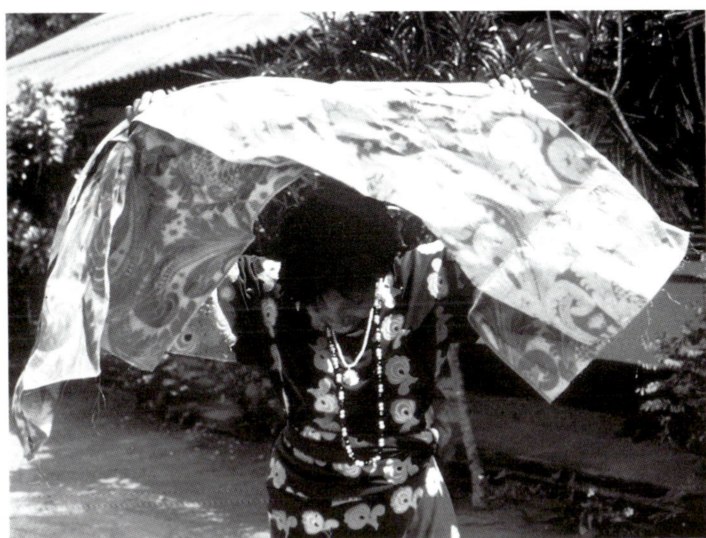

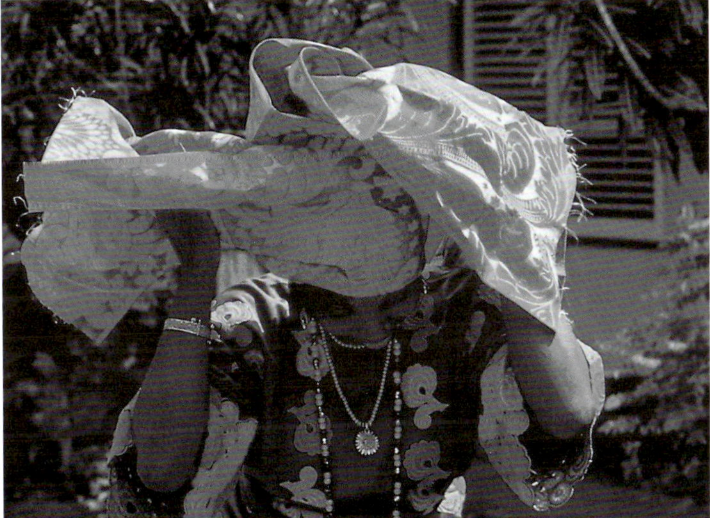

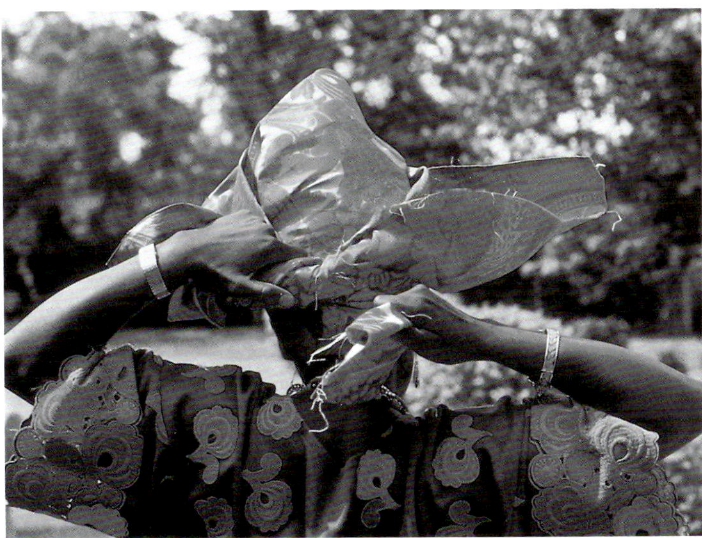

**Figures 7.3 – 7.6.** Steps in arranging one style of Yoruba headtie.

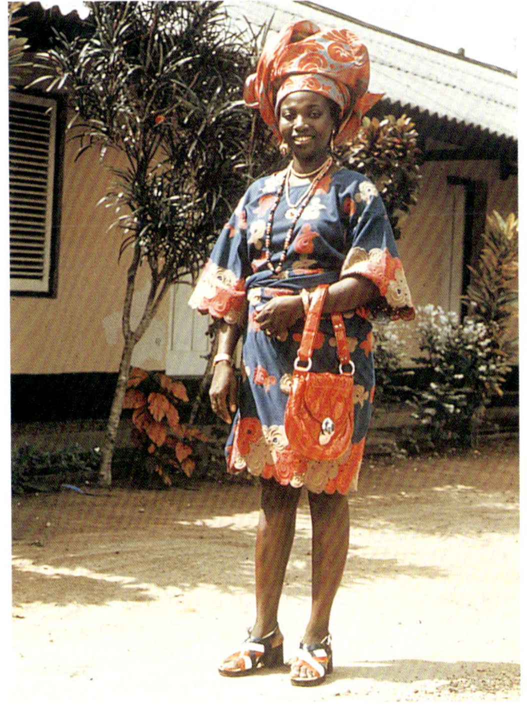

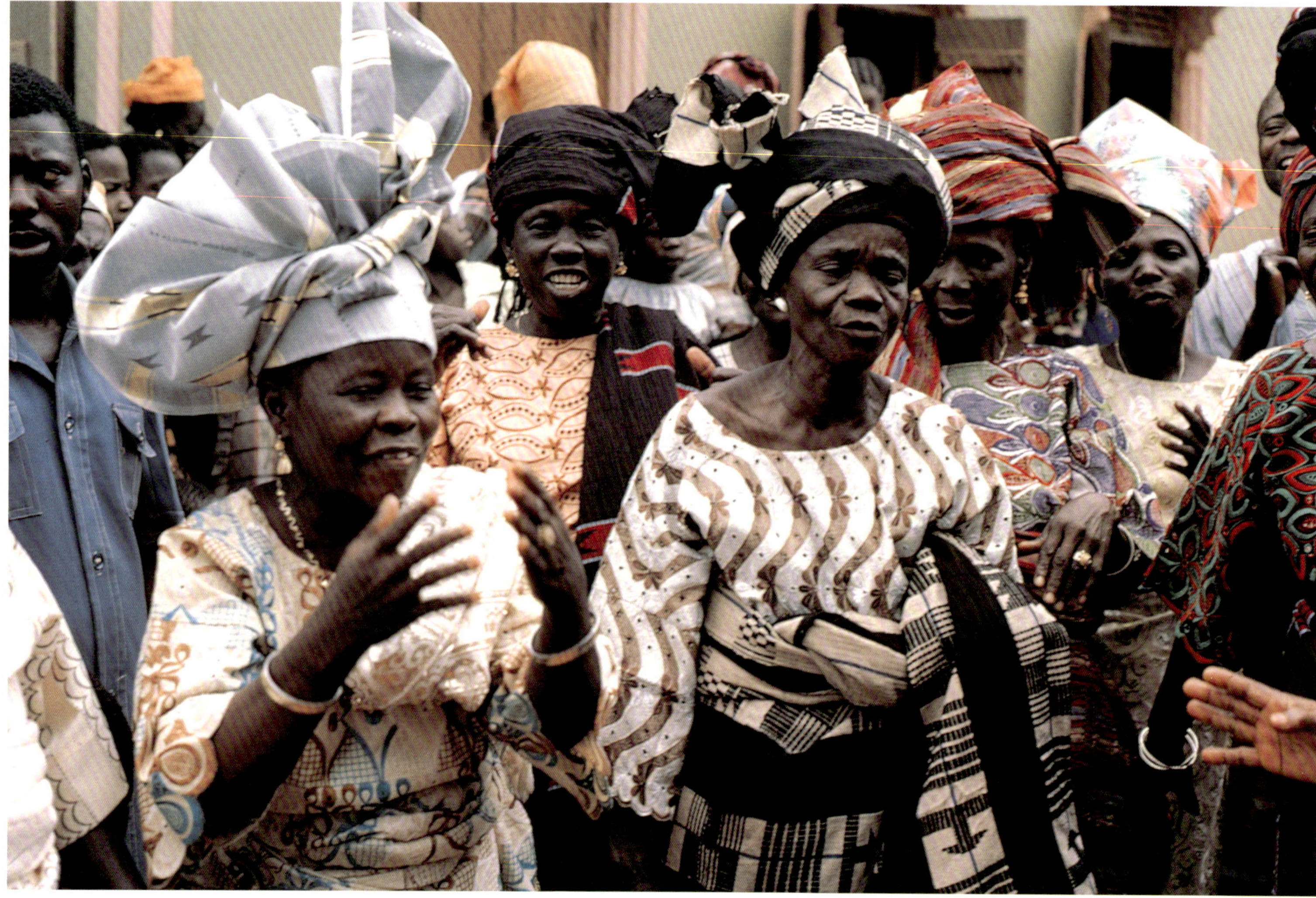

**Figure. 7.7**. Women wearing headties. Yoruba, Nigeria. Photograph by Henry John and Margaret Thompson Drewel, 1982. Slide no. YRB (A1992-028-05319). Eliot Elisofon Photographic Archives. National Museum of African Art.

headtie is worn in a more elaborate arrangement for a party than one would usually wear to church.

The source of fashion change can occasionally be identified. A prominent woman, such as the wife of a political leader, may arrange the *gèlè* cloth into a form that is admired and emulated to the extent that the shape will be named after her. Demonstrations of how to tie the latest fashion in headties have been featured on Nigerian television.

The patience and creativity illustrated by the process of arranging the headtie are further displayed in women's hair styles and in hats worn by men. Traditional women's hair styles are arranged by wrapping tiny strands of hair with shiny black thread or by meticulously braiding multiple sections in patterns known in the United States as "corn-rowing." Men's heads are often adorned with hats elaborately embroidered in colorful geometric patterns or in gold metallic threads.

To better understand the importance of headdressing in Yoruba culture, it is pertinent to consider philosophical principles underlying the place of the head in the Yoruba world view. In straightforward semantics, "head" is translated as *orí* in Yoruba. In other functional usages *orí* is, on the one hand, a spatial point of reference, and on the other, a spiritual concept. For example, a sentence like "Put it on the table" will be translated to the Yoruba language as "Put it on the head of the table."

In the Yoruba belief system, *orí* is the spiritual counterpart of the individual. It is believed to be the principle of predestination. In all essential ways, it is the spiritual representation of the physical head. Thus, the head that we see is a physical and symbolic manifestation of one we cannot see. It may be convenient to describe the physical (anatomical) head as an anthropomorphic symbol of the spiritual head. Yoruba believe that the visible head is transient, human, secular, imperfect, and limited. The one we cannot see is sacrosanct, eternal, spiritual, sacred, infallible, and immaculate. It is the symbol of fate, destiny, inspiration, aspiration, and the totality of life. It is believed that the malevolent spirits, who are thousands in number,[1] are always in constant war against humans, and only *orí* can subjugate the spirits' rebellion and counter their efforts, especially at the individual level. Thus, *ori,* the head, is a very important aspect of the belief system, often connected to Yoruba philosophical and cultural symbols.

In a recent work, Abiodun (1994) discusses *orí* in relation to *àse*, another concept in Yoruba philosophy. In the Yoruba world view, *àse*, like the Greek *logos*, is the principle of utterance and the power of irrevocability. Abiodun argues that the efficacy of *àse* depends largely on the will of one's *orí*. *Orí* is thus central to human existence and operations. In this context, it is understandable that the Yoruba seldom negotiate the price they pay in the beautification of their hair. A logical question must be added to Abiodun's observation, however. Given the cost of hair styling, the rigor of the process, and the aesthetic quality that it bestows on the individual, why then is it that the final product, the well-groomed, well-braided hair is often completely covered with the *gèlè,* the female headdress, or *filà*, the male headdress? We hypothesize that hair styling and hair grooming are beyond the realm of the aesthetic.

The concept of *orí* analyzed in the context of Yoruba rhetoric and indigenous verbal arts lends additional enlightenment to the subject of headdressing. *Ifá*, the oracular divinity which represents the principles of wisdom and philosophy provides an array of poetry celebrating the spiritual and secular significance of the head. In the works of scholars like William Bascom, E. M. Lijadu, and especially Wande Abimbola, the sacred poetry of *Ifá* has been used to explain the origin of the importance of the head among the Yoruba.

In *Ifá* poetry, as in folk beliefs, *orí* is said to be present during the creation of each individual and alone knows the future of each person. When the individual

A

*Orí mi yé, jà, jà fún mi*
*Édá mi yé o, jà, jà fún mi*
*Torì pé orí agbe a jà fún agbe*
*Orí Àlùkò a jà fún un*
*Elédàa mi o máse gbàgbé mi yé O*
*Ò bá mà jà o!*

*My head please fight for me*
*My creator/creature, please fight for me*
*Because it is the head of the Blue Touraco that fights for the Blue Touraco*[2]
*It is the head of aluko that fights for the bird Aluko*
*My creator, please do not forget me,*
*Please, do fight for me!*

B

*Ewúre ilé yìí, mo n relé oko*
*Àgùntàn ilé yìí, mo n relé oko.*
*Bée ní komodé ilé yìí sìn mí,*
*Bi wón bá sìn mí títí, won ó padà léhìn mi.*
*Sùgbón bée bá ní kórí mi sin mí,*
*Yóo sìn mí títí yóo moo tèlé mi kiri.*
*Òrìṣà bí orí ò sí omo lágbájá*
*E seá pé kórí mi ó mó padà léhin mi;*
*Ire lónìí, orí mi àfire.*

*Goats of this home, I am going to my husband's house, sheep of this house, I am going to my husband's house.*[3] *If you ask the youth of this home to accompany me even if they accompany me for a long time, they will later return. If you ask the elders of this home to accompany me, even if they accompany me for a long time, they will later return. But if you ask my head to accompany me, it will accompany me for a long time and keep going with me. There is no god like one's head, child of "Lagbaja" just pray that my head will not fail to accompany fortune today, my head, I say fortune.*

kneels down to voluntarily choose his or her own destiny, only an individual's *orí* is there to witness. Having sailed through *Òkun Ìgbàgbé* (the sacred Sea of Forgetfulness) the individual arrives on earth and forgets what he chose. But *orí* still knows. Individuals can solve no problems, nor resolve issues without their *orí* acting on their behalf. In the lyrics of the music by the celebrated Yoruba musician King Sunny Ade, this fact is articulated (see sidebar, A).

*Orí* is seen as the "guiding angel" in all human endeavors. Yoruba people believe that one's *orí* is the only spirit that an individual can totally rely on in seeing one through life, regardless of where or when. No matter how dangerous the journey may be, and be it real or metaphorical, only one's head can go all the way with one's self. On the ultimate journey, death, a person is accompanied only by one's *ori*. No other spirits benevolent or malevolent, can be constantly entrusted with the responsibility of seeing individuals through their difficulties. In Yoruba rhetoric, proverbs and aphorisms allude to the pertinence of *orí*, the head. These include the following:

1. *Orí l'onise*
   *Orí* is the dispenser of all propositions.

2. *Orí eni làwúre eni*
   One's head is the secret behind one's fate.

3. *Orí nìkàn ló le bá'ni d'Adó ìbìnnì*
   Only one's head is capable of accompanying one to Ado Ibinni.[2]

4. *Orí nìkàn ló le sílèkùn ayè bá tì*
   Only one's head can open the door when it is shut.
   (When all avenues close, one's *orí* is the lender of the last resort.)

In the tradition of Yoruba nuptial songs, a body of poetry chanted only by brides on the eve of their marriage ceremonies, almost every verse ends with the phrase, *"Ire lónìí, orí mi àfire"* (Fortune today, my head, I say fortune). This statement is made in the last line of the final verse which a bride usually chants before leaving her parents' home (see sidebar, B). This reaffirms the Yoruba belief that one's *orí* is the harbinger of one's fortune, and only it can be relied upon to lead one to a reasonable conclusion in one's life enterprises.[4]

Yoruba also believe that the *orí* is the custodian of individual secrecy. Nooter (1993) notes the existence of secrecy in various African traditions. Her book presents contributing articles focusing on multiple dimensions of secrecy in particular African societies, and specifically, on traditional practices. Among the Yoruba, it is often said,

*Orí eni l' alásìírí ẹni,* that is, "One's head is the envelope for one's secrets." It is therefore common to chide a person, particularly a young girl, who does not put on a headdress that *Asiri re o le bo,* "Your secret cannot be kept." In other words, there is a protective role of secret preservation believed to be played by the covering of the head. Here, a very thin line is drawn between the realm of physical appearance and its spiritual implication. While this may very well be an attempt to encourage a young girl to embrace a prevailing aesthetic value system, it has a lasting psycho-spiritual implication since the taboo has long been taken seriously by those in the traditional society.

## IMPLICATION

The discussion reveals that the concept *orí* is more than just the physical head for the Yoruba person. It is both a sacred and temporal symbol. This sacred entity has been referred to in literature as *orí inú* (inner head). Thus, the headdress is a covering for two separate but related entities: the physical head and the sacred head. When the hair is styled, it is primarily intended to honor the head. Dressing the head is therefore an extension of the honor, both spiritually and aesthetically. The head is like a temple or a shrine inside of which a spiritual entity resides. The Yoruba headdress, in addition to imparting aesthetic values, constructs a display that honors the spiritual capacity of the individual. Thus, the headdress is not only a recognition of devotion on the part of the person who wears it, but it also expresses respect to the ancestors who are believed to be ever-present with their relatives. Furthermore, since a respectful traditional ensemble (*aso t'o wuyi*) must be attended to from head to toe, the headdress is an expression of completeness, modesty, self respect, and reverence for others, especially on public occasions.

# STATUS AND ACCUMULATION

Becoming a person is a life-long process in most societies, and an individual's status and relationship to the community undergoes many changes throughout the life course. In African societies, an individual's status is both ascribed and achieved, and it is more fluid than previously recognized by outsiders. Ascribed status is often dependent on one's lineage, birth position in the family, and gender; these factors clearly affect an individual's access to cultural and material resources. Yet, within these constraints, individuals also make choices and accumulate status over their lifetime through their personal talents and achievements, their active participation in cultural institutions, and their acceptance or rejection of expected and chosen roles. As part of this ongoing process, people acquire hats and other objects of dress and adornment, along with the right to wear them. Dress becomes an objective emblem of status within the community. In everyday situations and on ceremonial occasions, headwear offers people the possibility of expressing and communicating their sense of self, their engagement in particular social roles, their accumulated status, and their relationships to others within their society.

Both the Lega and the Kuba peoples living in Zaire invest considerable time, energy, and value in the production of a variety of headwear and other objects of bodily adornment. The cultural history and the political and social organization of these two Zairian societies are quite different from one another, as is the repertoire of headwear through which they express their sense of cultural identity, their achievements, and their accumulated status. In Lega and Kuba societies, men and women accrue prestige throughout their adult lives by participating in titled associations. It is not simply a matter of birthright or the process of aging which allow the accumulation of status, but it is through a person's ability to engage, elicit, and actively build upon the support of others in their extended families and their community. Elisabeth Cameron's essay on Lega hats and Pat Darish and David Binkley's essay on Kuba hair styles situate the discussion of the aesthetic and symbolic importance of headwear within the societies that create and give value and meaning to these displays.

# 8 LEGA HATS: HIERARCHY AND STATUS

## ELISABETH L. CAMERON

The Lega[1] live in eastern Kivu Province, Zaire, a densely forested area close to the equator. They live by hunting and gathering, fishing, and limited slash-and-burn agriculture. They are made up of subgroups having unique but analogous histories and similar social and political lives. Local government is managed through limited patrilineal clans. The *bwami* association, however, cuts across territorial groups, clans, and lineages, creating a link between all Lega (Biebuyck 1972:10, 1973:37). *Bwami* also refers to the small cap worn by all society members. This essay examines how hats publicly mark hierarchy (which is expressed through a combination of lineage, personal prestige through elevation and rank, and accumulation of wealth) within *bwami* and Lega societies. In order to understand the role of hats among the Lega, an examination of *bwami* is essential.

### *BWAMI*

*Bwami* is an association open to all adult men and their wives. It is common knowledge who constitutes the membership, and some ceremonies take place in public; however, most initiations are open only to members of that grade or higher (Biebuyck, personal communication 1994). The primary purpose of *bwami* is to instruct the initiate in "wisdom and moral excellence" (Biebuyck 1973:91). It also fulfills political, economic, social, artistic, and religious roles in broader Lega society. *Bwami*, for men, is divided into five levels or grades — *kongabulumbu, kansilembo, ngandu, yananio, kindi*[2] — which are entered sequentially. The candidate for each level is initiated by members of that and higher levels. During initiation, level-specific wisdom is taught through the presentation of objects, dance, proverbs, and theater by specially appointed teachers. The initiate, in turn, distributes large quantities of meat and goods. At the end of the ceremony, the teachers give the initiate insignia of his new rank in *bwami,* which includes hats, belts, and other objects. The women's levels — *bombwa, bulonda, bunyamwa*[3] — are tied to the men's levels and their initiations occur concurrently.

Ninety-five percent of all Lega men are members of *bwami*; most, however, remain at the lower levels. It is the ambition of most Lega men to obtain the higher levels of *bwami* where they will enjoy social, political, and economic prominence. Few men, however, reach *kindi,* the highest *bwami* level (Biebuyck 1986:14; Biebuyck, personal communication 1994). Men join *bwami* through a variety of different means. The most prestigious way is personal desire to be a member. A man must have the enterprise to gather the necessary goods and recruit the needed support from both his clan and the *bwami* association. A *bwami* member can invite his son to join, or a man can be selected from within a kin-group to take the place of a relative who has moved to a higher level or died. In some circumstances, a man may be forced to join *bwami* as treatment prescribed by a diviner or because he broke *bwami* rules (Biebuyck 1973:85–86). In such a case, the expense of joining the association would have to be endured before the person was ready to assume the responsibility. It is important to recognize that without the support of relatives and other *bwami* members, a Lega man will not be able to join or advance in *bwami* (Biebuyck 1986:13–14).

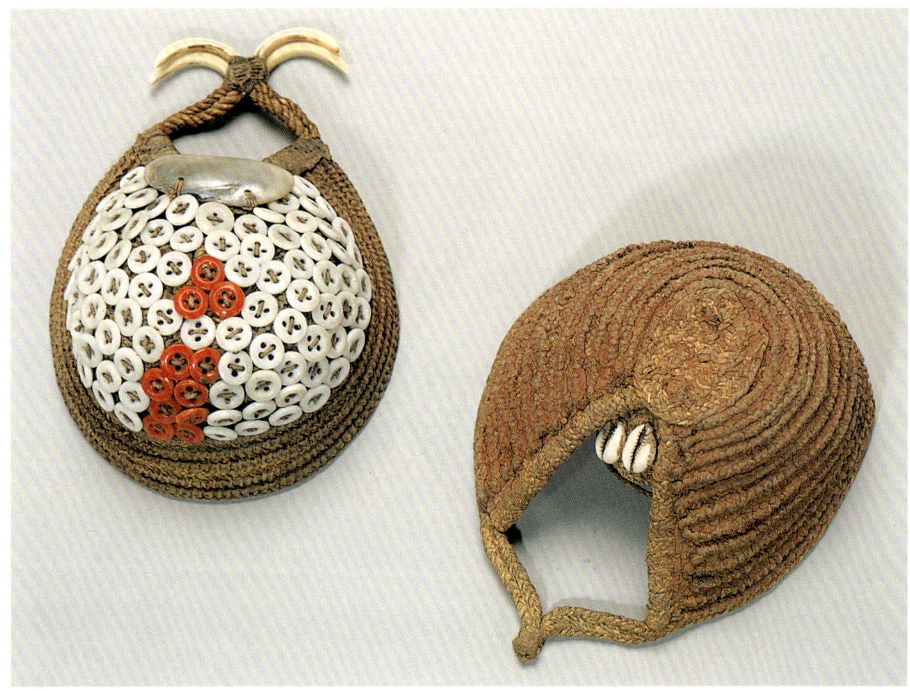

**Figure 8.1a, b.** Hats *(bwami)*. Lega, Zaire. a. Raffia, hyrax teeth, shell, buttons. NMNH E367,951; b. Raffia, clay. NMNH E379,058. H. of largest, 12.0 cm. Department of Anthropology, Smithsonian Institution. Photograph by Diane L. Nordeck. Caps *(bwami)*, hidden under a hat denoting *bwami* rank, are traditionally worn at all times by members of the association. The open slit *(kilingi)* is worn toward the front and is covered with an animal skin to hide the method of attaching the hat to the head. Figure 8.1a is elaborated with buttons and cowries and was used didactically in lower-level initiations.

The Lega have a noncentralized political structure, depending instead on clan, *bwami* membership, and personal qualities to provide stability (Biebuyck, personal communication 1994). While there is a village chief (Mulyumba 1968:2), his minimal authority is balanced by the influence of clan leaders and *bwami* officials. Even within *bwami,* authority is shared in the higher levels by all *kindi* initiates (Biebuyck 1973:93). *Kindi* initiates are almost always clan leaders, creating yet another link between clan and *bwami* (Yongolelo 1975:23).

*Bwami* and clan membership are important in this life and in the afterlife. At death, the Lega believe they go to live with the ancestors in Uchimu, a city divided into clans that are led by the original clan founder. The deceased keep their clan ranking as well as the final *bwami* grade they achieve in life. The living and dead interact through an ancestor cult in which the deceased's *bwami* rank is carefully observed. For example, a diviner may act as an intermediary between an ancestor and the living to communicate the ancestor's desires (e.g., a ceremony in his honor centered on drum playing). The drumming and related ceremonies are taken from *bwami* rituals of the appropriate level; participants, therefore, must have the same or higher grade as the deceased. This forces the larger *bwami* community to engage in, what is basically, a clan event (Mulyumba 1968:9–14).

## HATS AND *BWAMI*

The basic *bwami* hat for men is a cap made of fibers covered with a red powder and with an attached seed-pod (Fig. 8.1). It is presented to the initiate at the end of the *kongabulumbu* initiation. When a member reaches higher levels, he can attach four cowrie shells to this hat. In the past, the cap was worn by the *bwami* member at all times, although in the privacy of his house he was allowed to remove it to shave his head. The *bwami* member attached the hat with a string to a small tuft of hair left on the back of his head. Another larger hat showing rank within *bwami* is worn over the cap (Biebuyck, personal communication 1994; 1986:210). Currently, because of the persecution of *bwami* members, many initiates only wear the cap and other special hats for initiations and special ceremonies (Biebuyck, personal communication 1994).

In initiatory settings, the *bwami* cap can also be called *kilembo*, or "the thing being sought" (Biebuyck, personal communication 1994), because the initiate seeks both entry into *bwami* and the cap *bwami* which signifies his acceptance. The conceptual link between the larger society and the cap is seen in the shared name. Just as *bwami*, the society, must be treated respectfully, so must *bwami*, the cap. It cannot be allowed to touch the ground, an incident that would create ritual impurity (Biebuyck 1986:26), and must be treated with honor (Biebuyck 1973:69).

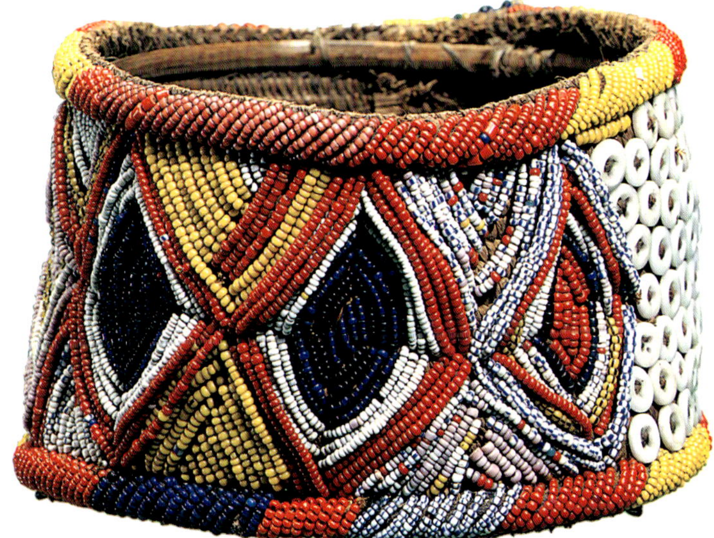

**Figure 8.2.** Hat *(lukunia)*. Lega, Zaire. Fiber, beads, wood, buttons. D. 19.0 cm. FMCH X94.29.4. Museum purchase, Jerome L. Joss Endowment Fund. This hat was worn by *kanyamwa* women (initiated wives of *kindi*-grade men), en route to and during high-level *bwami* ceremonies. These hats were originally decorated with cowrie shells; buttons began to replace cowries as early as the 1940s. The beaded pattern signifies a hat of recent manufacture.

High-ranking women in *bwami* receive diadems made of fiber and covered with beads, cowries, buttons, and occasionally, other materials (Figs. 8.2–8.4). Like the caps, they are worn on a daily basis and during ceremonies (Biebuyck 1986:63). For certain rituals, women are permitted to wear men's hats.

Hats are used during initiations to teach sayings and actions associated with them. As initiation objects, hats take on *masengo*, or "heaviness," a meaning understood only by *bwami* members of the appropriate level (Biebuyck 1976:338). The meaning of the hat is understood as a combination of the materials, the form of the hat, activities or theater involving the hat, and sayings related to the hat (Biebuyck 1973:146).

When a member dies, his hat is buried with him (Biebuyck, personal communication 1994). Other hats are placed on his grave along with the other insignia and initiation objects he controlled (Biebuyck 1973:105, 173; 1986:26–27). At the appropriate time, a kinsman removes the insignia and holds it until a clan member takes the deceased's place in *bwami*. If a *bwami* member should die away from home, the

**Figure 8.3**, below. Hat *(lukunia)*. Lega, Zaire. Beads, buttons, fiber. D. 19.0 cm. Private collection.

**Figure 8.4**, below right. Hat *(lukunia)*. Lega, Zaire. Buttons, fiber, wood. D. 20.0 cm. Private collection.

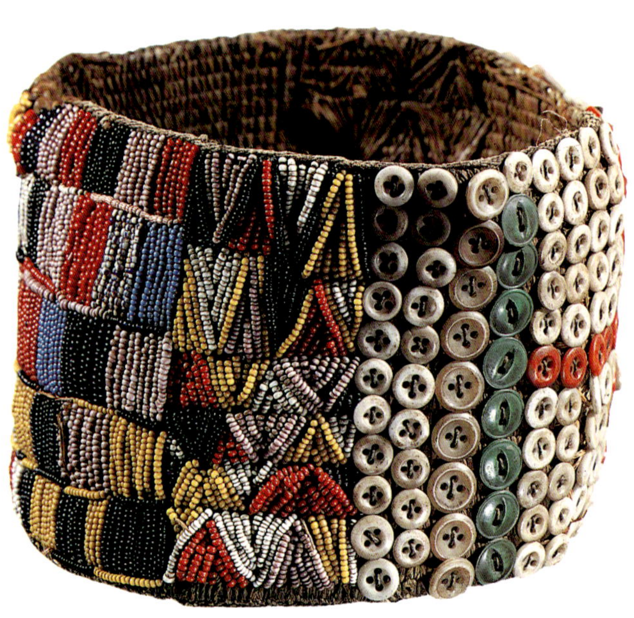

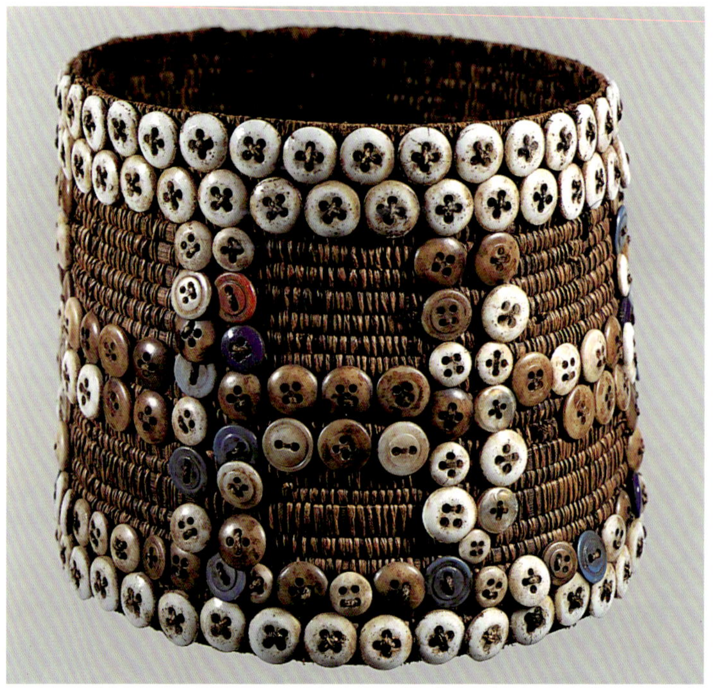

*bwami* hat is returned and buried in place of the body (Biebuyck 1986:170). The hat, therefore, not only represents *bwami* ideology and status, but also serves to bridge the gap between living and dead, keeping a balance within the clan and between *bwami* and clan (Biebuyck 1977:12).

The *bwami* cap is the basic hat worn by all male *bwami* members. It is a symbol of power, fame, and intelligence, and is coveted by all Lega men (Biebuyck 1973:189). The cap shows that the man wearing it, as Biebuyck says, "is capable, through appropriate initiatory experience, of supporting the mystic burden of the skullcap" (1973:69). Other *bwami* hats, generically called *kikumbi,* also carry a heavy charge of meaning and power.

The small feather hat *(idumbi;* Fig. 8.6) is used in all levels of male and female initiations." These are not the feather hats of war but the feather hats of dance" is a saying attached to the hats (Biebuyck and Van den Abbeele 1984:82; Biebuyck, personal communication 1994), stressing one of the original and basic functions of *bwami,* the keeping of peace (Biebuyck 1973:67, 129). During the lowest level initiation, *kongabulumbu,* the initiate's wife appears wearing a feather hat, standing on a stool and surrounded by shoulder bags filled with initiation objects. Here the hat's purpose is to give the woman a hint of future initiations and greatness (Biebuyck, personal communication 1994; 1977:14–15). In a women's *bombwa* initiation observed by Biebuyck, a feather hat was worn by a character representing Kingungungu, a poor beggar (1986:149). In *bulonda,* a woman wearing a feather hat represents Kiluku, a woman who seems to have the material goods for initiation, but does not have the moral requirements (Biebuyck 1977:15). During one *kindi* rite, two initiates appear with feather hats in their mouths (Biebuyck 1986:156–57).

The *yananio* initiate wears a hat made of black goat skin (Biebuyck 1973:Fig. 8.9). When reaching *lutumbo lwa yananio,* the highest subgrade within *yananio,* the initiate places a mussel shell on his hat as an emblem of his high rank (Biebuyck 1973:182). During *bwami* ceremonies, the hat is referred to with the proverb "a mwami [is] a Mr. Lusembe [Shell]; Mubinga [Dendrohyrax] dies because of Mbalo [Waxing moon]" (Biebuyck 1986:31). The shell carries many levels of meaning, but especially refers to the waxing moon, a public symbol of *bwami* rank, visible to all (Biebuyck 1986:24).[4]

Initiations for certain *bwami* levels are held in private, restricted to members of that level and higher. Most initiation objects are not seen by the public, and are only brought out and displayed during ceremonies when they are explained to the new initiate (Biebuyck 1981:120). The art, therefore, is "a hidden art," not readily accessible to the public but understood by the trained initiate (Biebuyck 1976:341). Conversely, some insignia, like hats, are public proclamations of rank and status within *bwami* (Biebuyck 1986:131). This is illustrated by the shell attached at the *yananio* level, referring to public acknowledgment of high-ranking *bwami* officials. While the hat revealing the rank of the wearer is visible to all, the *bwami* cap, symbolic of *bwami* esoterica, is kept hidden underneath. The hats, therefore, can be understood as a metaphor for the dual nature of *bwami,* both secret and public.

Not only do hats refer to the secret/public dichotomy, they also reveal the blending of gender in the higher ranks as the male takes on female characteristics and the female, in turn, becomes male. The *sawamazembe* hat worn at the *kindi* level duplicates a woman's *mazembe* hair style (Figs. 8.11, 8.12, 8.13; Biebuyck 1986:84). Attached to the front are *lubumba* shells that, as in *yananio* level hats, publicly proclaim the status of the wearer. The *muzombolo* hat worn by women of *bunyamwa* level, the highest female grade, is a long shaft topped with feathers and worn on top of the head (Fig. 8.14). The hat has a phallic shape (Biebuyck and Van den Abbeele 1984:82) that, paired with the *sawamazembe,* stresses the interdependency between the *kindi* initiate and his *bunyamwa*-level wife. In one *kindi* rite, women wear their husbands' *mukuba* hats. Biebuyck and Van den Abbeele note that this emphasizes the high-ranking women's "quasi-male status" (1984:84).[5]

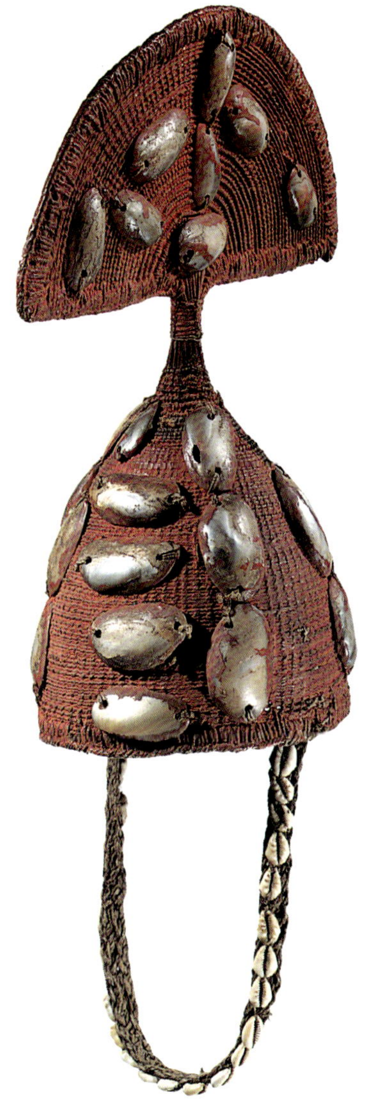

**Figure 8.5.** Hat. Lega, Zaire. Fiber, cowrie shells, shell, pigment. H. 49.0 cm. Private collection. Various objects, when attached to hats, carry specific meanings in *bwami* and can function as didactic devices used to instruct initiates in *bwami* esoterica.

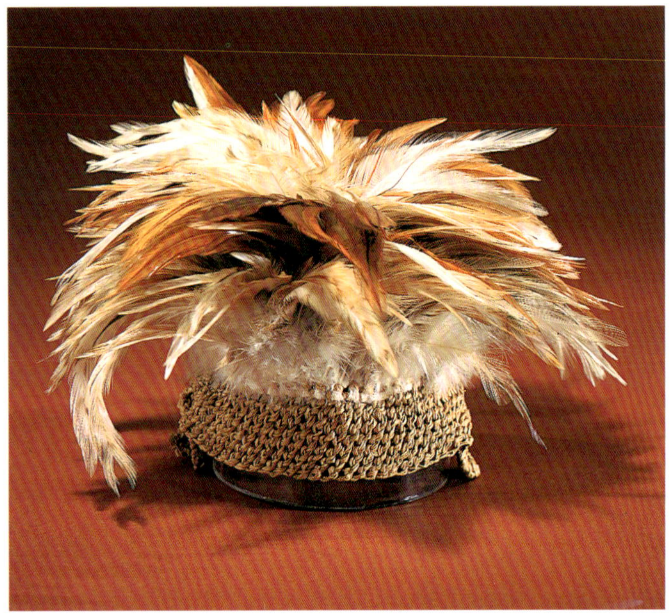

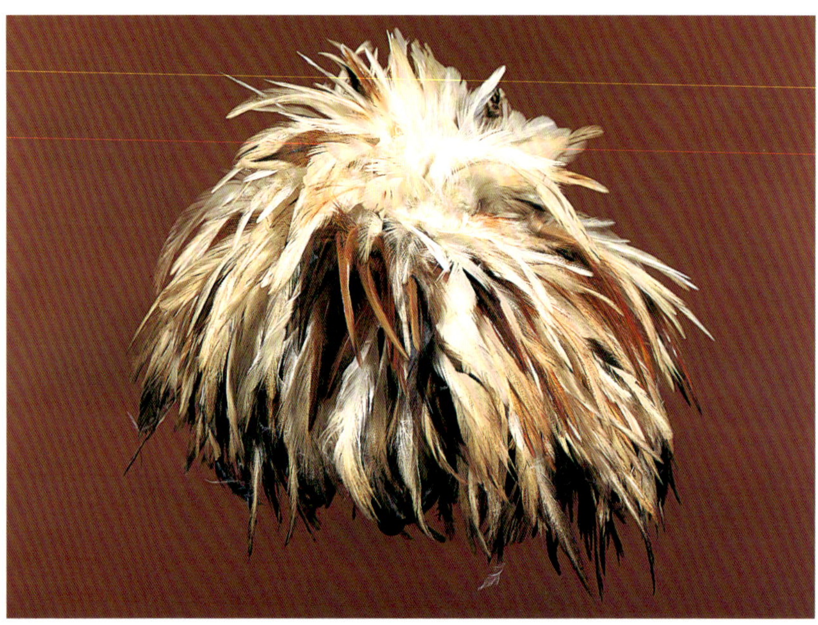

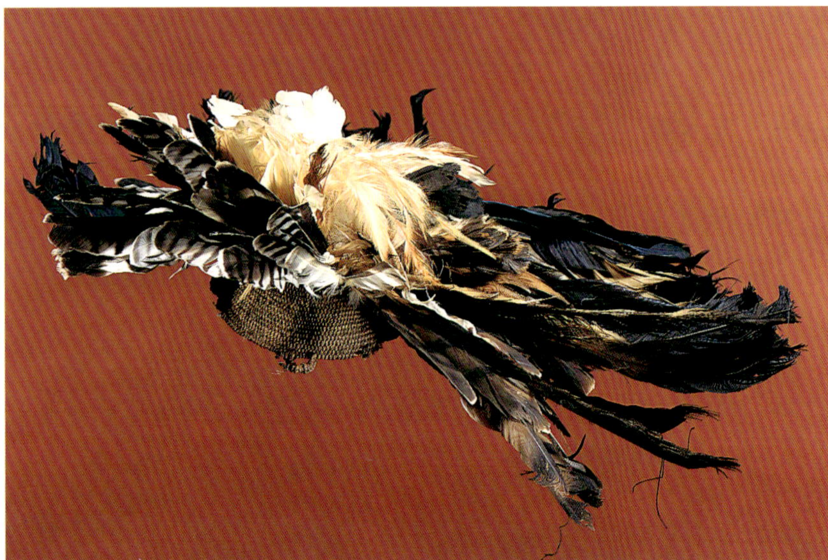

**Figure 8.6,** above left. Headdress *(idumbi).* Lega, Lualaba River, eastern Zaire. Fiber, feathers. H. 30.0 cm. FMCH X378.371. Museum purchase. This feather hat is worn by a young woman at the first initiation of a close male relative to show her future possibilities if she marries a *bwami* member. It is also used to instruct initiates.

**Figure 8.7,** above right. Headdress *(isala).* Lega, Lualaba River, eastern Zaire. Fiber, feathers. H. 20.0 cm. FMCH X378.372. Museum purchase. Hats made of a variety of feathers, including chicken, parrot, and guinea fowl, are used as dance paraphernalia in *bwami* contexts, but also appear outside of *bwami* in divination, hunting, and healing cults.

**Figure 8.8,** left. Headdress *(isala).* Lega, Lualaba River, eastern Zaire. Fiber, feathers. H. 17.0 cm. FMCH X378.377. Museum purchase.

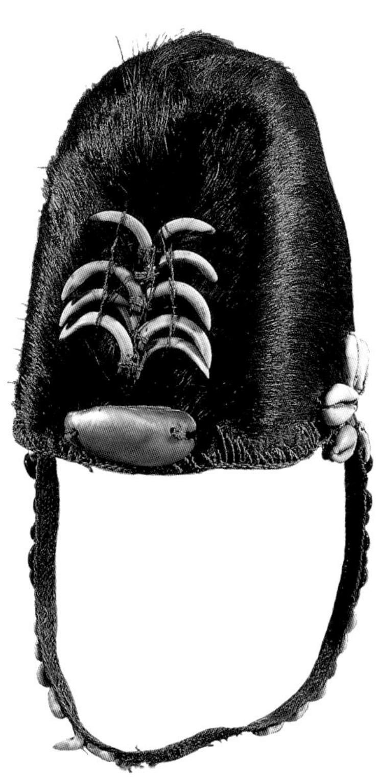

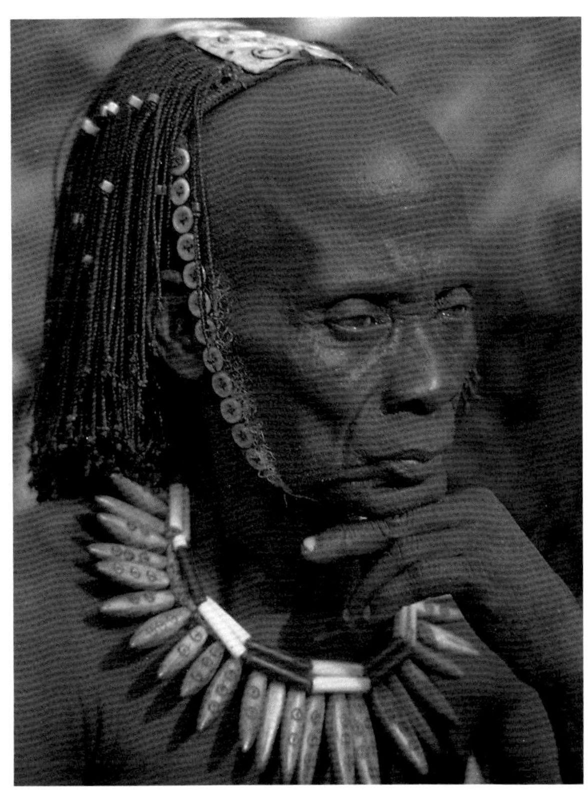

**Figure 8.9**, above. Headdress. Lega, Shabunda, Lualaba River, eastern Zaire. Goat hide, cowrie shells, teeth, fiber, buttons, shell. H. 33.0 cm. FMCH X378.395. Museum purchase. The black goat skin, mussel shell, and teeth on this hat signal that the wearer is of the *lutumbo lwa yananio* grade.

**Figure 8.10**, right. Hat. Lega, Zaire. Shells, cowrie shells, seed pods, tusk, fiber. H. 41.0 cm. Private collection.

**Figure 8.11**, above right. Man at a dance for a member reaching fourth grade (of five) in *bwami* society. Lega peoples, near Kalima, Zaire. Photograph by Eliot Elisofon, 1966. Slide no. F LGA 14.2 (5405). Eliot Elisofon Photographic Archives. National Museum of African Art.

**Figure 8.12**, far right. Men's hat. Lega, Zaire. Fiber, shells, seed pods. H. 33.0 cm. Private collection. The *sawamazembe* hat, worn by *lutumbo lwa kindi* men, copies a woman's elaborate hair style.

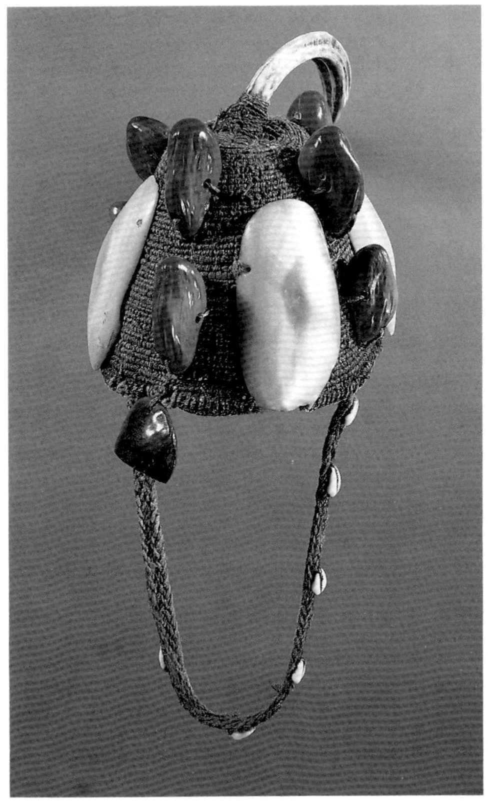

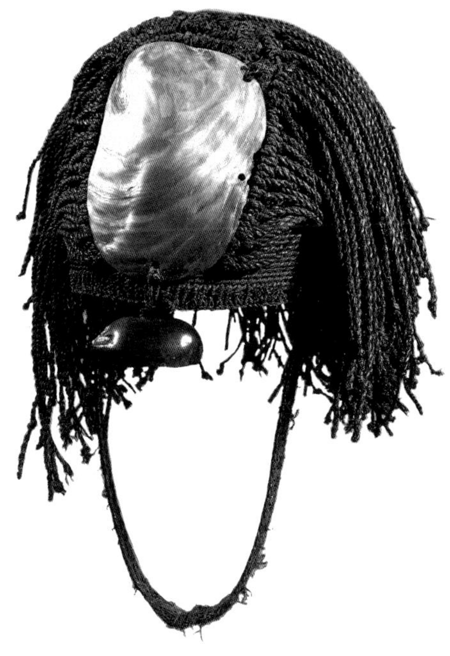

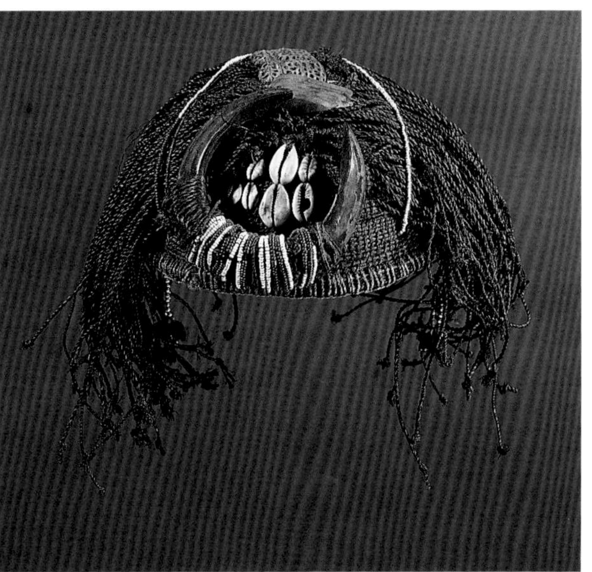

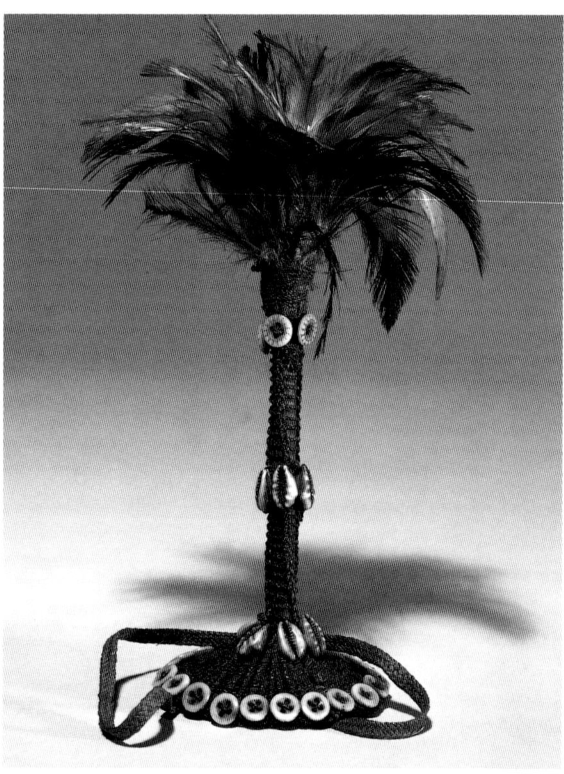

**Figure 8.13,** above left. Hat. Lega, Zaire. Fiber, cowrie shells, beads, tusks, shell, seed pods. H. 30.0 cm. Private collection.

**Figure 8.14,** above right. Hat. Lega, Zaire. Feathers, fiber, buttons, cowrie shells. H. 30.0 cm. Private collection. This phallic-shaped hat is worn by women in some *kindi* and *bunyamwa* ceremonies.

Members of the highest level of *kindi, lutumbo lwa kindi,* wear hats made of canvas covered with shells, cowries, and (more recently) buttons, and surmounted by an elephant tail (Biebuyck 1973:Fig. 8.15). The hat is called *mukuba wa maseza* (Biebuyck and van den Abbeele 1984:84) and is worn daily. The *mukuba* hat can be worn in the *ibugebuge* rite by the owner's *kanyamwa*-level wife. She wears her husband's hat, while in her hands she holds her own diadem, moving it back and forth. The rite signifies the danger of fighting and, again, the peacekeeping role of *bwami* (Biebuyck 1986:156).

Hats revealing status are made of skins and objects specific to rank. Animals are especially important in *bwami* symbolism (Figs. 8.16–8.18). Initiates refer to themselves as specific animals; for example, *kindi* initiates call themselves "Elephant-Tail-Folks," referring to the elephant tails in the *mukuba* headdress (Biebuyck 1986:101). Besides status, animals carry meanings. Rites themselves can be named after an animal that has symbolic significance in the ceremony (Figs. 8.19, 8.20; Biebuyck 1979:77). Finally, many animals are sacred and must be treated according to strict guidelines and distributed carefully according to *bwami* status (Biebuyck 1953:907).

The hornbill, occasionally attached to hats, is not symbolic of specific rank but has meaning within *bwami* esoterica (Fig. 8.21). The hornbill symbolizes the man who has high ambitions, but is unaware of the cost of attaining them. It also stands for a woman with the habit of wandering from home, and whose husband must go

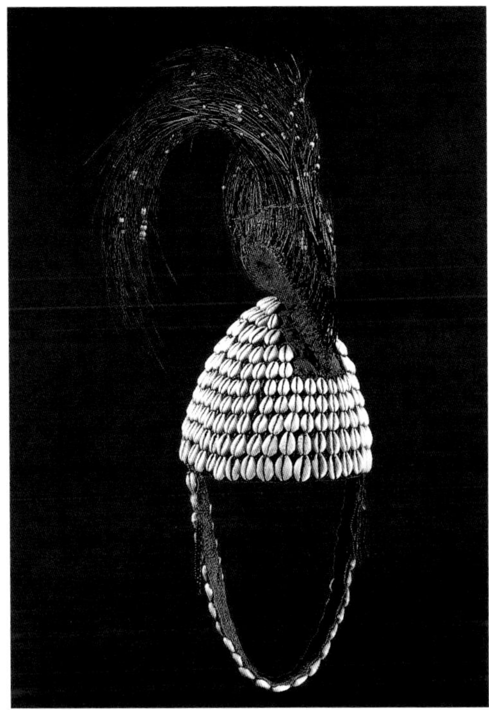

Figure 8.16, left. Hat *(mukuba wa bifungo)*. Lega, Zaire. Fiber, cowrie shells, beads, hide, elephant tail, string, vegetable fiber. H. 58.0 cm. Private collection.

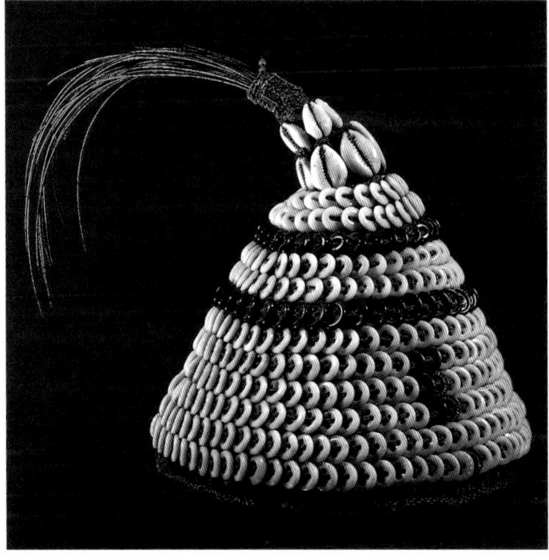

**Figure 8.15,** left. Hat. Lega, Zaire. Fiber, buttons, cowrie shells, elephant hair. H. 18.3 cm. FMCH X378.389. *Mukuba wa bifungo* is a hat worn by members of the highest *bwami* grade, *lutumbo lwa kindi.* The attached elephant hair refers to the association between *bwami*, especially the highest grade of *lutumbo lwa kindi*, and the elephant with its quiet, yet potentially destructive, strength. Buttons are used in place of cowrie shells.

**Figure 8.17,** below. Hat. Lega, Zaire. Fiber, cowrie shells, elephant tail, beads. H. 48.0 cm. Private collection.

and fetch her (Biebuyck 1973:189). This meaning derives from the male hornbill's habit of trapping the female and her chicks in a nest behind a wall of mud (Biebuyck 1986:93).

The pangolin is a sacred animal that is not hunted. If, however, a hunter finds a trapped pangolin or one already dead in the forest, he is obligated to take the pangolin to a *bwami* member who has the "Right of the Pangolin Knife." Anyone who does not follow these strict guidelines is sanctioned and often forced to leave their clan and village. Pangolins are rich in meaning, symbolizing power, family, and knowledge (Fig. 8.22; Biebuyck 1953:909–10). They are associated with the *ngandu, yananio,* and the lower levels of *kindi* (Biebuyck 1953:910). The scales of the small pangolin *(kabanga),* when attached to hats, symbolize piety and respect and call to mind Isamukulu, the "Great Old One" (Biebuyck 1973:190; personal communication 1994).

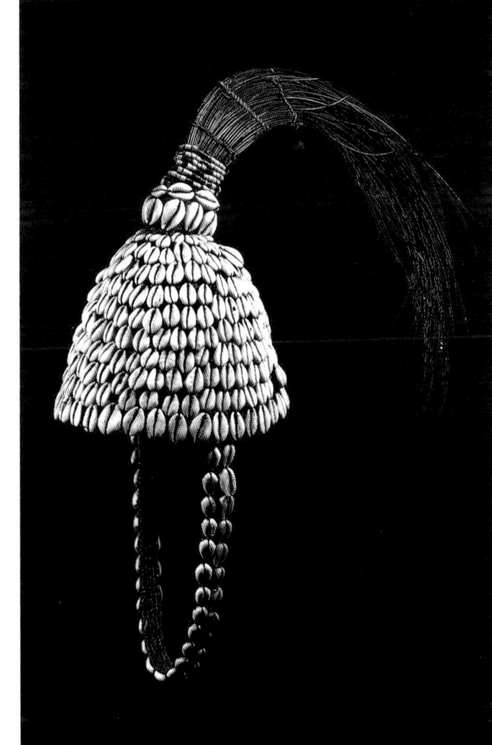

Elephants represent simultaneously all of *bwami* and the highest level of *kindi.* Aphorisms compare all *bwami* members to elephants: "*Bwami,* the stampeding of elephants; the place where it has passed cannot be forgotten" (Biebuyck 1973:127). Elephant products, however, are reserved for members of *kindi, bwami's* highest grade. *Kindi* hats can be made of elephant ears and adorned with elephant tails (Cameron 1992).

It is interesting to note that pangolins, symbolizing family and clan, are tied to lower grades of *bwami* where family is vitally important in acceptance and advancement. Elephants, however, symbolic of *bwami* itself, represent the highest level of *bwami* where the initiate must be able to draw on much broader levels of support. A proverb states "the pangolin is bigger than an elephant" (Biebuyck 1953:910), reveal-

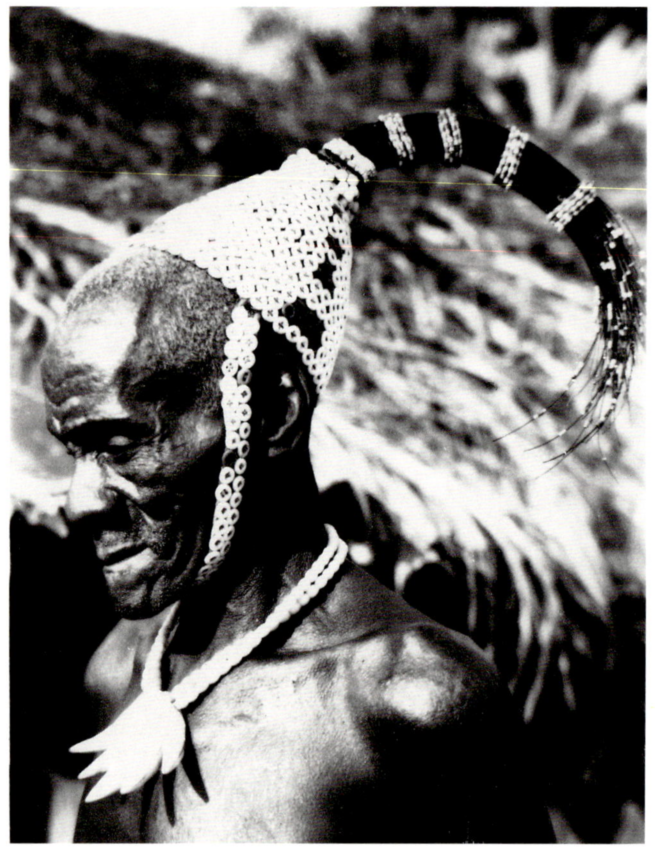

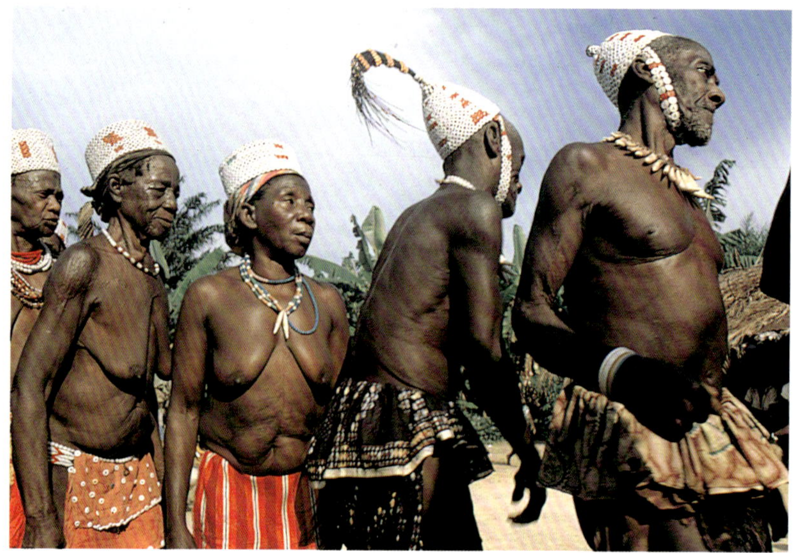

**Figure 8.18**, above. A *lutumbo lwa kindi*, a member of the highest grade in the *bwami* society, wearing an elephant tail hat. Lega peoples, Zaire. Photograph by Eliot Elisofon, 1966. Neg no. OA 71264, C-11, 26A. Eliot Elisofon Photographic Archives. National Museum of African Art.

**Figure 8.19**, above right. Wives of *kanyamwa* grade in *bwami* society. Dance for a person reaching the fourth (of five) grade. Lega peoples, Zaire. Photograph by Eliot Elisofon, 1966. Neg. no. OA 71264, C-11, 24A. Eliot Elisofon Photographic Archives. National Museum of African Art.

ing some rivalry between clan and *bwami*.

Hats and diadems are also used in combination with the display of other initiation objects. During *bele muno,* a part of *kindi* initiation, ivory and wood figures are rested against hats (Biebuyck 1986:58). Women's diadems also are used to support figures in the *kasumba* rite of women's *kanyamwa* level initiation (Biebuyck 1973:57, 203). Finally, in some initiations, anthropomorphic figures are made representing *bwami* members wearing insignia including hats (Biebuyck 1986:39).

## CONCLUSION

*Bwami,* both the association and the hat, represents for the Lega a noncentralized, but highly hierarchical, structure open to all circumcised men and their wives. The association, in combination with the local patrilineal clan structure, provides economic, political, and social structure for the Lega as a whole. *Bwami* also appears among the Lega's neighbors as both an initiatory noncentralized association and in a centralized leader or king.

Among the Sile, *bwami* has three grades: *bwami, buba'i,* and *ngandu.* For the *bwami* level, the main insignia is a hat of goat skin. The highest level, *ngandu,* has the

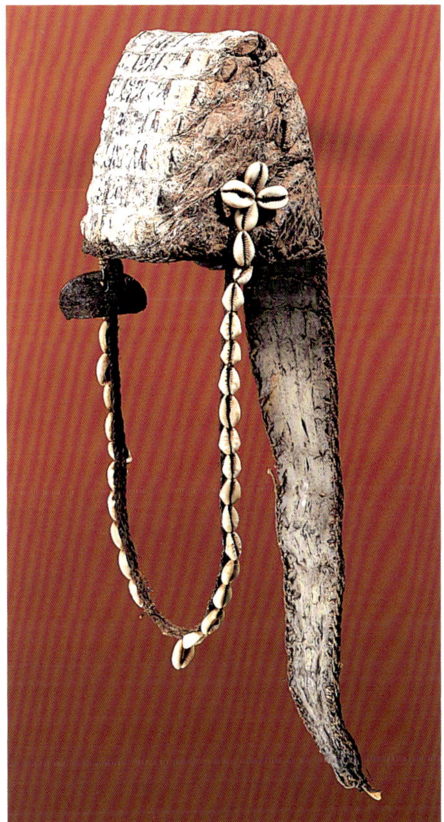

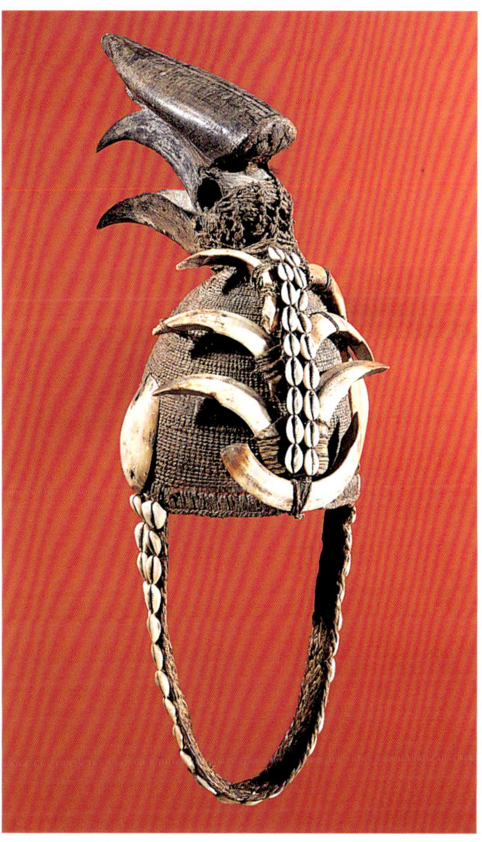

**Figure 8.20**, far left. Hat. Lega, Zaire. Crocodile skin, cowrie shells, fiber, teeth, skin. H. 44.0 cm. Private collection. *Kindi*-level *bwami* members often own a variety of hats like this one made of forest crocodile hide.

**Figure 8.21**, left. Hat. Lega, Zaire. Raffia, cowrie shells, shells, hornbill, glass beads. 48.5 cm. Private collection.

**Figure 8.22**, below. Hat. Lega, Zaire. Pangolin skin, cowrie shells, shell, seed pod, fiber. H. 35.7 cm. Private collection. In Lega myths, pangolins bring elements of culture, such as roof building, to the people. The real pangolin is considered a sacred animal, and its protection is guaranteed by strict laws; it is associated with *ngandu* and *yananio* grades.

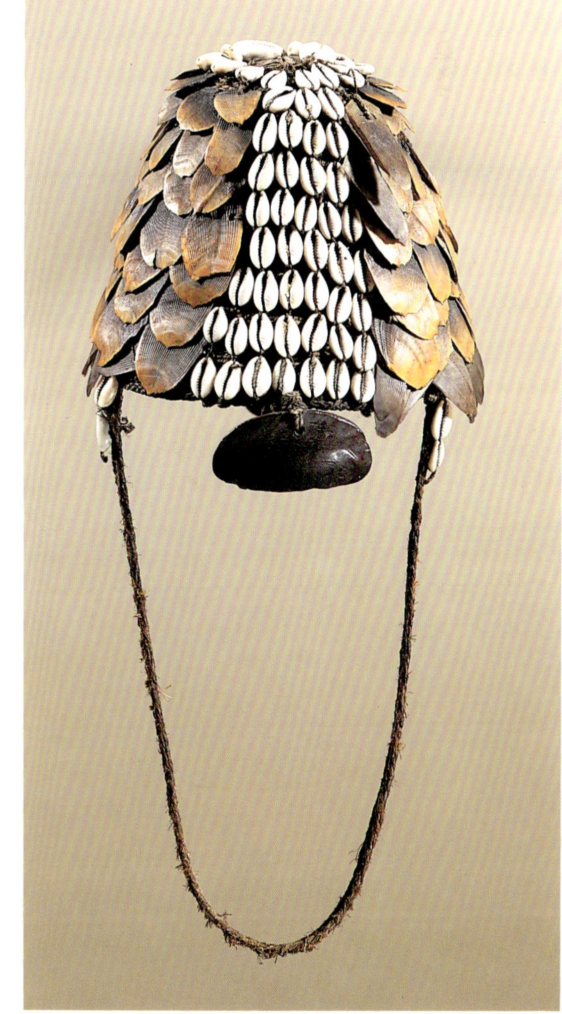

right to wear an antelope skin hat and to fulfill a judicial role in society (Mulyumba 1978:23–25). The most important form of Sile *bwami,* however, is *bwami bwa lusembe,* a centralized form of government investing final authority in a king (Mulyumba 1978:28). Many parallels occur between the *bwami* association and *bwami bwa lusembe,* including the use of identical paraphernalia and the similarity between *bwami* initiation rites and *bwami bwa lusembe* enthronement rituals.

Hats play an important role in centralized *bwami.* The Sile king wears a leopard skin cap with attached teeth and shells. Among the Nyindu, the king is given a *bwami* cap and then a hat symbolic of his royal status (Biebuyck 1986:220). According to myth, *bwami* began when a man needed money. He took off his hat and sold it to another man with the promise that if he never took the hat off and would instruct his people in the secrets of the hat, he would receive power and wealth (Biebuyck 1986:209–10). Whether centralized or noncentralized, hats play an important, public role in the authority of the wearer and in his search for wealth and power.

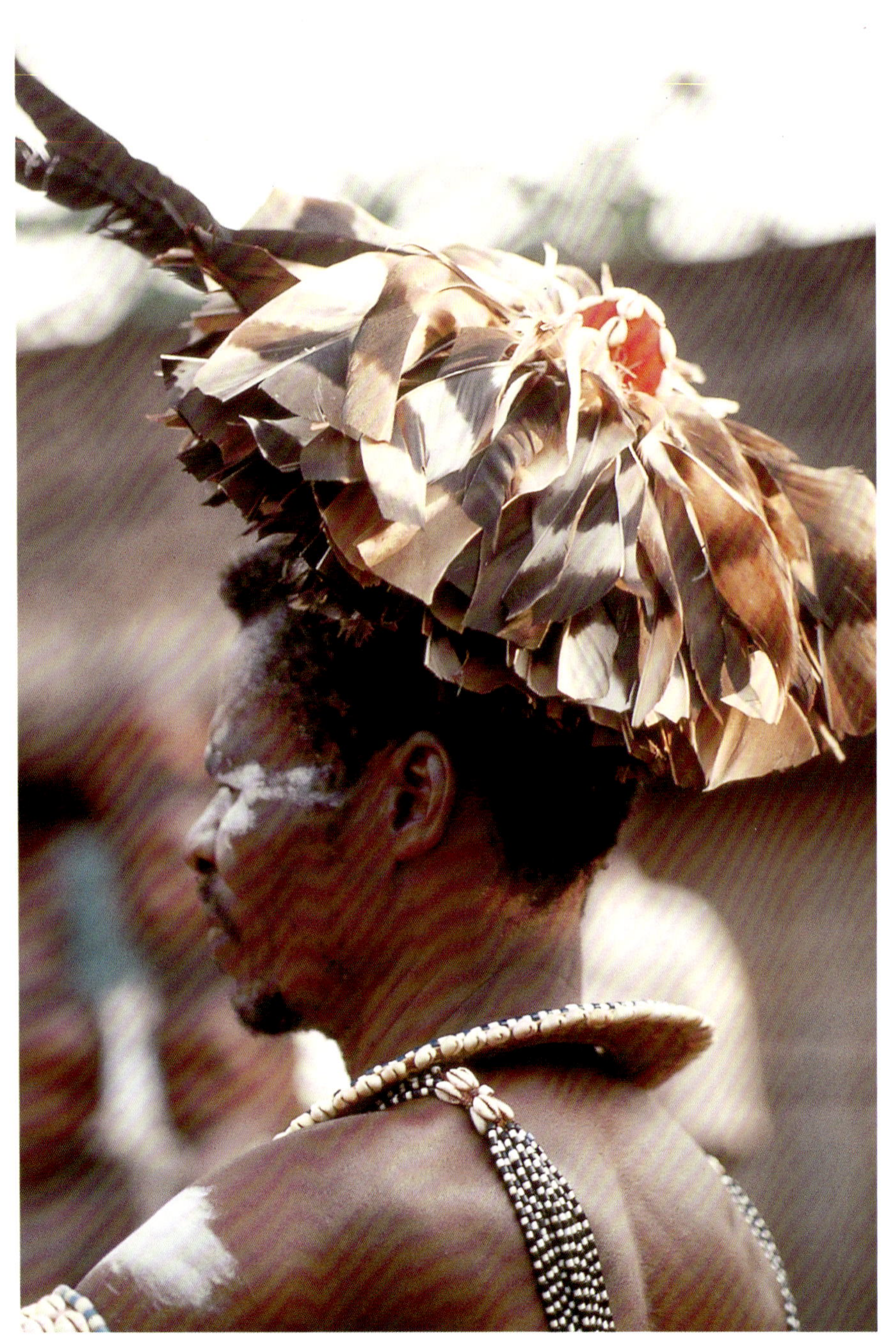

# 9 HEADDRESSES AND TITLEHOLDING AMONG THE KUBA

PATRICIA DARISH AND DAVID A. BINKLEY

> Had I not known it by any other way, the costume of the natives I met would have told me that I had entered a country far different from any I had yet seen. Well built and tall, every man wore a full skirt that reached below his knees. And on every head was perched a tiny conical hat — the lukete, . . . By every sign I knew that at last I was in the territory of the Bushongo; the tribe known to Europeans as Bakuba.
>
> (Herman Norden, *Fresh Tracks in the Belgian Congo,* 1925:222)

## LATE 19TH AND EARLY 20TH-CENTURY HAIR AND HAT STYLES

Late nineteenth and early twentieth-century explorers and travelers in Central Africa were fascinated with the varied ways Africans decorated their heads and bodies. Written accounts from the period are filled with detailed descriptions noting minute differences in hair styles, scarification patterns, deformation of teeth, and application of oils and pigments to the head and body. A fascinating colonial narrative on African bodies and their decoration was developed from accounts of the various voyages up the Congo (Zaire) River and its many tributaries. A characteristic example of this narrative is the journal of the missionary Samuel Norvell Lapsley (1893) who, together with William H. Sheppard, were the first missionaries sent by the American Presbyterian Congo Mission (APCM).[1] While aboard the steamer *Florida* on the Kasai River in March and April 1891, Lapsley described the changing landscape along the river banks as the steamer moved slowly upstream toward the future home of the APCM mission at Luebo.[2] From time to time, the steamer stopped at villages to take on firewood and provisions. On these occasions Lapsley also described the *bodyscape* of the differing populations he encountered delineating their hair styles, scarification patterns, body decoration and ornamentation (1893:160). On April 16, 1891 the *Florida* stopped at a Kuba village and Lapsley described the distinctive dress of the Bakuba.[3]

> There were larger crowds grouped around various parties from the steamer, buying chop in quantities for their respective messes. Nice looking people. . . . head shaved, except a chignon at the apex, and this topped by a natty little cap, fastened on with ivory or fancy brass hairpins, lady fashion (1893:160).[4]

**Opposite.** An eagle feather chief *(kum apoong)* wears a laket covered with the insignia of his office. Yele Ngongo. Photograph by David A. Binkley and Patricia Darish, 1989.

Many early twentieth-century accounts also record the distinctive dress of Kuba men and women in detail taking into account the treatment of the coiffure, the patterning of facial and body scarification, and the types of clothing worn (Torday and Joyce 1910; Torday 1925).[5] The written accounts of the Hungarian ethnographer Emil Torday describe the treatment of the head and hair of Bushoong and Ngongo men and women.[6] For Bushoong people living at the Kuba capital of Nsheng, Torday (1925:112) notes that both men and women shaved their heads except the men left a "thick tuft on the summit to which the cap was pinned." However, at the Ngongo capital of Misumba they let their hair grow and pulled it to the back of the head.[7] A distinct hairline was then sharply delineated by shaving the hair straight across the top of the forehead except for a sharp angle at the temples. A "crescent-shaped space" was also shaved on the back of the head from ear to ear leaving about one inch of hair below this line (Torday 1925:100). This distinctive hairline is clearly represented in Kuba woodcarving: palm wine cups in the shape of the human head, *ndop* figures of the paramount ruler, and wooden masks.

Other Kuba-affiliated groups created other distinctive treatments of the hair. Torday describes first-time expectant Ngongo mothers wearing a distinctive hair style that consisted of hair formed into a "round cap on the summit, flanked by two wings shaped like buffalo horns" (1925:100). He was told that this hair style was occasionally worn by elderly Kuba men. The frontispiece photograph of Torday's book, *On the Trail of the Bushongo,* depicts an elderly Isambo chief wearing this archaic hair style.[8]

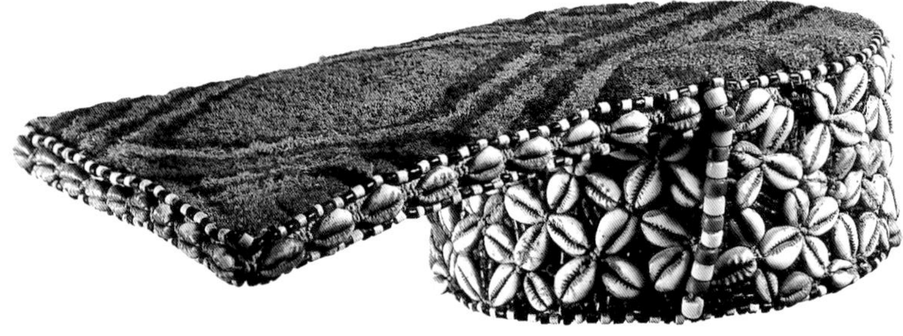

**Figure 9.1**. Hat *(shody)*. Kuba, Zaire. Raffia, cowrie shells, glass beads. H. 9.5 cm. Anonymous loan. The royal headdress known as *shody* is characterized by the horizontal extension of a visor. This distinctive headdress is always represented on the important carved wooden *ndop* figures of the Kuba paramount rulers. This headdress visor may also be related to the fiber combs worn by initiation novices in the central and northern Kuba regions (Cornet 1982:219).

Among Shoowa peoples living in the northern Kuba region, the headdresses of first-time expectant mothers were also extended with the addition of an elaborate horseshoe shaped headdress sculpted from *tool*, a red cosmetic powder which has long been important to the Kuba in both secular and ritual contexts.[9] *Tool* is created from a mixture of ground camwood and palm oil. The mixture is formed into balls or sculpted into various shapes and stored for future use. Torday notes that at the Ngongo capital of Misumba both men and women liberally covered their bodies and heads with *tool*. In the 1980s we occasionally met elderly Kuba women who still applied this cosmetic to their bodies regularly. Over an extended period of time its use imparted a distinctive reddish tonality to the skin.

Today, all Kuba periodically shave their heads for hygienic reasons. Men and women also shave their heads upon the death of members of their immediate family. In Southern Kuba culture, the heads of novices entering the forest initiation camp are shaved, symbolically suggesting their immature status (Binkley 1987b, 1990).[10] After a period of seclusion and instruction they are presented to the community in festive dances as adult members of society. On these occasions they wear long woven raffia

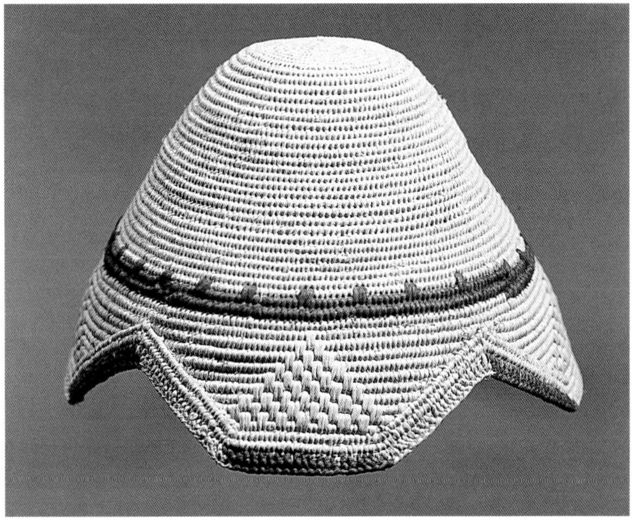

**Figure 9.2.** Hat. Kuba, Zaire. Raffia. H. 10.5 cm. Private collection. This is one of the most common forms of hats *(laket)* worn by adult men. A small, circular cap with a scalloped edge, this form is the foundation for more elaborate Kuba hat styles. This example is embellished with surface embroidery in a contrasting color which emphasizes the body and scalloped lobes or "ears" of the hat.

skirts and often a small conical hat *(laket)* that designates their newly achieved adult status (Fig. 9.2). In this regard, Kuba hats have been associated, at least in early twentieth century literature, with the acculturation of young men.[11] The successful completion of initiation was also considered a prerequisite for marriage. The American missionary William H. Sheppard (1917:132) notes that

> [b]efore a man takes his wife he must, bearing a present, proceed to King Lukenga, seek an audience, and have the king with his own hands place the hat on his head and run the pin through. No young man is permitted to wear a hat or marry a girl, it matters not how many days' journey he lives from the capital, until he sees the king and receives the blessing by the hat process.[12]

## KUBA HATS AND TITLEHOLDING

The emphasis on titleholding and the competition for and the subsequent prestige that accrues to titleholders is a dominant aspect of Kuba culture (Vansina 1964, 1978; Binkley 1987a). Kuba hats are important visual manifestations of Kuba ideas about ethnicity and leadership. Each titled position has emblems, symbols, and praise names associated with it. Titleholding is dominated by men; there are only two titles held by women. For men, the importance of distinguishing headgear has remained constant throughout the twentieth century. Even for men who choose Western-style clothing, the *laket* is often worn as a symbol of cultural identity and as a principal means by which a man can declare his titled position.

For special occasions the wearing of the *laket* is still imperative. This is especially true at funeral dances or dances held in conjunction with initiation rituals. On

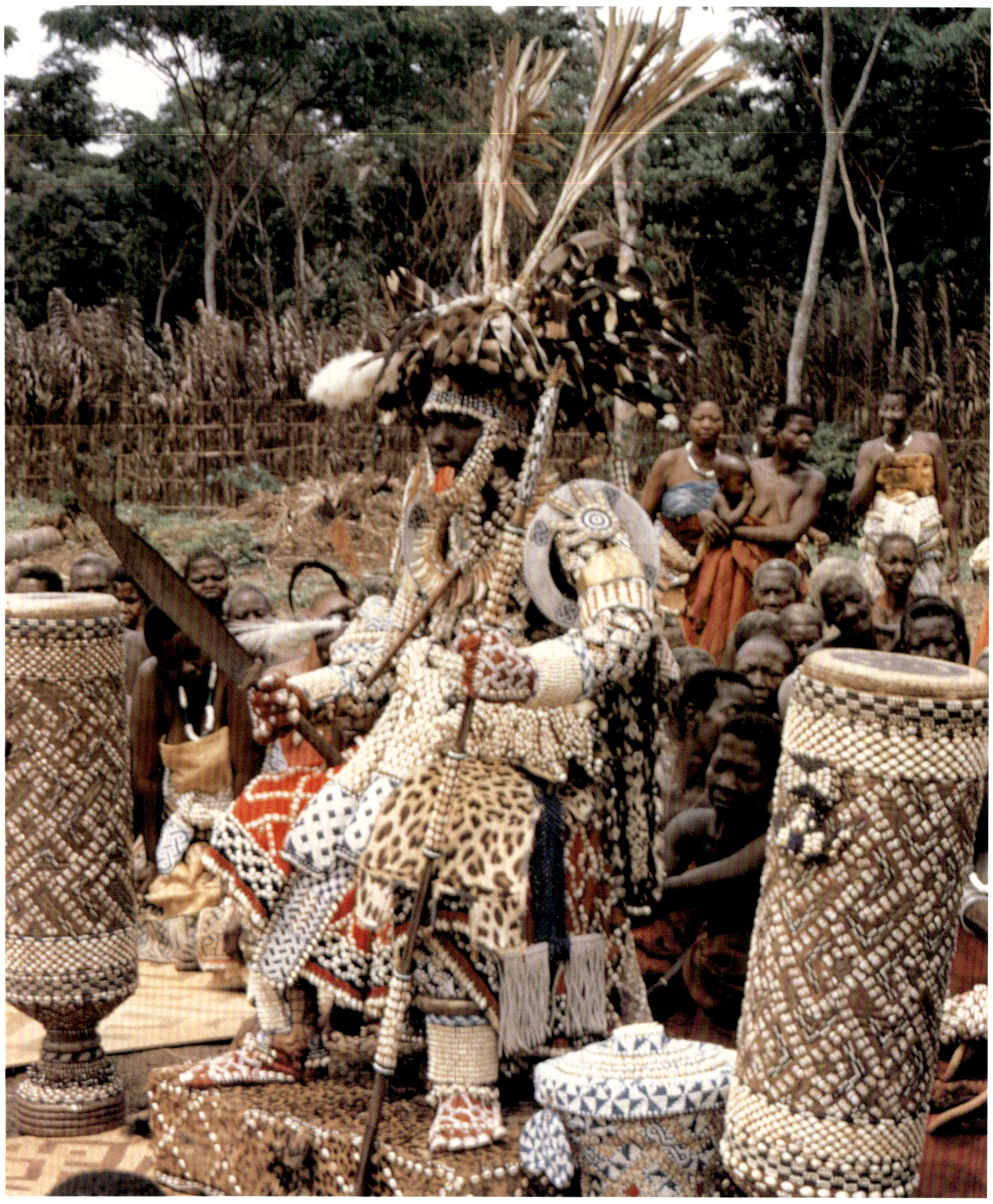

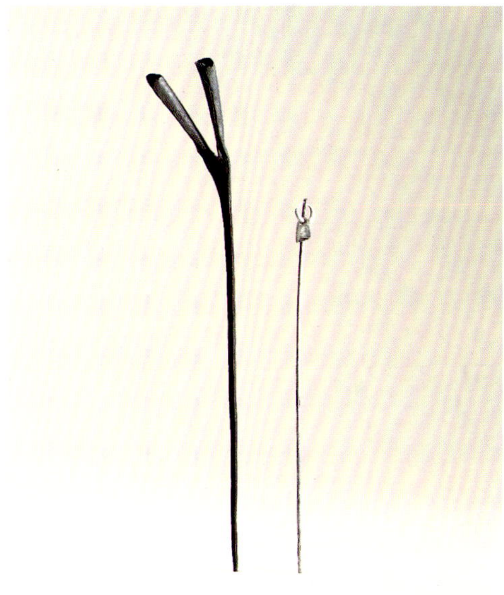

**Figure 9.3a**, above left. Featherholder. Kuba, Zaire. Iron. Some hat pins also serve as featherholders. They may hold two or more feathers. This example was acquired from a Kuba soldier. **Figure 9.3b**, above right. Hat pin *(ndwong angwoong).* Kuba, Zaire. Iron, brass, aluminum. Private collection. The most common hat pins are made of iron and aluminum, or entirely of brass. A miniature bell is affixed to the end of the pin by a ring. Pins made from brass clearly articulate a person's elevated rank even when they are worn with a common everyday *laket.*

**Figure 9.4**, opposite. Kuba *nyim* (king) Kot a Mbweeky III, in state dress with royal drums at Mushenge, Zaire. Photograph by Eliot Elisofon, 1971. Slide no. C KBA 2 (2139). Eliot Elisofon Photographic Archives. National Museum of African Art.

these occasions, the *laket* becomes a means by which the individual can display those particular emblems that articulate one's social standing. One of the most visible emblems of elevated rank is the wearing of a brass hat pin. Hat pins are made of iron and aluminum or entirely of brass. A miniature bell is affixed to the end of the pin by a ring.[13] Nineteenth-century travelers to the Kuba region note that among the prerogatives of the paramount ruler was the right to wear brass. This included not only brass jewelry but also brass hat pins.[14] Even today, hat pins made of brass clearly articulate a person's elevated rank.[15] Non-titled or low-ranking titled officials display hat pins made of iron and aluminum. The hat pin is usually worn so that the bell is suspended just above the center of the forehead (Fig. 9.3).

Some high-ranking Kuba men wear two hat pins. One is typically of brass with a miniature bell; the other, often in a different style, is worn at right angles to the first with the decorated end positioned over the right ear of the wearer.[16] The wearing of two pins has been explained as indicating an individual who is a personal acquaintance of the Kuba paramount ruler *(nyim).*

The most visible insignia of titleholding associated with hats and headdresses is the specific bird feather *(lashal)* worn by each titleholder. Each title is associated with a particular bird whose characteristics the titleholder is thought to share. The highest titled officials in the region are eagle feather chiefs *(kum apoong)* who have the right to wear eagle feathers in their hats and headdresses. Eagles are thought to be the most powerful birds in the daytime sky. Directly below the rank of chief is the *kikaam,* who is chief of the initiation society and wears an owl feather in his hat. Owls are considered to be the rulers of the forest and the night sky. Other titles include the *cik'l,* who wears a parrot feather, and the titleholders *mbeem* and *mbyeeng* who are permitted to wear guinea fowl feathers in their *laket* (Vansina 1964:126–8, Binkley 1987a:77–9).[17]

The angle of the feather as it is worn on the hat is also significant. *Kum apoong* wear one or more eagle feathers standing vertically in their hats or headdresses while Kuba soldiers *(iyol)* may wear eagle feathers, but they are worn horizontally in the hat. For the highest titled officials such as *kum apoong,* multiples of different feathers are worn on their most elaborate headdresses. It is the accumulative nature of Kuba costuming, encompassing not only feathers but beads, shell, brass, and copper which is characteristic of Kuba royal display at the highest level (Fig. 9.4).

## KUBA HATS: SHAPES OF AUTHORITY

A basic Kuba man's hat *(laket)* is essentially a small, domed cap worn on the crown of the head and held in place with a metal hat pin. All Kuba hats are created from undyed raffia fiber using the basketry technique of coiling. The circular shape of the basic *laket* is completed with a scalloped edge of four projections called "ears" *(mato;* Cornet 1982:213). The *laket* is worn so that one of the ears is always squarely centered on the

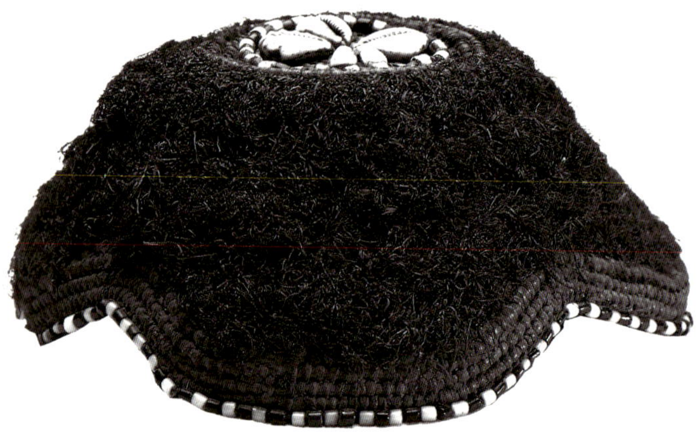

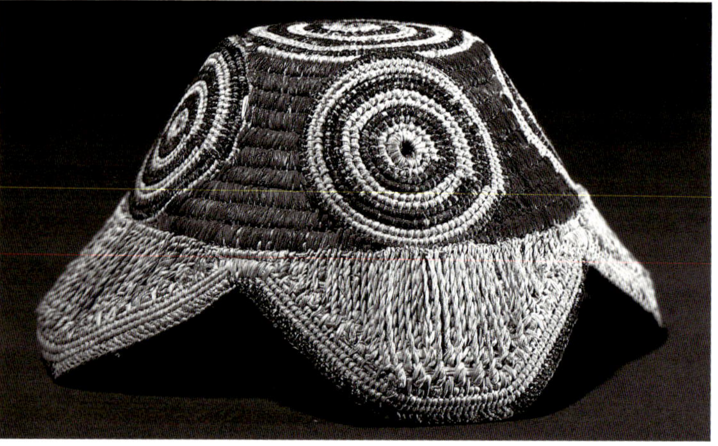

**Figure 9.5**, above left. Hat *(laket)*. Kuba, Zaire. Raffia, cowrie shells, glass beads. H. 8.0 cm. Private collection. A variation of the basic Kuba hat *(laket)*. The surface is decorated with embroidered cut-pile and the flat dome of the hat is adorned with a quatre-foil of cowries encircled by black and white beads. The edges of the hat are outlined with black, blue, and yellow beads.

**Figure 9.6**, above, right. Hat *(laket mishiing)*. Kuba, Zaire. Raffia. H. 9.5 cm. Private collection. This is a variation of a common Kuba hat known as *laket mishiing. Laket mishiing* are recognized by the addition of "strings" or *mishiing* to the scalloped lower edges or "ears" of the hat. Four smaller coils are sewn over the coiled foundation of the hat.

**Figure 9.7a,** below left. Hat *(laket mishiing)*. Kuba, Zaire. Raffia. H. 11.5 cm. Private collection. A variation of the coiling technique is seen in this version of *laket mishiing* or "hat with strings." The foundation coils include decorative openwork between rows of coiling which is enhanced by contrasting colors of surface embroidery. **Figure 9.7b,** below right. Hat *(laket mishiing ingyeeng)*. Kuba, Zaire. Raffia. H. 13.0 cm. Private collection. Known to the Bushoong as *laket lishaash ingyeeng*, this hat is in form a doubling of the hat known as *laket mishiing*; the style represents one small "hat with strings" sitting atop another one. The right to wear this hat is limited to two important community titleholders, the *mbeem* and the *mbyeeng*.

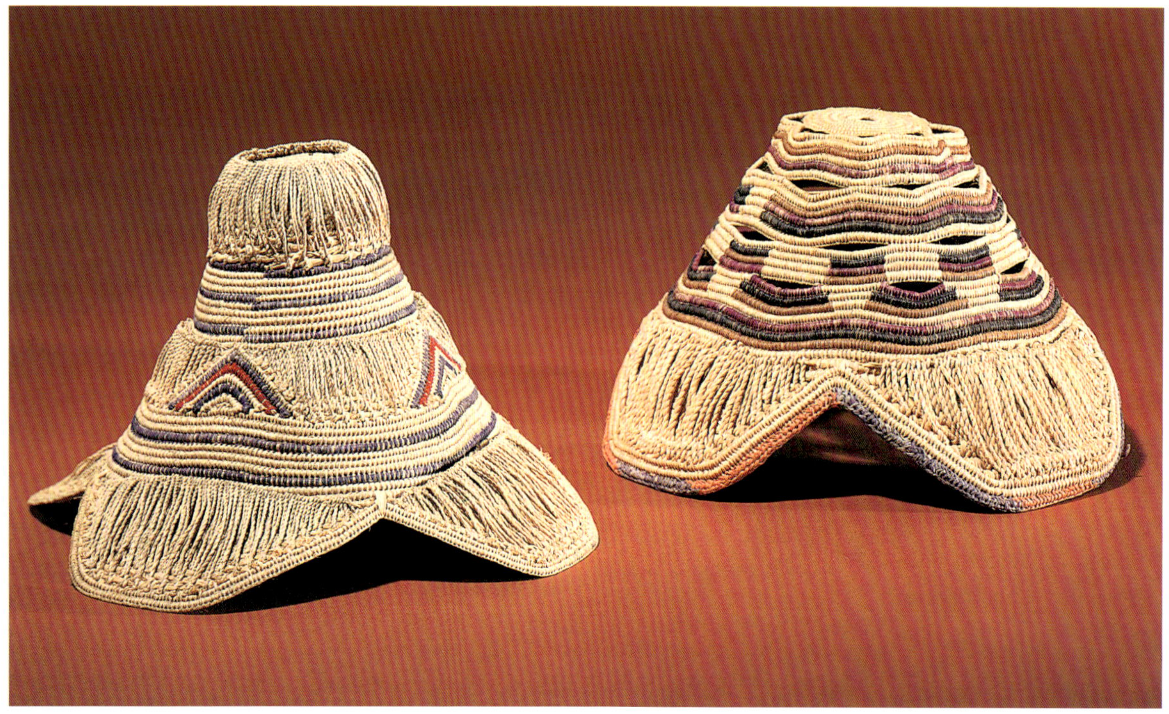

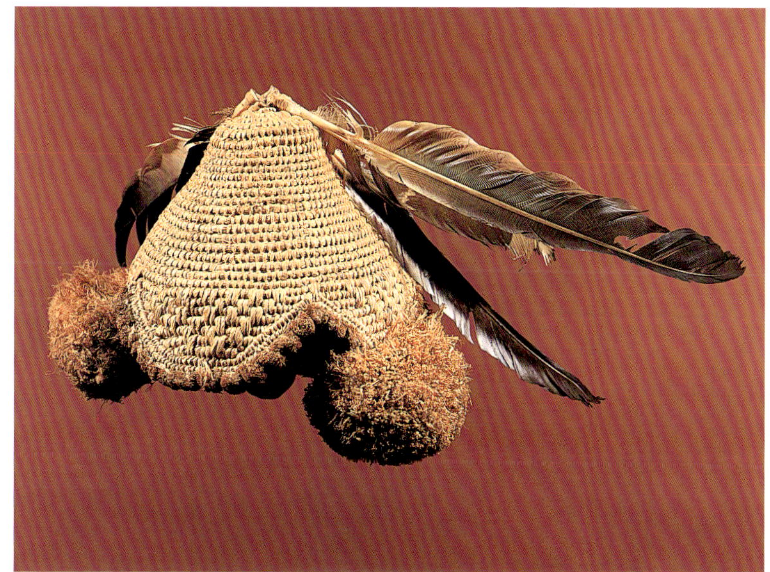

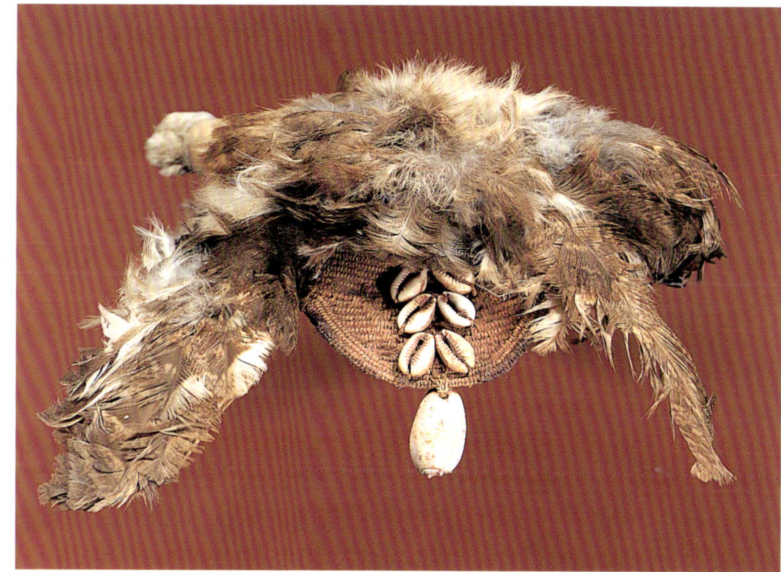

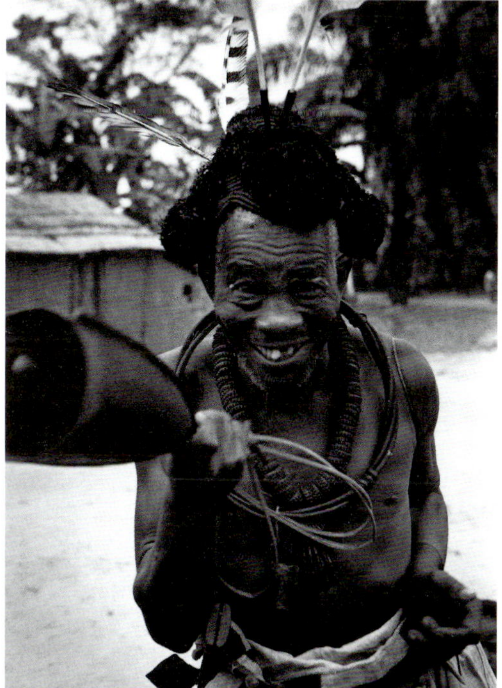

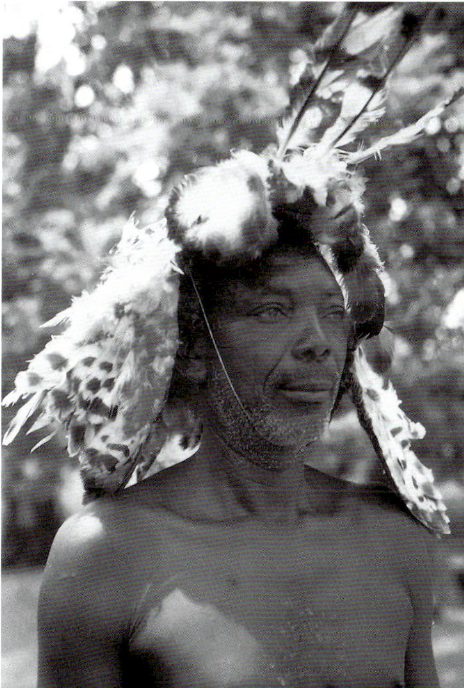

**Figure 9.8**, above left. Hat. Kuba, Zaire. Raffia, feathers. H. 25.0 cm. Private collection. This type of hat is only worn by titled soldiers *(iyol)*. Stylistically it relates to the basic *laket* form, but is often more coarsely sewn and includes larger "ears" which are trimmed with four large round tufts or poms of raffia. Together with village chiefs, titleholders of the *iyol* class have the right to wear eagle feathers.

**Figure 9.9**, far left. Kumuashibuanga, a Northern Kete titled soldier. Bansueba, 1981. Photograph by David A. Binkley and Patricia Darish.

**Figure 9.10**, above right. Hat. Kuba, Zaire. Raffia, feathers, cowrie shells, shell. H. 8.0 cm. Private collection. This hat is part of the extensive regalia worn by Kuba soldiers. A conical *laket* forms the support foundation for the body of an eagle whose wings hang down on either side of the wearer's head.

**Figure 9.11,** left. A Bushoong soldier wearing a hat embellished with the feathered body of an eagle. Shongaam, 1981. Photograph by David A. Binkley and Patricia Darish.

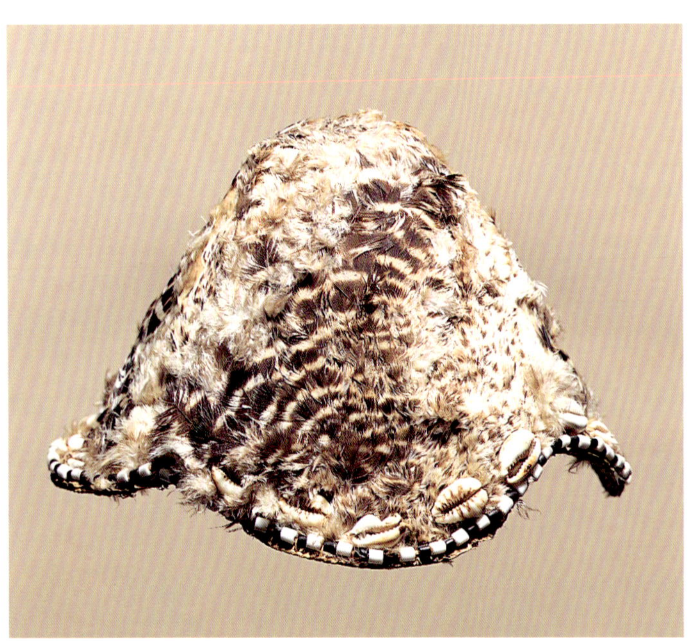

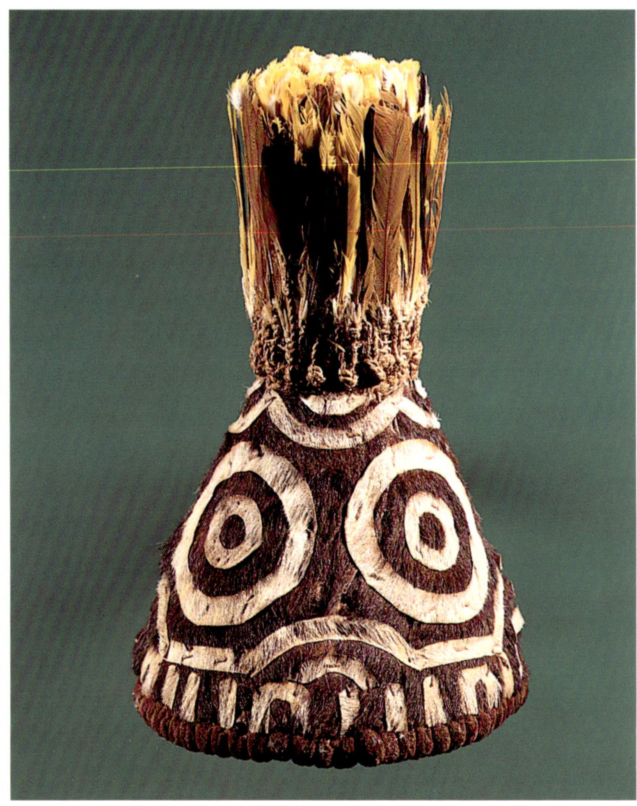

**Figure 9.12**, left. Hat. Kuba, Zaire. Raffia, feathers, cowrie shells, glass beads. H. 11.5 cm. Private collection. Hats that are covered with eagle feather down and bordered with cowrie shells and beads are the prerogative of village chiefs throughout the Kuba area.

**Figure 9.13**, right. Hat *(lapuum)*. Kuba, Zaire. Raffia, feathers, hide. H. 23 cm. Collection of Craig A. Subler. The hat known as *lapuum* is reserved for the *nyim* and senior male titleholders. The coiled foundation of the hat is covered with animal skin and appliqued designs, also cut from skins. The top of the hat is usually completed with red feathers from the gray parrot, symbols of the highest ranked titleholders. The use of yellow feathers here is unusual.

face with a hat pin running through the hair from the front to the back of the hat.

The many surface textures and patterns of the *laket* reflect the variations possible with the coiling technique and the skillful manipulation of the hatmaker, who is a male specialist. Surface embroidery also changes the color and texture of the *laket.* The *laket* is often embellished with embroidery in a contrasting color which emphasizes the circular dome and body of the cap.[18] Surface embroidery in a contrasting color also wraps the coiling to decorate and delineate the widest circumference of the hat and accent the hat's bottom edges. In addition, the ears of the hat provide another area for surface design; they are often embroidered with split or spaced stitches to create an embroidered pattern of a triangular shape. This design is usually sewn in a neutral color, although a contrasting thread color can also be used. These accents of overlaid embroidery can be seen on the examples of ordinary hats. Another common feature is the addition of *mishiing* or "strings" to each of the four ears. For this, the quadrant of each ear is oversewn with two to three tightly spaced rows of twisted raffia thread, adding a sculptural quality to the hat. Both the basic *laket* with surface embroidery and the *laket mishiing* are the most common hats worn by titled and non-titled adult men (Figs. 9.5, 9.6, 9.7).

Many variations of the basic *laket* are possible given the versatility of the coiling technique. Another hat style known as *laket lishaash ingyeeng* is a creative doubling of the ordinary form of *laket mishiing*; the hat represents one *laket mishiing*

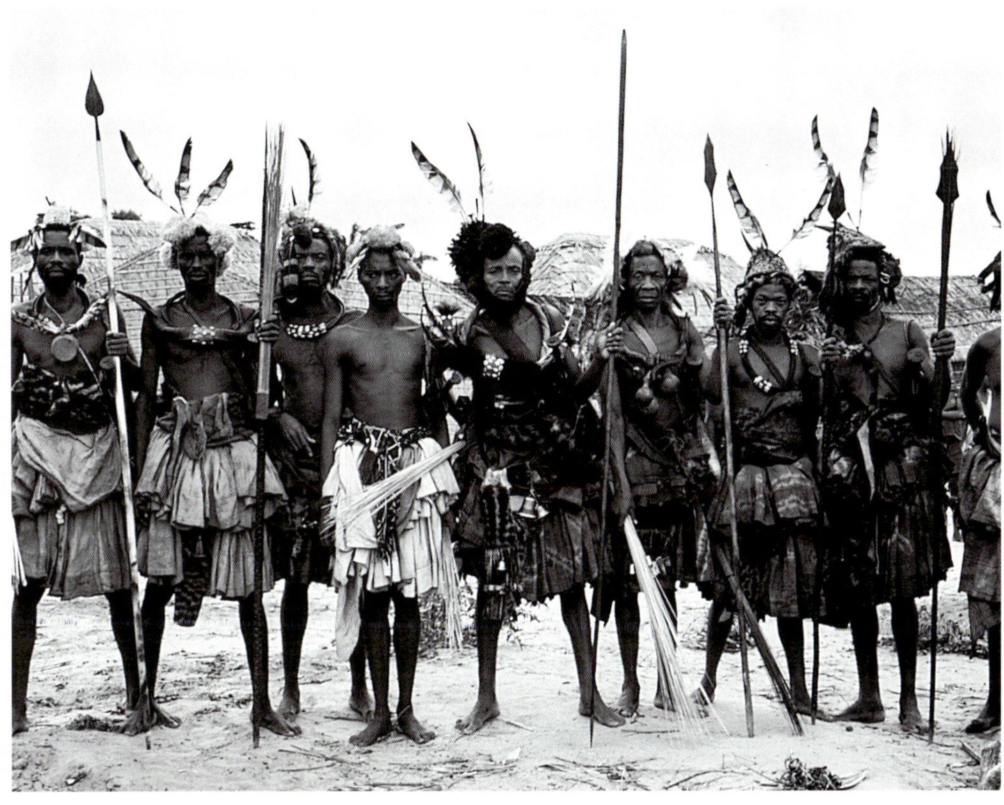

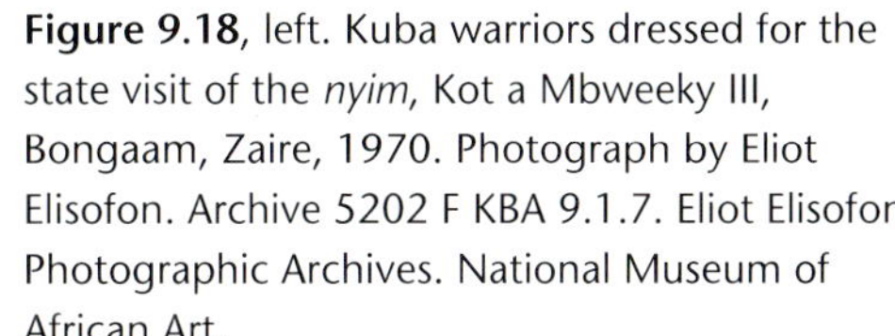

**Figure 9.18**, left. Kuba warriors dressed for the state visit of the *nyim*, Kot a Mbweeky III, Bongaam, Zaire, 1970. Photograph by Eliot Elisofon. Archive 5202 F KBA 9.1.7. Eliot Elisofon Photographic Archives. National Museum of African Art.

**Figure 9.20**, below. Hat. Kuba, Zaire. Raffia. H. 9.5 cm. Private collection. Hats with bills are rarely seen in the Kuba area. This example covered with cut-pile is certainly based upon a Western prototype and clearly demonstrates the innovative nature of Kuba hatmakers.

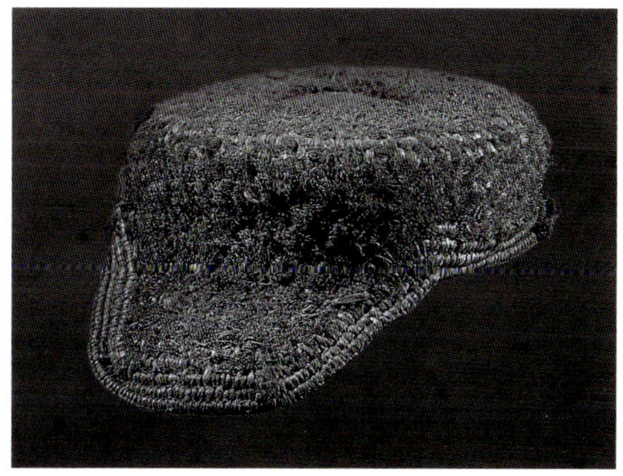

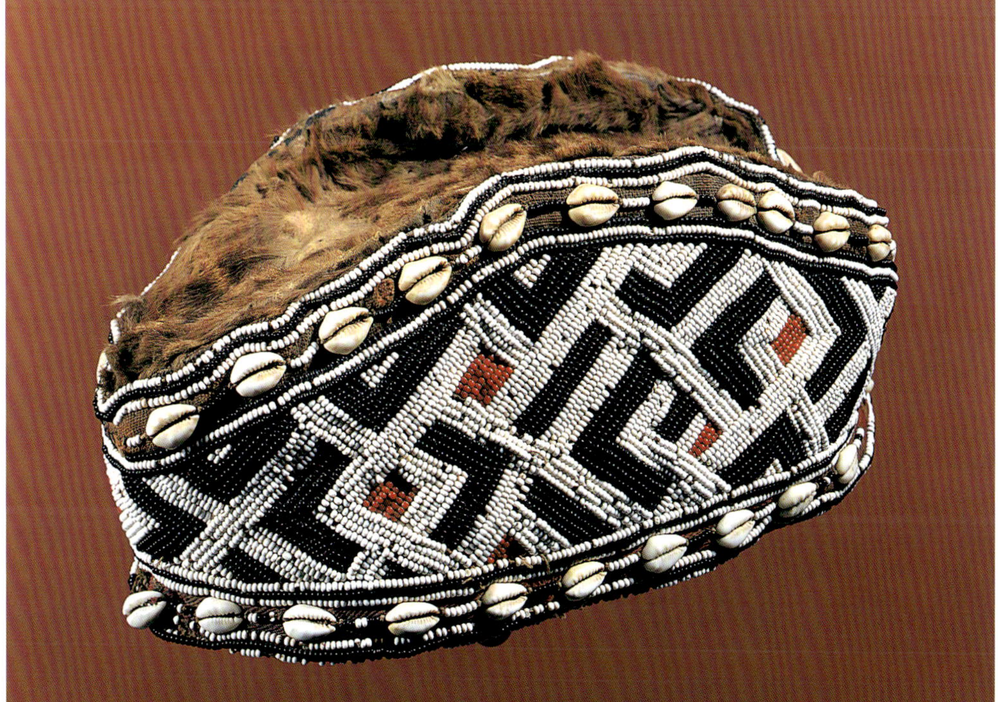

**Figure 9.19**, left. Hat. Kuba, Zaire. Raffia, cloth, glass beads, cowrie shells, fur. H. 12.0 cm. Collection of Robert Alan Friedman. This hat is a variation of the style made of leopard skin worn by the president of Zaire, Mobutu Sese Seko, as well as by titleholders including the current Kuba paramount ruler. President Mobutu's image wearing this hat and a spotted ascot was widely displayed in Zaire on postage stamps and photographs in government and commercial buildings. Hats and regalia displaying leopard and other spotted cat fur are important symbols of chieftanship throughout Central Africa.

Based on a European military hat, similar styles were worn by the "Tirailleurs Sénégalais" (West Africans serving in the French colonial army) in the 1950s (Echenberg 1991:124). A similar style of leopard skin hat was also popular among Belgian women during the same era (Marc Leo Felix, personal communication, 1994).

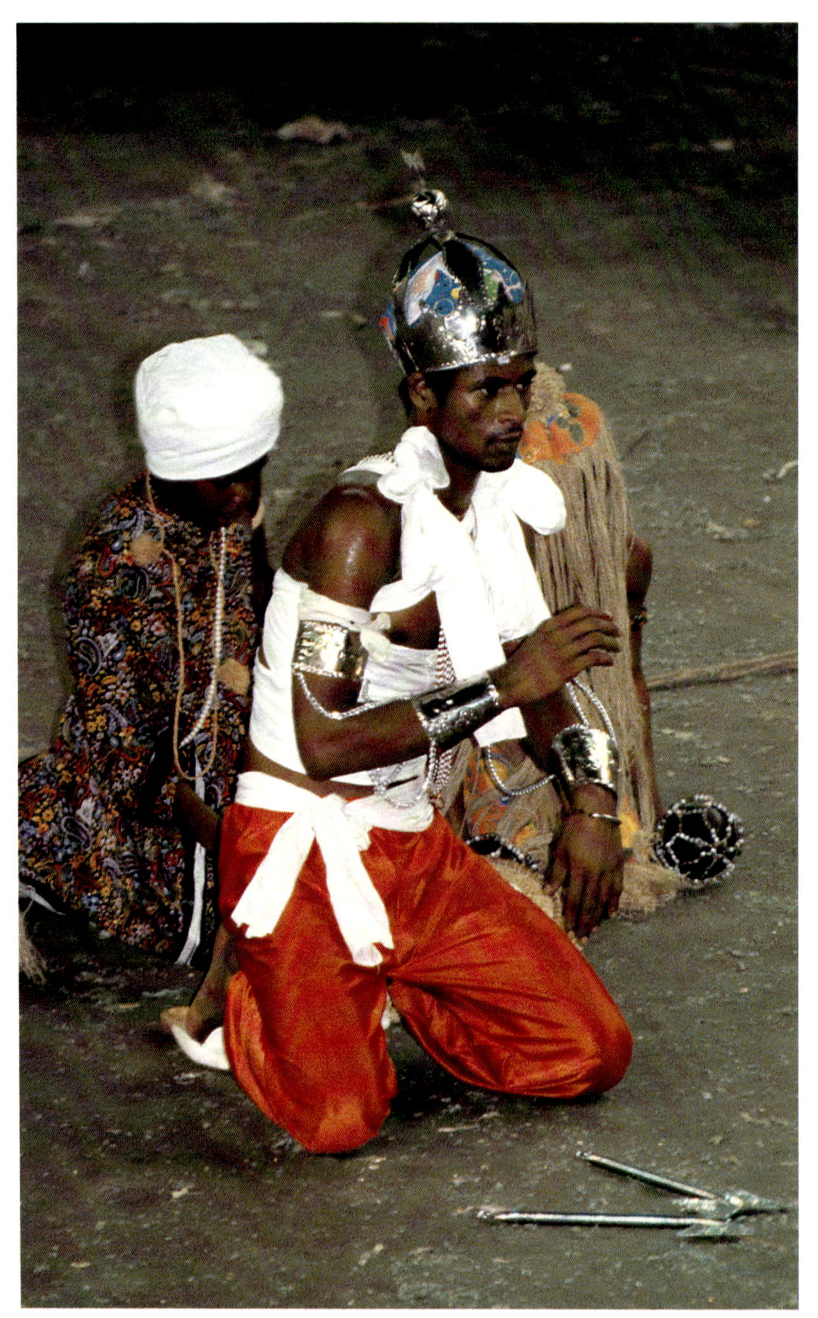

# 10 TRANSATLANTIC INFLUENCES IN HEADWEAR

CHRISTINE MULLEN KREAMER

African styles of dress and personal adornment have had a significant impact on the Western fashion world. When Kwame Nkrumah chose to wear *kente* cloth at Ghana's independence day celebrations in 1957 and on subsequent visits to the United Nations, he brought into public view a Ghanaian-based fashion that held then, and holds today, considerable political and cultural significance. Worn by traditional chiefs and men of status in southern Ghana, *kente* cloth is associated with political and social prominence. K*ente* cloth has become a symbol of African empowerment. These associations are not lost on African-Americans, or on other Americans from diverse ethnic and racial backgrounds, who have incorporated *kente* cloth into various modes of dress.

## CONTEMPORARY FASHION

*Kente*-inspired fashions include handbags, shirts, shorts, ensembles, and hats (Fig. 10.1). These may be made entirely with *kente* cloth, or strips and smaller pieces may be used as decorative accents. The popularity of Ghanaian narrow-strip weaving has made *kente* cloth not only recognized, but *the* name for a variety of cloth from other parts of Africa. *Kente* — whether it is hand-woven in Ghana on traditional narrow-strip looms, or machine-made by workers in factories in Côte d'Ivoire and New Jersey — has become the symbol *par excellence* for cloth that is immediately recognizable as African. Its association, in Ghana and the United States, as a prestige cloth worn by Ghanaian royals and individuals of high status makes *kente* cloth an appropriate material for high fashion and its more popularized off-shoots. In the United States, strips of *kente* cloth are worn draped over the shoulders by ministers as part of liturgical garb and by African-American politicians as a link with the African homeland. It is wrapped around the waist as belts; it is sewn into shoulder bags and back-

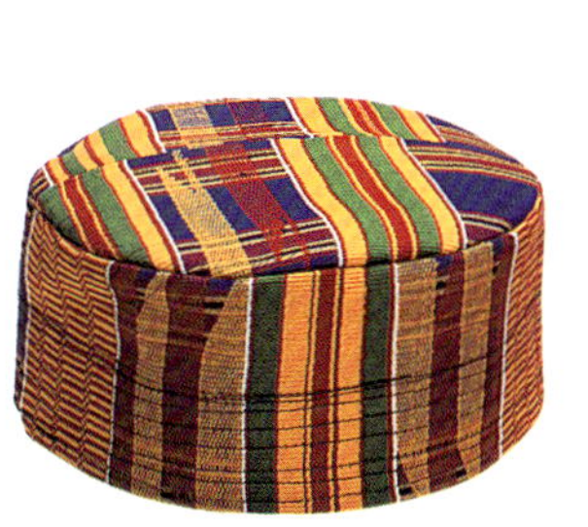

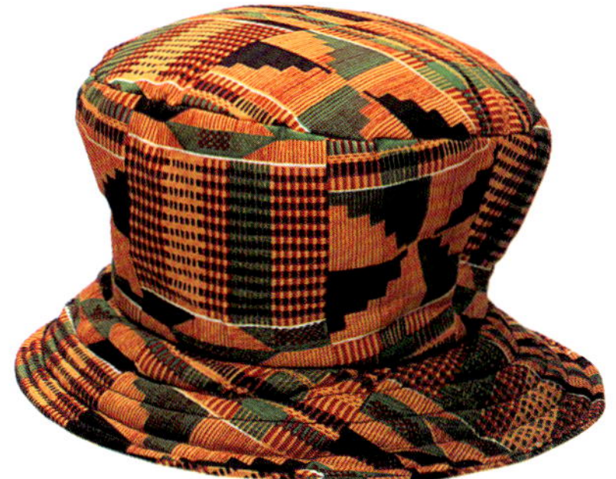

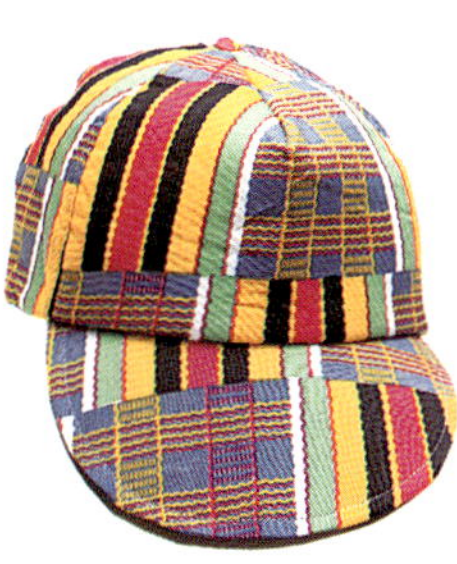

**Figure 10.1**, left. *Kente* cloth hats. United States. Cotton cloth. a. FMCH X94.28.2; b. X94.28.1; c. X94.26.2. Greatest height: 14.0 cm. Museum purchase. Southern Ghana's colorful, narrow-strip woven cloth called *kente* has provided inspiration for a wide variety of popular attire including hats. These hats draw on a number of styles including the American baseball hat, the Tanzanian cap, and a fanciful "Mad Hatter" style hat that may be related to Jamaican Rastafarianism. While some of the *kente* cloth clothing available for sale in the United States is tailored from narrow-strip cloth woven in Ghana, broad-loom, machine-made *kente* (manufactured in Africa, Europe, and the United States) has expanded the possibilities of using the fabric for articles of clothing as well as fashion accents.

**Opposite.** Individuals representing Xangô and Omolu from the Carnaval group "Mestiço da África." Salvador da Bahia. Brazil. Photograph by Doran H. Ross, 1981.

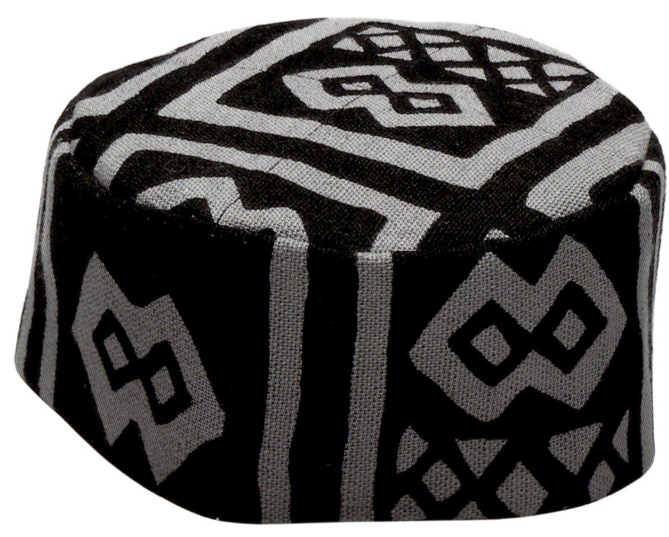

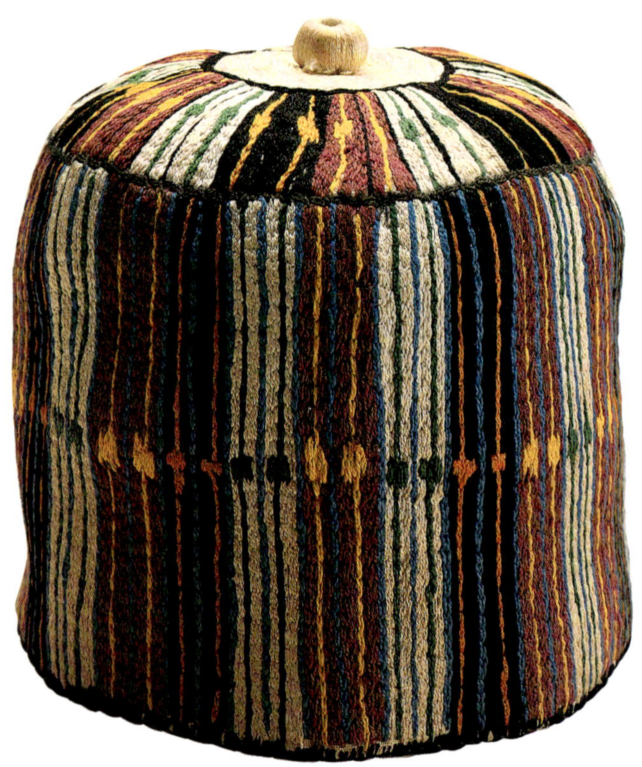

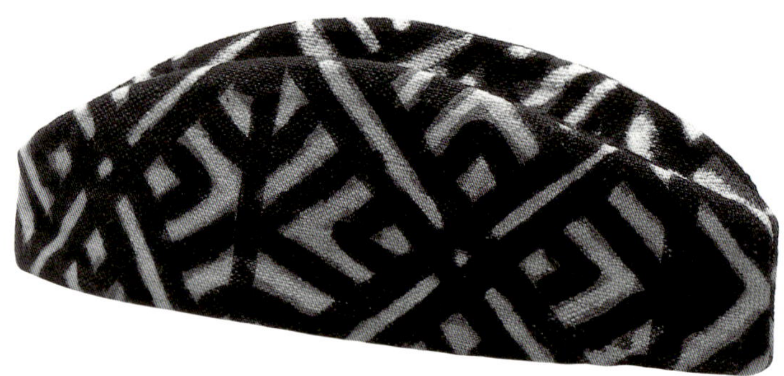

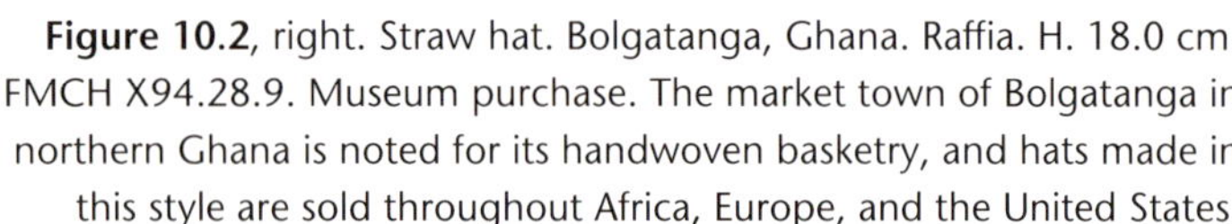

**Figure 10.2**, right. Straw hat. Bolgatanga, Ghana. Raffia. H. 18.0 cm. FMCH X94.28.9. Museum purchase. The market town of Bolgatanga in northern Ghana is noted for its handwoven basketry, and hats made in this style are sold throughout Africa, Europe, and the United States.

**Figure 10.3**, above right. Embroidered hat. Hausa, Nigeria. Cotton. H. 17.0 cm. FMCH X89.119. Museum purchase, Manus Fund.

**Figure 10.4**, above. Mud-cloth hats. a. United States. Cotton, polyester. H. 8.0 cm. X94.28.13. Museum purchase; b. Bamana, Mali. Mud-cloth, cotton. H. 9.0 cm. FMCH X94.28.12. Museum purchase. The traditional mud-dyed cloth of the Bamana of Mali, *bogolanfini,* has been transformed into a wide range of contemporary fashions. Mud-cloth headwear includes American-style baseball caps, as well as Islamic-inspired skull caps.

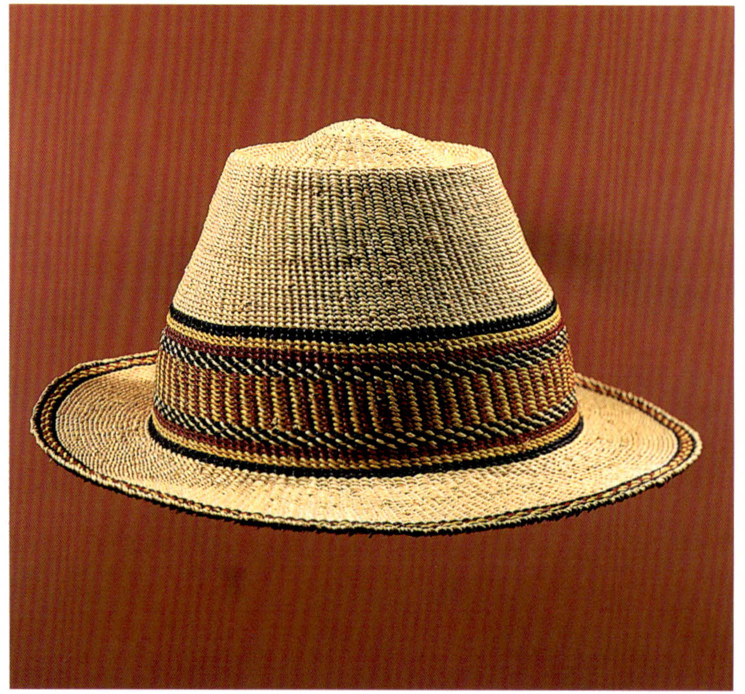

packs carried by trendy young adults; it is tailored into caps and baseball caps worn by young men; and it is sewn into high-fashion ensembles and separates.

Kwame Nkrumah's high-visibility introduction of *kente* cloth on a global, public level in the late 1950s was met in the 1960s in the United States by a growing interest in African-inspired dress. Some of this impetus came from Peace Corps volunteers returning from two-year assignments in Africa, who were exposed to African fashions. In those politically charged times, colorful tunic-style *dashiki* shirts for men and kaftans for women became part of the liberal fashion scene for college students and young adults, suggesting, perhaps, a measure of political awareness and growing support for the black power movement.

**Figure 10.5a,b**, below. McCall's pattern P473, front and back. Paper. H. 21.5 cm. Anonymous loan. A full range of patterns for African-inspired ensembles and separates is available through McCall's Fashions.

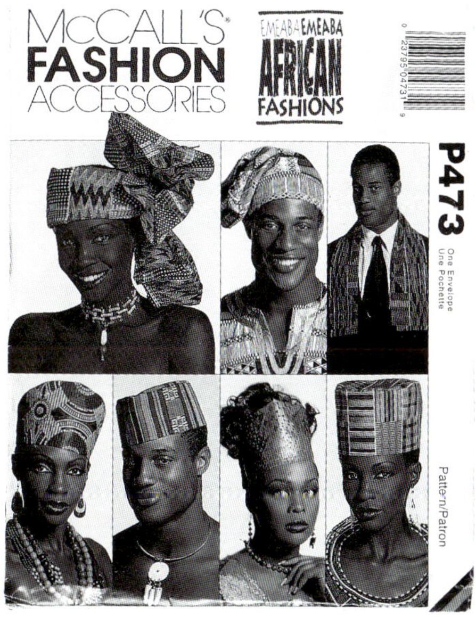


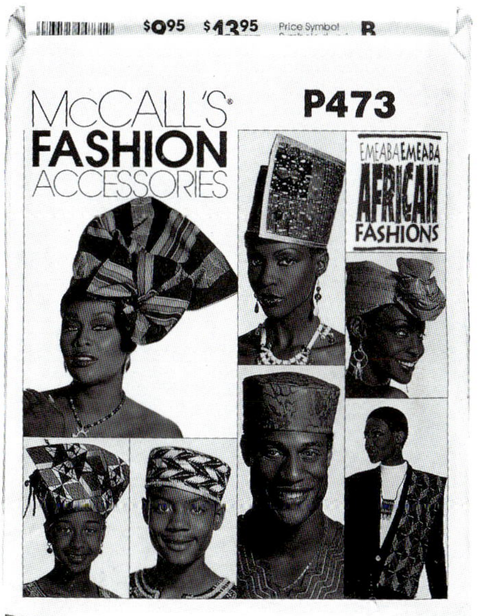


The story of *kente's* rise to prominence in the American fashion industry is one that has been repeated — with varying degrees of intensity and success — by a considerable number of African-inspired fashions. Among the more long-established headwear from Africa available for sale in the United States is the wide-brimmed Bolgatanga basketry hat (Fig. 10.2). The Bolgatanga basket industry in northern Ghana produces a wide range of containers, fans, and broad-brimmed hats for sale in local, regional, and international markets. Bolgatanga wares are sturdy and decorated attractively with alternating bands of red, yellow, black, and other colors. The shape and subdued colors seem to appeal to Western as well as African markets, for the hats are popular throughout West Africa as well as in shops and street stalls in the United States. In northern Ghana, these basketry hats are worn by men as they work in the fields or make their way across the hot savanna landscape to the village market. In the United States, men and women purchase them for wall decorations or hats.

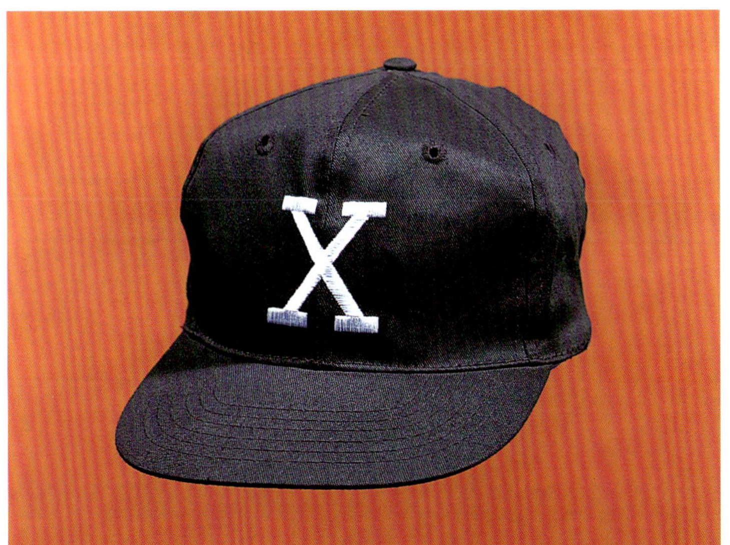


**Figure 10**. Malcolm X baseball hat. Cotton, polyester, plastic. H. 13.0 cm. Lent by Frances Tabbush.

Africa's association with the Islamic faith may have prompted the popularity of caps among African-American men in the past few decades. Although today, a wide range of caps are imported from Africa and the Middle East, the original model from Africa was probably the embroidered Hausa-style cap brought in by Nigerian traders. White cloth caps, decorated with

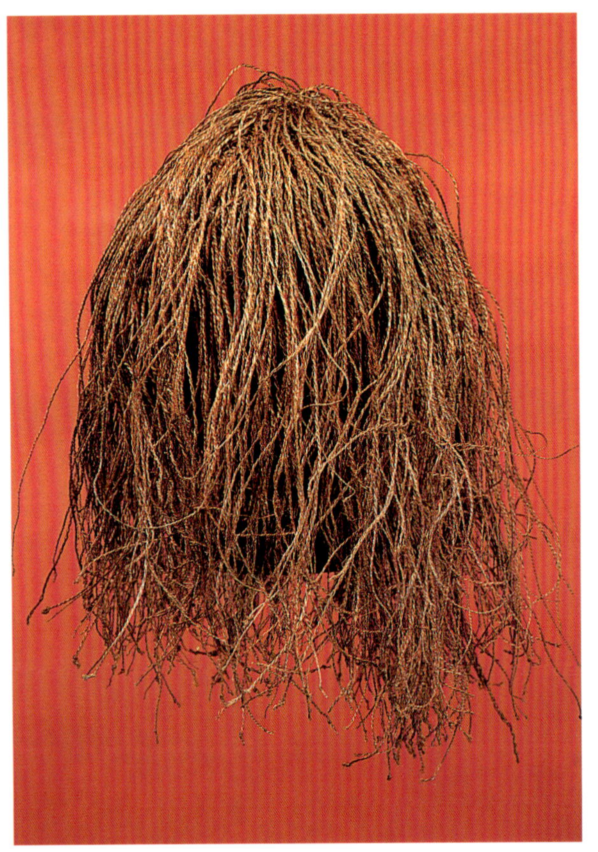

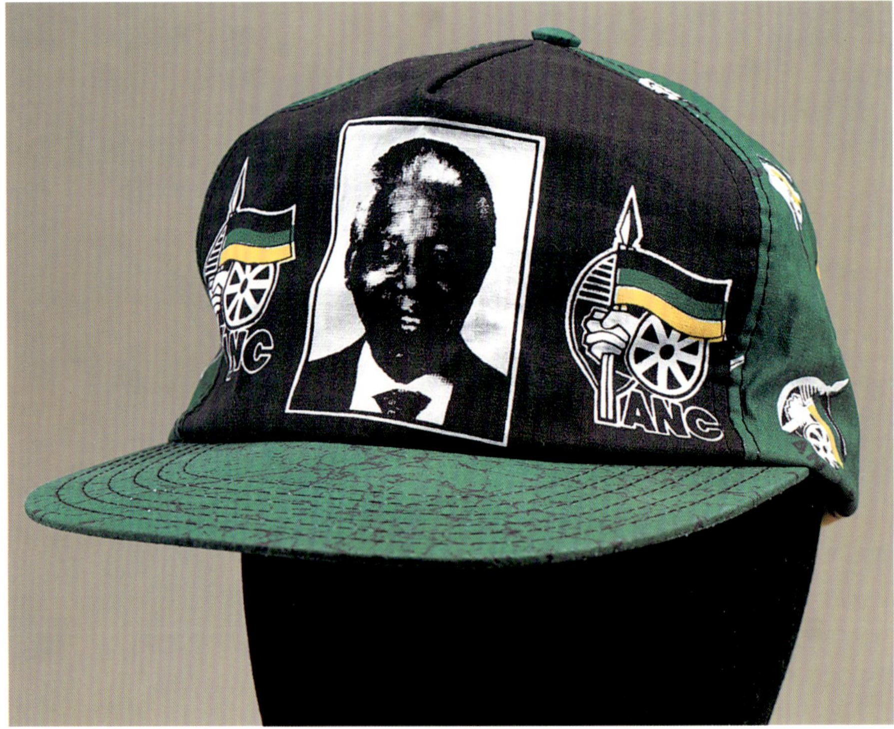


**Figure 10.7**, above. "Peter Tosh" wig. Rastafari, Zimbabwe. Sisal. H. 46.0 cm. Lent by Owen Moore. Following a successful performance in Zimbabwe of reggae superstar Peter Tosh, this style of wig began to appear in the local markets. Throughout much of Africa, reggae is a popular musical form and the faces of Bob Marley, Jimmy Cliff, and other reggae masters adorn tee shirts, caps, and posters.

**Figure 10.8**, above right. Baseball cap. South Africa. Cotton, polyester, plastic. H. 12.5 cm. FMCH X94.26.1. Museum purchase. This cap combines baseball imagery with a political promotion for Nelson Mandela and the African National Congress for the April 27, 1994 election.

white embroidered designs, are called *marafia* (Heathcote 1975:54). Still popular in Nigeria today, this style of cap is the precursor to more ornate and colorful varieties now being made in Nigeria (Fig. 10.3). The embroidered hat industry is sizeable in northern Nigeria, involving numerous people, from suppliers of material to artists and craftspeople.

Originally the work of men, the embroidered hat industry is now so viable in Nigeria that young boys and women are also participating in the work. Embroidered patterns range from references to elements of daily life — grains of corn, growing beans, ram's intestines, and pestles — to the natural environment, such as rainbow lizards and silk-cotton trees — to Islamic geometric designs from mosque architecture (Heathcote 1975: 58). The hats include close-fitting beenie-shaped caps and caps of a more rectangular shape that sit on top of the head rather than flat against the skull.

The influences go both ways. Leather caps, popularized in the United States in 1986 by the Eddie Murphy film *The Golden Child*, appear to draw on the Islamic caps as a model. These leather caps found their way to many West African cities where they were popular among the youth for some years during the late 1980s. In the United States, the leather model was combined with strips of *kente* that adorned the top or sides of the caps.

**Figure 10.9**, below left. Crown. United States. Velveteen, cotton, gold braid, paint. H. 13.0 cm. FMCH X94.28.16. Museum purchase. The importance of Egypt in the history of African civilizations is undeniable. These forms of headwear evoke a connection with Egypt, as does the wide range of Egyptian-influenced jewelry and clothing popular in contemporary fashion.

**Figure 10.10**, below right. Crown. United States. Cotton. H. 10.0 cm. FMCH X94.28.17. Museum purchase.

**Figure 10.11**, bottom. Hat. United States. Cotton, metal thread. H. 11.5 cm. FMCH X94.28.11. Museum purchase. The star-and-crescent motif is common in Islamic-inspired designs.

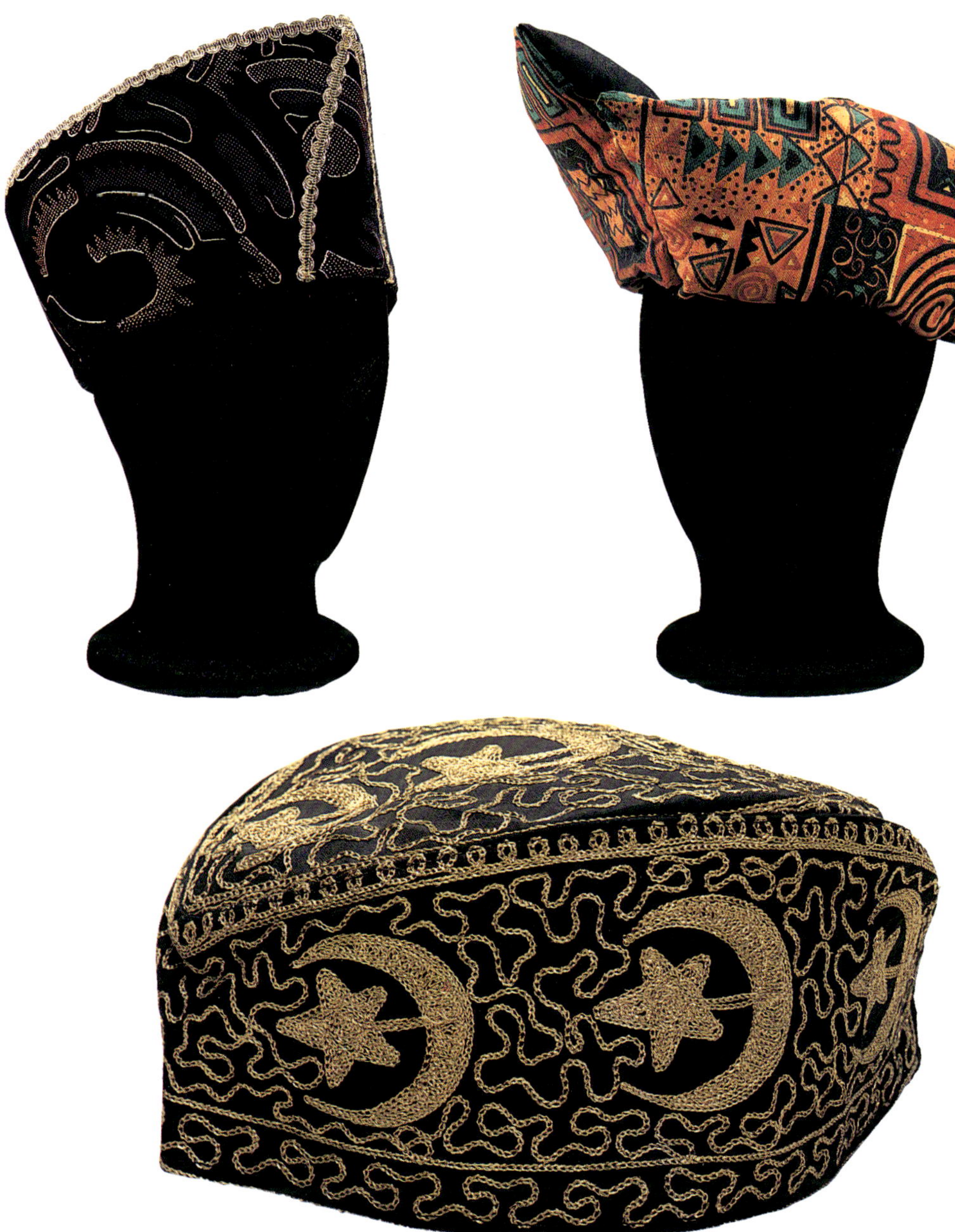

In addition to caps made of *kente*, hats made from Bamana mud-cloth called *bogolanfini* (Fig. 10.4) are now in vogue, sold along side *kente* caps. In their more traditional contexts in Mali, mud-dyed cloth caps with intricate geometric patterns are worn by men and women for major life transitions — birth, excision, marriage, and death. The geometric designs refer to common household objects, the flora and fauna of the surrounding environment, and Bamana cultural heroes, folk epics, songs, and proverbs with many of the motifs serving "as mnemonic devices or cues, which trigger broader reflections about the nature of life and aesthetics" (Aherne 1992:11). The cloth itself, and the technique of making it, have been incorporated into the work of a number of contemporary artists in Mali, such as the Groupe Bogolan Kasobane and Ismael Diabate (ibid.:15).

Malian mud-cloths are part of a growing urban fashion statement in Mali, where examples of the cloth and clothing tailored from it are purchased by Malians and tourists from other parts of West Africa, Europe, and America. The Malian clothing designer, Chris Seydou, created *bogolan* clothing in a predominantly European style. Realizing that more traditional mud-cloth designs were too complicated and visually saturated to suit European fashion tastes, Seydou began designing his own version of machine-printed fabrics with one or two predominant motifs that he uses in his international clothing line (Victoria

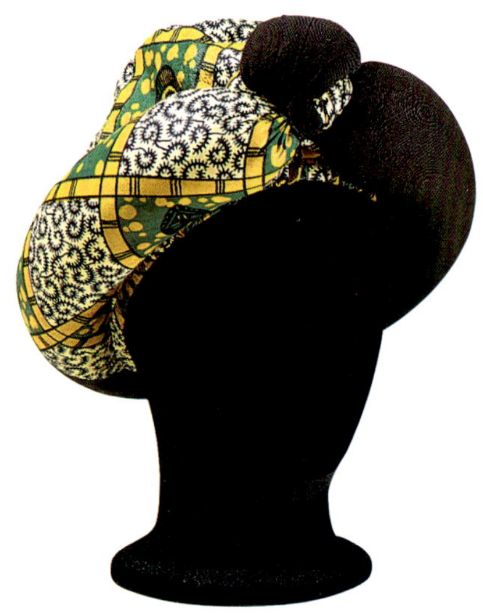

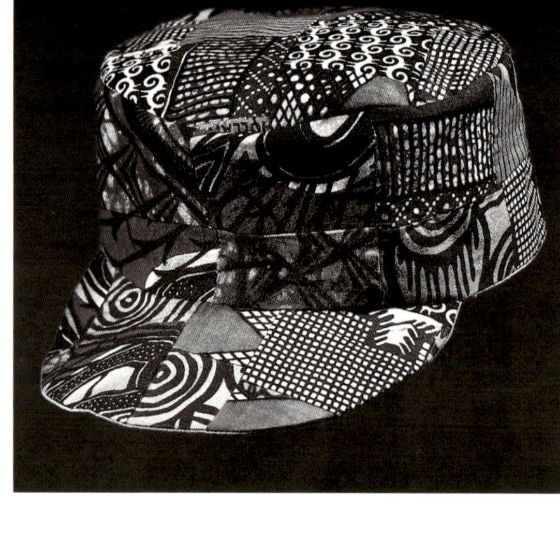

**Figure 10.13,** left. Baseball hat. Senegal, West Africa. Cotton, thread. H. 10.0 cm. FMCH X94.30.1. Museum purchase. In Senegal, patchwork cloth is commonly identified with the *Bay Fal*, a subgroup in the Muride Muslim brotherhood. In the 1980s, *Bay Fal* patchwork gained popular appeal and began to be used in urban areas to make hats, shirts, blouses, and trousers. Among the Ewe of southern Togo and Ghana, patchwork cloth called *asana* began as a way to recycle scraps of cloth, but now reflects the prestige of one who is able to purchase a variety of cloths and have them cut up, sewn together, and tailored into ensembles.

**Figure 10.12,** above. Cap with "halo." United States. Cotton, elastic. H. 16.5 cm. FMCH X94.28.18a,b. Museum purchase.

Rovine, personal communication 1994). Although Seydou's creations are on the high end of the fashion scale, Malian mud-cloth fashions (especially hats, vests, and bags) are available in shops, boutiques, and street stalls selling African-inspired clothing and accessories.

The availability and diversity of African-inspired clothing and accessories is clearly growing. Major retailers are capturing some of the market with small sections of their stores devoted to African and African-inspired fashions and accessories. J.C. Penney has a complete line of clothing, jewelry, and housewares (sheets, dishes, placemats, and napkins) that recall African designs, including Ghanaian *kente* and Malian mud-cloth patterns. Independent street vendors maintain a ready supply of items from or inspired by Africa. The Harlem Textile Works, among other fabric design shops, is creating a line of sheets and other household items derived from Bamana *bogolanfini* mud-cloth patterns. For those handy with a sewing machine, McCall's patterns offer low-cost options for creating elaborate headwear, shirts, dresses and jackets of African design (Fig. 10.5). Headties, *kente*-inspired caps, and tall, cylindrical caps complement flowing West African-style gowns and chic tunic and trouser

**Figure 10.14,** below. Hats. a. Collection of Owen Moore; b. Rasta "tam." Guatemala. Cotton. H. 16.5 cm. FMCH X94.28.4; c. Collection of Owen Moore; d. Baseball cap. Taiwan. Cotton, plastic. FMCH X94.28.3. Museum purchase. In the United States, the impact of Jamaican reggae music and Rastafarian religious beliefs on the popular culture has created a market for distinctive knit caps and oversized baseball caps that evoke the "Rasta" style.

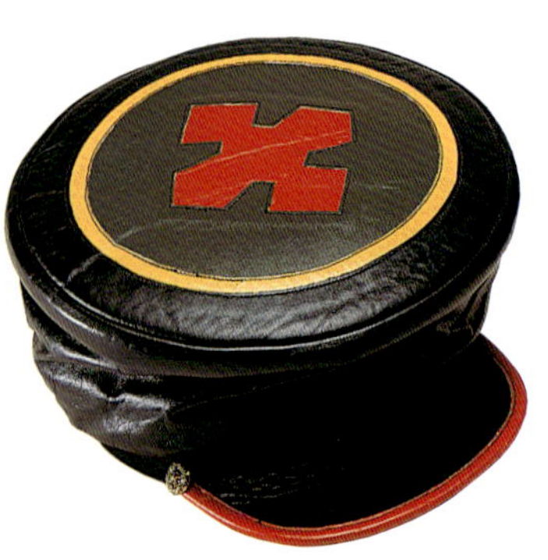

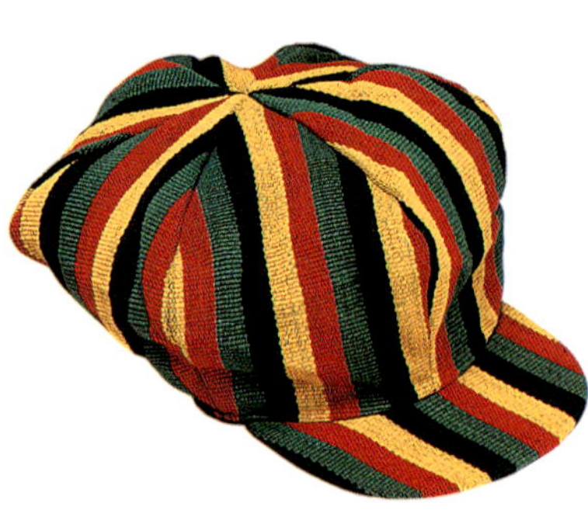

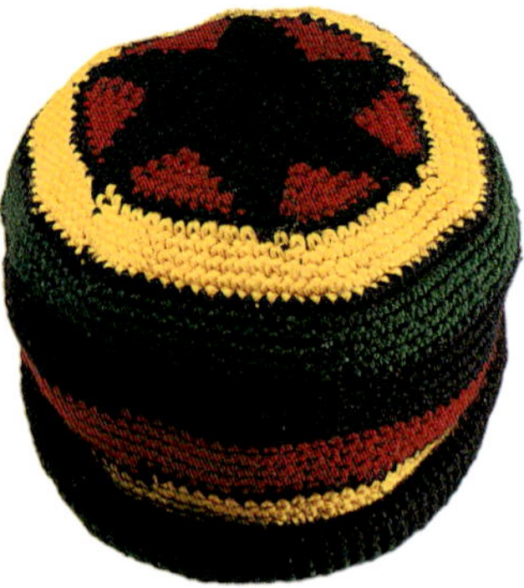

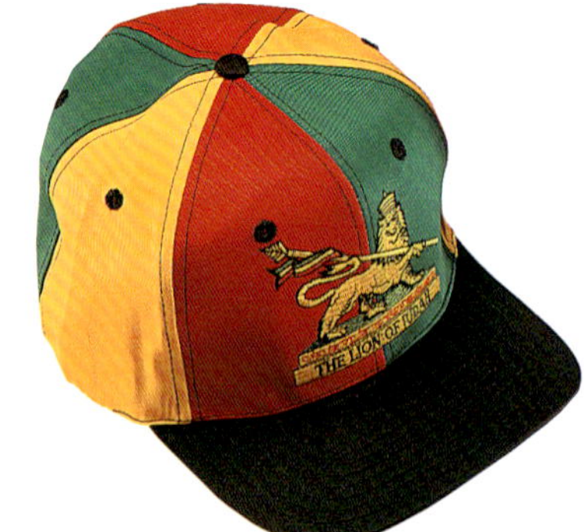

sets inspired largely by West African fashions and embroidered decorations.

Popular international figures can inspire headwear made in Africa. The success of Spike Lee's 1992 film *Malcolm X* starring Denzel Washington, created a market in the United States for Malcolm X tee shirts, baseball caps, and other items; these soon made their way to Africa's big cities where both imported and locally made "Malcolm X wear" was bought by fashion-conscious, politically aware youths (Fig. 10.6). Similarly, the multicolored "Kenya bag" in the 1977 Woody Allen film *Annie Hall* led to a boom in production and export of similar bags from Kenya. Although long made and used by Kikuyu women, the woven fiber bags became a big business that led to innovations (e.g., leather straps, leather flap closures) and experiments in color that catered to the tastes of the export market. Along with a wide range of "ethnic" jewelry and accessories from Africa, Kenya bags, woven baskets from Bolgatanga in northern Ghana, leather pouches and bags made in Togo, Niger, Mali, and Burkina Faso, and several styles of headwear were sold in major cities throughout the United States. Following the appearance in Zimbabwe of reggae superstar Peter Tosh, markets were flooded with Tosh-inspired hats of Zimbabwe manufacture (Fig. 10.7).

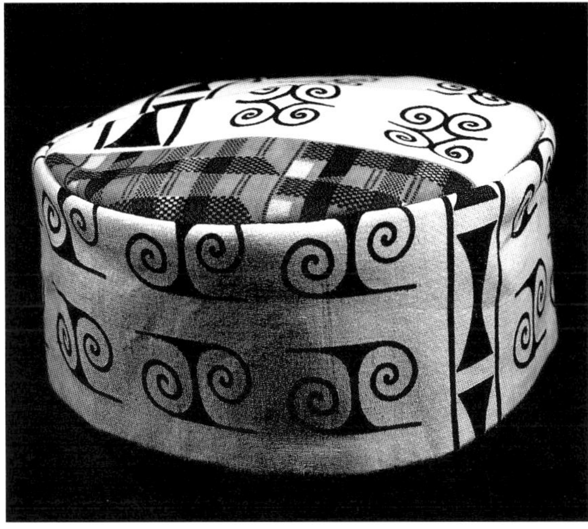

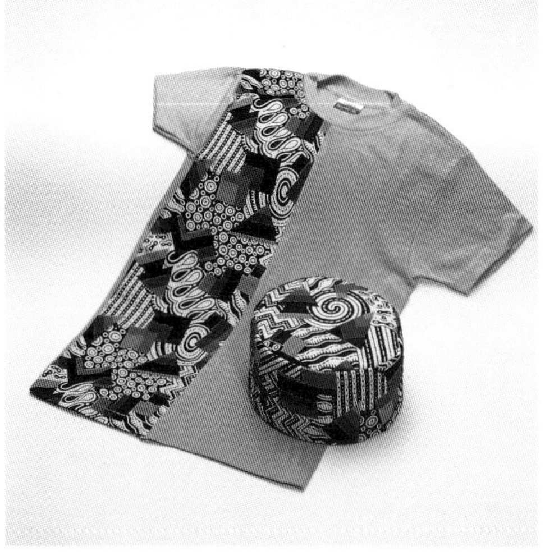

**Figure 10.15**, above left. *Kofia*-style hat with *adinkra* and *kente* patterns. United States. Cotton. H. 8.5 cm. FMCH X94.28.14. Museum purchase. This cap incorporates decorative motifs inspired by *adinkra* stamp patterns of the Asante of Ghana, West Africa. These patterns, which may be abstract curvilinear patterns or representations of stools, fowl, and other items, refer to proverbial sayings that are part of southern Ghanaian discourse. This hat was purchased at the African Marketplace in Los Angeles.

**Figure 10.16**, above. Child's *kofia*-style hat with matching tee shirt. United States. Cotton, polyester. H. 17.0 cm. FMCH X94.28.20a,b. Museum purchase.

Indeed, popular culture has played a significant role in shaping fashion trends. American-style baseball caps have made their way to clothing markets in Africa, inspiring locally made varieties that advertise popular beers and soft drinks, annual festivals, and political parties. The ANC baseball cap (Fig. 10.8) suggests a sustained, if not growing popularity in Africa for this American-inspired headwear. The baseball cap is the new model for headwear made from African or African-inspired fabrics. Among the more popular items today available for sale on the streets and in specialty boutiques of Africa are *kente* and mud-cloth baseball caps.

A selection of hats purchased at the African Marketplace in Los Angeles by the Fowler Museum of Cultural History specifically for this exhibition offers an excellent case study for the range of African-influenced headwear available for sale in a major American city. A quick review of some of these hats reveals affinities with Egypt (Figs. 10.9–10.12), African Islam, Senegal (Fig. 10.13), Jamaican Rastafarianism (Fig. 10.14), and with Swahili and Ghana in combination (Figs. 10.15, 10.16). This eclectic mix may suggest the extent to which actual African forms (as well as the notion of Africa) have captured the imaginations of clothing designers and their clients. Regardless of their faithfulness to African styles of headwear, the inventiveness of forms and the growing popularity of such hats suggests a conscious desire by the wearer to be linked with the African homeland and to celebrate with respect and pride African influences within and outside the continent.

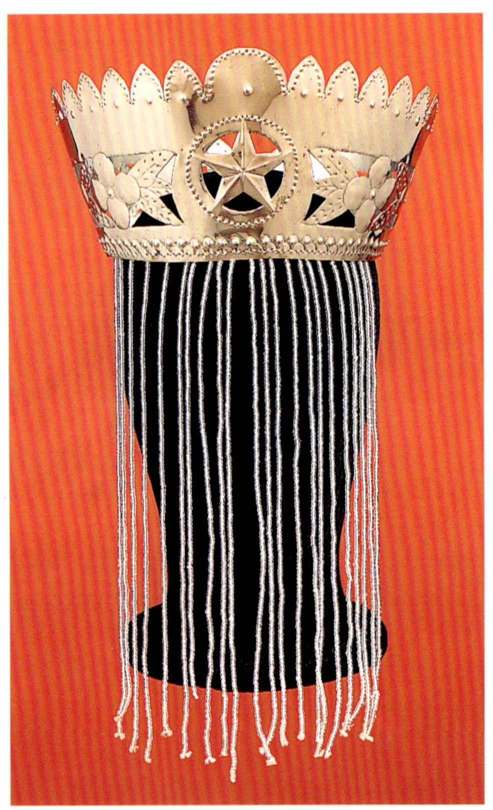

**Figure 10.17**. Crown *(ade)*. Salvador da Bahia. Brazil. Tin, glass beads. H. 38.0 cm. FMCH X83.536a. Museum purchase. The Afro-Brazilian *Candomblé* religion uses and manipulates imagery and symbols derived from the religious beliefs and practices of the Yoruba of southwestern Nigeria. The liturgical dress of *Candomblé* religious leaders alludes to the powers and preferences of particular gods and goddesses *(orixás)*. This openwork tin crown and white beaded fringe veil is part of the ritual costume for a priestess of Yemanjá, the goddess of water and purity.

## LITURGICAL DRESS

Along with African influences on contemporary fashion, music, cuisine, and oratory, African religious beliefs have also survived the long journey across the Atlantic. In terms of practice, as well as in the forms of ritual dress and religious regalia, African spiritual beliefs are clearly present beyond Africa's shores.

Religious beliefs and practices of the Yoruba of southwestern Nigeria, the Ewe of Benin and Togo, and the Kongo of Zaire have been points of inspiration and departure for religions in the Americas. The Afro-Cuban *Lucumi* and Afro-Brazilian *Candomblé*, religions that took shape during and after the slave trade in the eighteenth and nineteenth centuries, have reorganized and reshaped Yoruba practices in the Americas. The result is the creation of new, distinct, and dynamic religions practiced not just in Cuba and Brazil, but in the United States as well.

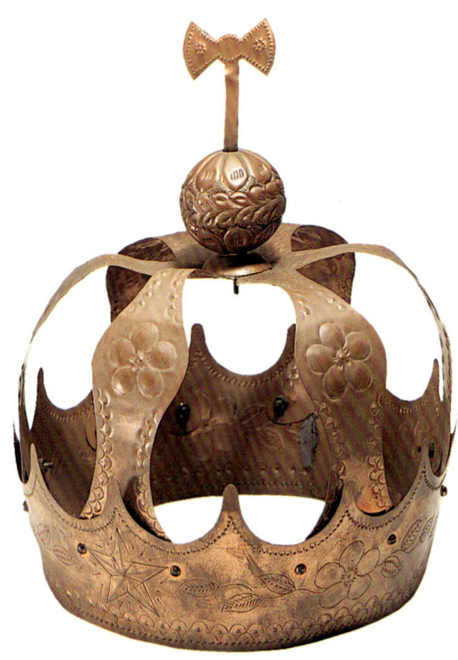

**Figure 10.18**, right. Crown. Salvador da Bahia. Brazil. Copper. H. 25.0 cm. FMCH X83.516. The double-axe form on top and the red color of the copper indicate that this crown is for the Orixá Xangô, god of thunder and lightening.

Both *Lucumi* and *Candomblé* use crowns, a practice that recalls the sacred crowns of Yoruba obas (kings) who, as religious leaders and political rulers, are thought to be descendants of *orixás* or deities. In the case of Afro-Cuban religion, some of the forms of religious paraphernalia derive from the colonial past, such as thrones, altars, and dress, but are invested with new religious relevance. Brown points out that female initiates who dress up as *orixás* wear formal garments "as crowned palace royalty reposing under lavish cloth thrones of satin, velvet, lame and lace. Their . . . ensembles include shimmering pasteboard crowns encrusted with cowries and iconographic details" (D. Brown 1993:47)).

In Brazilian *Candomblé*, initiates are similarly dressed in formal gowns in anticipation of manifesting an *orixá* during a possession trance (Omari 1984:pl. II). An openwork tin crown and white beaded fringe veil (Fig 10.17) is a part of the ritual costume for the Orixá Yemanjá. The entire ensemble includes a flowing white cotton and synthetic lace skirt and a blouse with openwork bodice and sleeves. Yemanjá, the goddess of water and purity and the mother of most *orixás*, is associated with the colors shimmering white, crystal blue, or green. The crown, linked to Yoruba chiefly crowns, "represents Yemanjá's sovereignty over the sea and, according to some, all water" (Omari 1984:21, 32).

The copper crown for Xangô (the Yoruba thunder deity, Shango; Fig. 10.18) is another example of a liturgical vestment used in Afro-Brazilian *Candomblé*. During ritual invocations, initiates who are possessed by Xangô exhibit the rapid and warriorlike movements of this proud and aggressive deity, whose preferred colors are red and white. The importance of these religious garments cannot be overstated. In discussing *Lucumi* liturgical dress, Flores-Pena (1994:13) states:

> The garment highlights the whole consecration ceremony and becomes one of the most beautiful memories of one's religious life. The clothing becomes for the initiate a "garment of glory." Once a person dons it, the outfit transforms him or her into a new being.

Offering a blend of Yoruba deities and Catholic saints, and a generous mix of local innovation combined with historic specificity, African-influenced religions in the Americas are "innovative transformations wrought on New World soil" (D. Brown 1989:10) that emphasize the dynamism and creative ingenuity of expressive culture. Yoruba-inspired deities and ritual paraphernalia are used and transformed in the Afro-Brazilian *Candomblé* and Afro-Cuban *Lucumi* religions. Brazilian carnivals are replete with references to African heritage in the costumes and artifacts worn and carried by participants. African-inspired masks from West and Central Africa are popular in carnival masquerades, but they are used alongside other forms, and some are a combination of elements invented by Brazilian artists.

Africa, as an influential presence in the Americas, is proclaimed in food, music, religious beliefs and practices, oral traditions, artistic expression, and contemporary fashion, to name a few. More than simply "retentions" or the passive "survivals" of expressive culture from the African continent, African-influenced cultural forms in the Americas are dynamic, creative, and inspired recastings that form part of the very fabric of life in the Americas today.

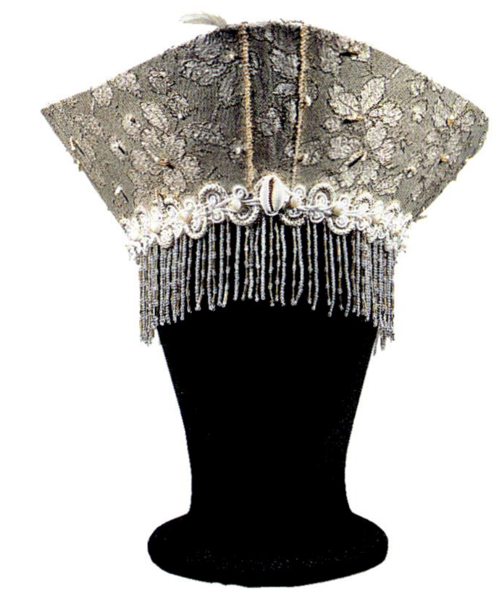

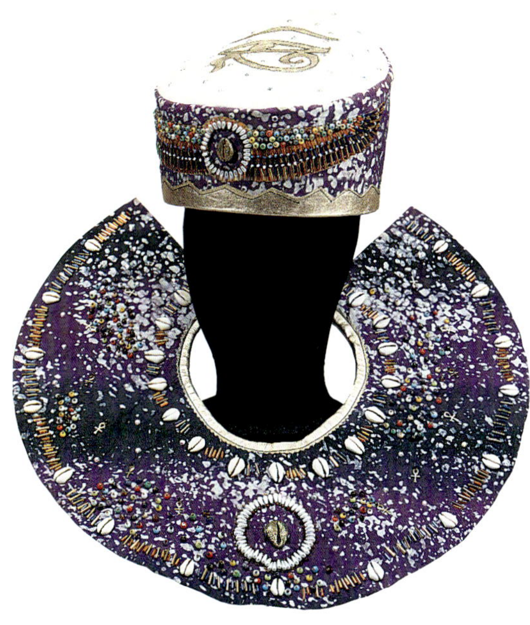

**Figure 10.19**, top. Crown. Synthetic cloth, glass beads, cardboard, cowrie shell, feather. H.14.0 cm. with fringe. Created by Los Angeles artist, Litina Egungun, 1994. Influenced by Zulu hat styles. Collection of the artist.

**Figure 10.20**, above. Crown and collar. Synthetic cloth, sequins, glass beads. H 17.0 cm. Inspired by Egyptian motifs and the crown of Nefertiti. Created by Los Angeles artist, Litina Egungun, 1994. Collection of the artist.

# NOTES

## CHAPTER 1

1. This current exhibition builds upon an exhibition I curated in 1988 for the University of Missouri-Kansas City Gallery of Art titled *Dressing the Head More Than a Matter of Taste,* which included more than eighty African hats in the collections of the Smithsonian's National Museum of Natural History and the National Museum of African Art and the Fowler Museum of Cultural History.

2. For a brief historical overview of traditional approaches to the study of African material culture and a discussion of the recent paradigmatic shift to a focus on human agency and the constituting capacity of objects, see Hardin and Arnoldi, "Introduction: Efficacy and Objects" in *Contemporary Approaches to the Study of African Material Culture* (in press). For approaches to the meaning of objects exchanged and circulated as commodities, see Appadurai, ed., *The Social Life of Things: Commodities in Cultural Perspective.* Cambridge: Cambridge University Press, 1986.

With few exceptions objects rarely have agency in and of themselves, however their production and use effects the constitution and transformation of people and social situations. Recent research on several categories of African objects including Yoruba crowns, Bamana *boliw,* the Golden Stool of the Ashanti, and Kongo *minkisi* strongly suggests that these objects might indeed fall into a different category and might be perceived to have agency.

3. This exhibition and the introductory essay were inspired by Daniel Biebuyck's essay in the catalogue for the 1984 exhibition *Power of Headdresses: A Cross-Cultural Study of Forms and Functions.* In his introductory essay Biebuyck lays out a comprehensive approach to the study of headwear, draws together disparate sources on dress and headwear, and examines the multiple functions of headwear worldwide. Many excellent studies of dress and headgear in Africa have been undertaken in recent years by art historians, historians and anthropologists and a number of these studies are cited throughout this catalogue.

4. Studies of the body have been important in anthropology and sociology since the nineteenth century (for more recent approaches see Blacking 1977; Bourdieu 1977; Brain 1979; Comaroff 1985; Desjarlais 1992; Douglas 1970; Ebin 1979; Jackson 1983; Jackson and Karp 1990; Locke 1993; Mason 1994; Mauss 1979; Polhemus 1975; B. Turner 1984, 1991; T. Turner 1980.

5. The film clip appears in the new permanent exhibition of African Cultures at the Field Museum in Chicago. "Hausa style" robes and caps have regularly been imported into Grassfields chiefdoms. Chiefs, like King Njoya, also attracted Hausa tailors and embroiderers to their capitals. These artists in turn taught local artists the techniques and patterns and a local industry producing Hausa style robes and embroidered caps flourishes in these chiefdoms (Christraud Geary, personal communication 1994).

## CHAPTER 3

1. Combs. Back row, left to right: a. Akan, Akuapem?, Ghana, wood, X87.1678; b. Somalia, wood, X79.344; c. Zaire, reed, bamboo, anonymous loan; d. Zaire, ivory, X67.720; e. Zaire? Angola? wood, metal, X77.1323; f. Tutsi, Rwanda, wood, 379.637; g. Zaire, brass, iron, X65.8987. Front row, left to right: h. Nande, Zaire, wood, metal, 392.146; i. Lega, Zaire, ivory, 378.542; j. Pende, Zaire, wood, X67.709; k. Luba, Zaire, wood, copper wire, 382.182; l. Asante, Ghana, wood, X92.179; m. Baule, Côte d'Ivoire, ivory, X87.1470; n. Yaka, Kwango River, Zaire, wood, X67.703; o. Susu, Cowakry, Guinea, bamboo, X64.1456.

2. Hairpins. Left to right: a. Zaire, ivory, X67.815; b. Zaire, ivory, X65.10063; c. Zaire, ivory, X67.799; d. Zaire, ivory, X67.818; e. Zaire, ivory, X67. 738; f. Zande, Sudan, Zaire, ivory X67.767; g. Mangbetu, Zaire, ivory, X65.10036; h. Mangbetu, Zaire, ivory, X67.767; i. Zaire, wood, X67.782; j. Kuba, Kasai, Zaire, aluminum, anonymous loan; k. Zaire, iron, copper, X65.10059; l. Zaire, copper, X65.10058; m. Zaire, copper, X65.10056; n. Zaire, iron, X65.10060; o. Republic of Congo, iron, X65.8468; p. Kuba, Zaire, aluminum, X94.37.1, anonymous gift; q.–s. Kuba, Zaire, ivory, anonymous loan; t. Zaire, ivory, X67.800; u. Zaire, ivory, X67.801; v. Southeast Africa, ivory, wood? X67.937; w. Southeast Africa, ivory, wood? X67.936 (front); x. Mangbetu, Zaire, ivory, X67.765.

## CHAPTER 4

1. In 1985 Dr. Christine Conte, anthropologist, collected these "Hausa" hats as part of a larger collection of hats, textiles, and baskets for the Department of Anthropology, Smithsonian Institution in Niger. She documented the production processes and marketing practices surrounding the hats and worked extensively with the artists, market people, and consumers to identify and record the meanings of design motifs used on the hats.

## CHAPTER 5

1. Other colors common in Zulu beadwork — such as black, pink, green, red, and yellow —

have favorable as well as unfavorable associations (Conner and Pelrine 1983:12) that require context-specific research in order to elucidate the message imbedded in a particular combination of beads.

2. Virginia-Lee Webb (1992:59) illustrates a tall, conical headdress with a simple white beaded band below in an 1870s black-and-white photograph by J.E. Middlebrook titled "A Study in Hairdressing."

3. The military cap's red and black coloring is consistent with the uniform and is replicated in carved representations of that uniform in Baule figure sculpture. Ravenhill (1980:24) illustrates a carved wood Baule figure wearing the *képi* and military coat that repeats the red and black color scheme of the regulation uniform.

4. Garrard (1989:91) illustrates a Baule seated figure wearing a pith helmet, with traces of gold leafing remaining on the carving.

5. For example, in the case of Kota/-Mahongwe reliquary bundles containing, among other materials, human bones, stones, and monkey skulls.

6. The hat was collected by Theodore Roosevelt, as part of the Smithsonian Africa Expedition to East Africa, led in 1909 by Edmund Heller in collaboration with Roosevelt and in conjunction with the Universal Film Manufacturing Company. The expedition collected a total of 113 mammals, 126 birds, 11 reptiles, 2 insects, and 16 ethnological specimens.

7. Given the similarity of materials for the headdresses worn by both men and women and lack of collection information about this particular Bidjogo headdress, it is difficult to state with certainty whether this headdress was worn by a male *canhocas* or a female *defunto*.

8. They are repaired and maintained for a period of weeks, after which the hardened shell is broken off. Now that these mud-plastered hair styles have captured the imagination of Western museums and private collectors, the coiffures are carefully shaved off, and thus preserved for sale on the art market.

## CHAPTER 6

1. Historically, turban cloths were dyed at several locations in northern Nigeria and it has been considered a prestige cloth for a very long time.

## CHAPTER 7

1. See the works of Wande Abimbola *in Ijinle Ohun Enu Ife, Apa Keji,* Glasgow: Collins, 1969; *Ifa: An Exposition of Ifa Literary Corpus,* Ibadan: O. U. P., 1976; and Mary H. Nooter, Secrecy: *An African Art that Conceals and Reveals,* New York: The Museum of African Art, 1993.

2. The blue touraco *(agbe)* and the *aluko* are two popular birds among the Yoruba. They are considered to be sacred. In Yoruba oral literature (poetry, songs, folklore, etc.) they are often spoken of together. The colors of their feathers are distinct and contrasting. The *agbe* is indigo blue, and the *aluko* is brownish-red.

3. The mythical, most distant place imaginable, or the final journey.

4. The use of goats and sheep in this context is metaphoric. It is used to express notions of everybody.

5. Barber's work (1991) speaks to the contextual pardigms of Ekun Iyawo.

## CHAPTER 8

1. In this essay on Lega hats, I am deeply indebted to Daniel Biebuyck. His writings over the years have been an example for the student of African art and anthropology of thoroughness of research and presentation. He has consistently written on basic issues in African art history well ahead of other scholars. He also graciously helped me with basic information for this essay, as well as reading a draft, looking at hat photographs, and providing the information for the captions. I look forward to his future extensive publication on Lega hats and the entire system of insignia and paraphernalia.

2. Biebuyck 1973:74–82. These are the basic grades for the Lega. Each Lega subgroup has a slightly different subset of these levels. In some areas, for example, *ngandu* is the highest grade. The listing of levels has been recorded by many scholars (Delhaise 1909:xv; de Kun 1966:74). In all the listings there is generally a consistency in grades, especially in the higher levels.

3. The women's and the men's grades are tied together: *bombwa/ngandu, bulonda/yananio, bunyamwa/kindi* (Biebuyck 1986:12).

4. The idea behind the proverb is that *lutumbo lwa yaninio* is like the moon, represented by the shell, seen and known by all.

5. Biebuyck and Van den Abbeele (1984:82) discuss the *muzombolo* hat and the implications of its maleness.

## CHAPTER 9

1. Lapsley's journal published in 1893 is among the earliest published descriptions of Kuba costuming. See *Life and Letters of Samuel Norvell Lapsley, Missionary to the Congo Valley, West Africa. 1866–1892,* Richmond, Va.: 1893. Lapsley's journal and letters were published shortly after his death at Underhill mission station on the lower Congo (Zaire) River on March 26, 1892.

2. Luebo is located at the southern edge of the Kuba territory east of the Kasai River and its convergence with the Lulua River.

3. The village may have been Bena Makima which is still a large village on the Kasai. The Kuba form a kingdom comprising more than seventeen distinct ethnic groups who reside in south-central Zaire. While the origins and languages of these groups differ, they are culturally similar. For the history of the politically dominant Kuba group, the Bushoong, see Vansina 1964, 1978.

4. See also Sheppard 1917:132.

5. Distinctive facial decoration was also employed by the Kuba. According to Torday and

Joyce (1910; Torday 1925), the upper incisor teeth of Bushoong and Ngongo men and women were removed at puberty. Kuba scarification patterns on the heads of men and women were relegated to small marks between the eye and the ear. However, the Ngongo often decorated their temples with scarification patterns in the form of concentric circles. Extensive scarification patterns were applied to the abdomen and thighs of women. By the early 1980s, these elaborate forms were only visible on elderly women. See Torday and Joyce (1910:159–63) for illustrations of scarification patterns and deformation of teeth.

6. The Ngongo live to the east of the Bushoong.

7. This must have also been a popular style for some Bushoong peoples since Torday illustrates a Bushoong woman wearing the identical style he describes for the Ngongo (1925: facing page 144).

8. The Isambo are a Kuba-related group who moved to the east of the Kuba area and reside at Lusambo near the upper Sankuru River. See the discussion of Isambo in Vansina 1978:66, 165.

9. *Tool*, a Bushoong term, is often referred to in art historical literature as *tukula,* a Kongo term. See Vansina 1978:287.

10. In the forest initiation camp some novices are selected to hold titled positions. These titles in part mirror community titleholding. During public dances novices wear special headbands and necklaces that denote the title of each novice.

11. Torday (1925) notes that following initiation rituals, the novices are considered adults and are allowed to wear the *laket.* See also Vansina 1955; Binkely 1987b, 1990; Darish 1990.

12. This would certainly only be true for the Bushoong proper or the Bushoong designated as *matoon* living in the southern part of the Kuba area.

13. This form of hat pin is called *ndwoong angwoong.* On iron pins the bell and ring are made of aluminum. The miniature bell does not have a clapper.

14. Moments before Sheppard's initial meeting with the Kuba ruler in April 1891, a Kuba elder noticed that a member of Sheppard's party wore "an old brass button tied by a string around the neck. . . ." Sheppard noted that "Very politely they removed it, saying, 'Only the king can wear brass or copper'" (1917:106). See also Vansina (1978:65, 191, 352, n. 78).

15. Torday notes that "only members of the royal family and the representative of the smiths are allowed to have these pins made of brass" (1925:179–80).

16. Two typical examples of these hat pins can be seen in Cornet (1982:220, fig. 270).

17. There are other feathers identified with other titles in the political hierarchy.

18. Popular patterns embroidered over the body of the cap are *mbish akot* ("back of the *kot* skirt") and *ikash intaan* ("lion's paw").

19. Torday noted this latter characteristic when he visited Misumba in 1907. Two styles of *laket* were popular among Ngongo men (1925:112).

20. In 1982 we inventoried and photographed the hats of a Shoowa eagle feather chief whose collection consisted of seven examples: one with an eagle down covering, one *kupash* (covered with beads and cowries), five regular *laket,* including the one he was wearing.

# BIBLIOGRAPHY


Abimbola, Wande
1969 *Ijinle Ohun Enu Ife, Apakeji*. Glasgow: Collins.
1973 "The Yoruba concept of human personality." *La Notion de Personne en Afrique Noire*, 73–90. Germaine Dieterlen, ed. Paris: C.N.R.S.
1976 *Ifa: An Exposition of Ifa Literary Corpus*. Ibadan: O.U.P.

Abiodun, Rowland
1994 "Understanding Yoruba Art and Aesthetics: The concept of Ase." *African Arts* 27(3):68–78, notes 102–103.

Abiodun, Rowland and John Henry Drewal
1991 *Yoruba: Art and Aesthetics*. New York: Center for African Art.

Adamson, Joy
1967 *The Peoples of Kenya*. New York: Harcourt, Brace and World, Inc.

Addis Ababa University
1988 *Visitors' Manual*. Addis Ababa: Institute of Ethiopian Studies.

Aherne, Tavy D.
1992 *Nakunte Diarra: Bogolanfini Artist of the Beledogou*. Bloomington: Indiana University Press.

Alagoa, Ebiegberi Joe
1971 "The Niger Delta States and Their Neighbors to c. 1800." In *History of West Africa, Vol 1*, 269–303. J. F. Ade Ajayi and Michael Crowder, eds. London: Longman.

Appadurai, Arjun, ed.
1986 *The Social Life of Things: Commodities in Cultural Perspective*. Cambridge: Cambridge University Press.

Arens, W. and Ivan Karp
1989 "Introduction." In *Creativity of Power: Cosmology and Action in African Societies*, xi–xxix. W. Arens and I. Karp, eds. Washington, D. C.: Smithsonian Institution Press.

Arkell, A. J.
1956 "The Making of Mail at Omdurman." *Kush: Journal of the Sudan Antiquities Service* 4:83–84.

Barber, Karin
1991 *I Could Speak Until Tomorrow: Oriki and the Past in a Yoruba Town*. Washington, D. C.: Smithsonian Institution Press.

Barley, Nigel
1988 *Foreheads of the Dead: An Anthropological View of Kalabari Ancestral Screens*. Washington, D. C.: Smithsonian Institution Press.

Bascom, William R.
1969 *The Yoruba of Southern Nigeria*. New York: Holt, Rinehart and Winston.

Bedaux, Roger M. A.
1988 "Tellem and Dogon Material Culture." *African Arts* 21(4):38–45, 90–91.

Beidelman, T. O.
1972 "The Kaguru House." *Anthropos* 67:690–707.
1993 *Moral Imagination in Kaguru Modes of Thought*. Washington, D. C.: Smithsonian Institution Press.

Beier, Ulli
1982 *Yoruba Beaded Crowns: Sacred Regalia of the Olokuku of Okuku*. London: Ethnographica.

Berns, Marla C.
1985 "Decorated Gourds of Northeastern Nigeria." *African Arts* 19(1):28–45, notes 86–87.
1986 Art and History in the Lower Gongola Valley, Northeastern Nigeria. Ph.D. dissertation, University of California at Los Angeles.

Berns, Marla and Barbara Rubin Hudson
1986 *The Essential Gourd: Art and History in Northeastern Nigeria*. Los Angeles: Museum of Cultural History.

Biebuyck, Daniel P.
1953 "Repartition et droits du pangolin chez les Balega." *Zaire* 7:899–935.
1972 "The Kindi Aristocrats and Their Art among the Lega." In *African Art and Leadership*, 7–20. D. Fraser and H. Cole, eds. Madison: University of Wisconsin Press.
1973 *Lega Culture: Art, Initiation, and Moral Philosophy among a Central African People*. Berkeley: University of California Press.
1976 "The Decline of Lega Sculptural Art." In *Ethnic and Tourist Arts: Cultural Expressions from the Fourth World*, 334–39. N. Graburn, ed. Berkeley: University of California Press.
1977 *Symbolism of a Lega Stool*. Philadelphia: ISHI Publications.
1979 "The Frog and Other Animals in Lega Art and Initiation." *Africa-Tervuren* 25:76–84.
1981 "Plurifrontal Figurines in Lega Art (Zaire)." In *The Shape of the Past: Studies in Honor of Franklin D. Murphy*, 115–27. G. Buccellati and Ch. Speroni, eds. Berkeley: University of California Press.
1982 "Lega Dress as Cultural Artifact." *African Arts* 15(3):59–65, 92.
1986 *The Arts of Zaire: Volume II: Eastern Zaire: The Ritual and Artistic Context of Voluntary Associations*. Berkeley: University of California Press.

Biebuyck, Daniel and Nelly Van den Abbeele
1984 *The Power of Headdresses: A Cross-Cultural Study of Form and Functions*. Ghent: Snoeck-Ducaju en Zoon and Brussels: Tendi S.A.

Binkley, David A.
1987a "Avatar of Power: Southern Kuba

Masquerade Figures in a Funerary Context." *Africa* 57(1):75–97.

1987b A View from the Forest: The Power of Southern Kuba Initiation Masks. Ph.D. dissertation, Indiana University.

1990 "Masks, Space and Gender in Southern Kuba Initiation Ritual." In *Iowa Studies in African Art,* 3:157–176. Iowa City: University of Iowa.

1992 "The Teeth of the Nyim: The Elephant and Ivory in Kuba Art." In *Elephant: The Animal and its Ivory in African Culture,* 277–291. Doran H. Ross, ed. Los Angeles: Fowler Museum of Cultural History.

Bivar, A. D. H.

1964 *Nigerian Panoply: Arms and Armour of the Northern Region*. Lagos: Department of Antiquities, Federal Republic of Nigeria.

Blacking, John, ed.

1977 *The Anthropology of the Body*. London: Academic Press.

Blier, Suzanne

1987 *The Anatomy of Architecture: Ontology and Metaphor in Batammaliba Architectural Expression*. New York: Cambridge University Press.

Bourdieu, Pierre

1977 *Outline of a Theory of Practice*. Richard Nice, trans. Cambridge: Cambridge University Press.

Bourgeois, Arthur P.

1982 "Yaka and Suku Leadership Headgear." *African Arts* 15(3):30–35, 92.

Brain, Robert

1979 *The Decorated Body*. New York: Harper and Row.

Bravmann, René

1983 *African Islam*. Washington: Smithsonian Institution Press.

Brown, David H.

1989 Garden in the Machine: Afro-Cuban Sacred Art and Performance in Urban New Jersey and New York. Ph.D. dissertation, Yale University.

1993 "Thrones of the *Orichas:* Afro-Cuban Altars in New Jersey, New York and Havana." *African Arts* 26(4):44–59, 85–87.

Brown, H. D.

1944 "The Nkumu of the Tumba: Ritual Chieftainship on the Middle Congo." *Africa* 14(8):431–447.

Brown, Jean

1986 "The Pokot." In *Tribal Traditions of Kenya*. Esther Bockhoff and Nancy I. Fleming, eds. Cleveland: The Cleveland Museum of Natural History.

Bryant, Alfred T.

1967 *The Zulu People As They Were Before the White Man Came*. New York: Negro Universities Press (reprint from 1949).

Buxton, David

1970 *The Abyssininans*. London: Thames and Hudson.

Cameron, Elisabeth

1992 "The Stampeding of Elephants: Elephant Imprints on Lega thought." In *Elephant: The Animal and Its Ivory in African Culture,* 295–305. Doran H. Ross, ed. Los Angeles: Fowler Museum of Cultural History.

Cannizzo, Jeanne

1989 *Into the Heart of Africa*. Toronto: Royal Ontario Museum.

Casajus, Dominique

1987 *La Tente dans la Solitude: La Société et les Morts chez les Touaregs Kel Ferwan*. Paris: C.N.R.S.

Chappel, T. J. H.

1977 *Gourds in North-Eastern Nigeria*. London: Ethnographica.

Cissé, Youssouf

1973 "Signes graphiques, représentations, concepts et tests relatifs à la personne chez les Malinké et les Bambara du Mali." *La Notion de personne en Afrique Noire,* 131–180. Germaine Dieterlen, ed. Paris: C.N.R.S.

Claudot-Hawad, Helene

1993 *Les Touaregs: Portrait en fragments*. Aix-en-Provence: Edisud.

Cole, Herbert M.

1974 "Vital Arts in Northern Kenya." *African Arts* 7(2):12–23, note 82.

1979 "Living Art Among the Samburu." In *The Fabrics of Culture: The Anthropology of Clothing and Adornment,* 87–102. Justine Cordwell and Ronald Schwartz, eds. New York: Mouton Publishers.

1989 *Icons: Ideals and Power in the Art of Africa*. Washington, D. C.: Smithsonian Institution Press.

Cole, Herbert M. and Chike Aniakor

1984 *Igbo Arts: Community and Cosmos*. Los Angeles: Museum of Cultural History.

Cole, Herbert M. and Doran H. Ross

1977 The Arts of Ghana. Los Angeles: Museum of Cultural History.

Colvin, Lucie Gallistel

1981 *Historical Dictionary of Senegal 23*. Metuchen, New Jersey: Scarecrow Press.

Comaroff, Jean

1985 *Body of Power, Spirit of Resistance: The Culture and History of a South African People*. Chicago: University of Chicago Press.

Comaroff, John and Jean

1992 *Ethnography and the Historical Imagination*. Boulder, Colorado: Westview Press.

Conner, Michael and Diane Pelrine

1983 *The Geometric Vision: Arts of the Zulu*. Purdue: Department of Creative Arts.

Cordwell, Justine

1952 Some Aesthetic Aspects of Yoruba and Benin Cultures. Ph.D dissertation, Northwestern University.

Cornet, Joseph

1982 *Art Royal Kuba*. Milan: Edizioni Sipiel.

Daly, M. Catherine

1987 "Iria Bo Appearance at Kalabari Funerals." *African Arts* 21(1):58–61, note 86.

Darish, Patricia J.

1989 "Dressing for the Next Life: Raffia Textile Production and Use among the Kuba of

Zaire." In *Cloth and Human Experience*. Annette Weiner and Jane Schneider, eds. Washington, D. C.: Smithsonian Institution Press.

1990 "Dressing for Success: Ritual Occasions and Ceremonial Raffia Dress Among the Kuba of South-central Zaire." In *Iowa Studies in African Art* 3: 179–191. Iowa City: University of Iowa.

Darteville, Edmound
1953 "Les 'Nzimbu:' Monnai du Royayume de Congo." *Bulletins et Memoires de la Société Royale Belge d'Anthropologie et de Prehistoire* 1. (Nouvelle serie), Brussels.

David, N.
1976 "History of Crops and Peoples in North Cameroon to A.D. 1900." In *Origins of African Plant Domestication,* 223–267. J. M. J. DeWet and B. L. Stemler, eds. The Hague: Mouton.

d' Azevedo, Warren
1962 "Uses of the Past in Gola Discourse." *Journal of African History* 3(1):11–34.
1975 "Sources of Gola Artistry."The *Traditional Artist in African Societies,* 28–340. Warren d'Azevedo, ed. Bloomington: Indiana University Press.

Decalo, Samuel
1979 *Historical Dictionary of Niger 20.* Metuchen, New Jersey: Scarecrow Press.

de Kun, M.
"L'Art Lega." *Africa-Tervuren* 12(3–4):69–99.

Delhaise, Le Commandant
1909 *Les Warega*. Brussels: Albert de Wit.

Desjarlais, Robert R.
1992 *Body and Emotion: The Aesthetics of Illness and Healing in the Nepal Himalayas.* Philadelphia: University of Pennsylvania Press.

de Sousberghe, Leon
1958 *L'Art Pende*. Brussels: Editions J. Duculot.

Dewey, William
1993 *Sleeping Beauties: The Jerome L. Joss Collection of African Headrests at UCLA.* Los Angeles: Fowler Museum of Cultural History.

Dike, Kenneth
1956 *Trade and Politics in the Niger Delta.* Oxford: Clarendon Press.

Douglas, Mary
1970 *Natural Symbols*. Revised in 1982. New York: Pantheon Books.

Drewal, Henry John
1977 *Traditional Art of the Nigerian People.* Washington, D. C.: Museum of African Art.

Drewal, Henry John, John Pemberton III, and Rowland Abiodun
1989 "Yoruba: Nine Centuries of African Art and Thought." *African Arts* 23(1);68–77, note 104.

Drewal, John Henry and John Pemberton III
1989 *Yoruba: Nine Centuries of African Art and Thought*. New York: Harry N. Abrams, Inc.

Drewal, Margaret Thompson
1977 "Projections from the top in Yoruba Art." *African Arts* 11(1):43–49, notes 91–92.
1992 *Yoruba Ritual: Performers, Play and Agency.* Bloomington: Indiana University Press.

Duquette, Danielle Gallois
1979 "Woman Power and Initiation in the Bissagos Islands." *African Arts* 12(3):31–35, 93.

Ebin, Victoria
1979 *The Body Decorated*. London: Thames and Hudson.

Echenberg, Myron
1991 *Colonial Conscripts. The Tirailleurs Sénégalais in French West Africa, 1857–1960*. Portsmouth, New Hampshire and London: Heinemann.

Eicher, Joanne and Tonye Victor Erekosima
1987 "Kalabari Funerals: Celebration and Display." *African Arts* 21(1):38–45, notes 87–88.
1988 Kalabari Headdresses of Power. Paper presented at the African Studies Association annual meeting.
1989 "Kalabari Funeral Rooms as Handicraft and Ephemeral Art." In *Man Does Not Go Naked: Testilen und Handwerk aus afrikanischen und anderen Ländern*. Basel: Ethnologisches Seminar der Universität und Museum für Volkerkunde.

Engard, Ronald K.
1989 "Dance and Power in Bafut [Cameroon]." In *Creativity of Power: Cosmology and Action in African Societies,* 129–164. W. Arens and Ivan Karp, eds. Washington, D. C.: Smithsonian Institution Press.

Erekosima, Tonye Victor
1988 Reply to Nigel Barley. Unpublished manuscript.

Erekosima, Tonye Victor and Joanne Eicher
1981 Kalabari Men's Dress: A Sophisticated African Response to Culture Contact. Paper presented at the African Studies Association annual meeting.

Euba, Titi
1985 "The Ooni of Ife's Are Crown and the Concept of the Divine Head." *The Nigeria Magazine* 53(1):1–18.

Ezra, Kate
1988 *Art of the Dogon*. New York: The Metropolitan Museum of Art.

Fischer, Eberhard and Hans Himmelheber
1975 *Das Gold in der Kunst Westafrikas*. Zurich: Museum Rietburg.

Fisher, Angela
1984 *Africa Adorned*. New York: Harry N. Abrams, Inc.

Flores-Pena, Ysamur and Roberta J.Evanchuk
1994 *Santeria Garments and Altars: Speaking Without a Voice*. Jackson: University Press of Mississippi.

Fortes, Meyer
1973 "On the Concept of the Person among the Tallensi." *La Notion de personne en Afrique Noire,* 283–320. Germaine Dieterlen, ed. Paris: C.N.R.S.

Fourneau, J. and L. Kravetz
1954 "Le pagne sur le côte de Guinée et au Congo du XV siècle à nos jours."

*Bulletin, Institut d'Etudes Centrafricans,* N.S. Nos. 7, 8:52–1. Brazzaville.

Fynn, Henry Francis
1969 *The Diary of Henry Francis Fynn.* James Stuart and D. McK. Malcolm, eds. Piertermaritzburg: Shuter and Shooter.

Garrard, Timothy F.
1989 *Gold of Africa: Jewelry and Ornaments from Ghana, Côte d'Ivoire, Mali and Senegal.* Geneva: Barbier-Muller Museum and Prestel-Verlag, Munich.

Geary, Christraud
1988 *Images from Bamum: German Colonial Photography at the Court of King Njoya.* Washington, D. C.: National Museum of African Art.

Gebauer, Paul
1979 *Art of Cameroon.* Portland: The Portland Art Museum in association with the Metropolitan Museum of Art, New York.

Gibson, Gordon
1956 "Double Descent and its Correlates among the Herero of Ngamiland." *American Anthropologist* 58:109–139.
1962 "Bridewealth and Forms of Exchange among the Herero." *Markets in Africa,* 617–639. Paul Bohannan and George Dalton, eds. Evanston: Northwestern University Press.

Gibson, Gordon D. and Cecilia R. McGurk
1977 "High Status Caps of the Kongo and Mbundu Peoples." *Textile Museum Journal* 4(4):71–96.

Giddens, Anthony
1990 *Central Problem in Social Theory: Action, Structure and Contradiction in Social Analysis.* Berkeley and Los Angeles: University of California Press.

Gilbert, Michelle
1989 "Sources of Power in Akuropon-Akuapem: Ambiguity in Classification." In *Creativity of Power: Cosmology and Action in African Societies,* 59–90. W. Arens and Ivan Karp, eds. Washington, D. C.: Smithsonian Institution Press.

Goldschmidt, Walter
1976 *Culture and Behavior of the Sebei: A Study in Continuity and Adaptation.* Berkeley: University of California Press.

Gulliver, P. H.
1952 "The Karamajong Cluster." *Africa* 22(1):1–22.

Gulliver, Pamela and P. H. Gulliver
1953 *The Central Hilo-Hamites.* East Central Africa, part 7. London: International African Institute.

Hallpike, C. R.
1978 "Social Hair." In *The Body Reader: Social Aspects of the Human Body,* 134–148. Ted Polhemus, ed. New York: Pantheon Books.

Hardin, Kris and Mary Jo Arnoldi
In press "Introduction: Efficacy and Objects." In *Contemporary Approaches to the Study of African Material Culture.* M. J. Arnoldi, C. Geary, and K. Hardin, eds. Bloomington: Indiana University Press.

Hardin, Kris
1993 *The Aesthetics of Action: Continuity and Change in a West African Town.* Washington, D. C.: Smithsonian Institution Press.

Heathcote, David
1975 "Hausa Hand-Embroidered Caps." *The Nigerian Field* 40(2):54–73.
1976 *The Arts of the Hausa.* Kent: World of Islam Festival Publishing Company, Ltd.

Herbert, Eugenia
1993 *Iron, Gender and Power Rituals of Transformation in African Societies.* Bloomington: Indiana University Press.

Hilton-Simpson, M. N.
1911 *Land and Peoples of the Kasai.* London: Constable and Company Limited.

Hogben, S. J. and A. H. M. Kirk-Greene
1966 *The Emirates of Northern Nigeria: A Preliminary Survey of Their Historical Traditions.* London: Oxford University Press.

Horton, Robin
1965 *Kalabari Sculpture.* Lagos: Department of Antiquities, Federal Republic of Nigeria.

Houlberg, Marilyn Hammersley
1979 "Social Hair: Tradition and Change in Yoruba Hairstyles in Southwestern Nigeria." In *The Fabrics of Culture: The Anthropology of Clothing and Adornment,* 349–398. Justine Cordwell and Ronald Schwartz, eds. New York: Mouton Publishers.

Jackson, Michael
1977 *The Kuranko Dimensions of Social Reality in a West African Tribe.* New York: St Martins Press.
1983 "Knowledge of the Body." *Man* (N.S.) 18(2):327–345.

Jackson, Michael and Ivan Karp
1990 "Introduction." In *Personhood and Agency: The Experience of Self and Other in African Cultures, 15–30.* Michael Jackson and Ivan Karp, eds. Uppsala: Uppsala University.

Johnson, Samuel
1921 *The History of the Yorubas.* Lagos, Nigeria: C.S.S. Bookshops.

Johnston, Harry A.
1908 *George Grenfell and the Congo.* 2 vols. London: Hutchinson and Co.

Jones, G. I.
1963 *The Trading States of the Oil Rivers: A Study of Political Development in Eastern Nigeria.* London: Oxford University Press.

Jones, Lisa
1994 *Bulletproof Diva: Tales of Race, Sex and Hair.* New York: Doubleday.

Karp, Ivan
1990 "Power and Capacity in Iteso Rituals of Possession." In *Personhood and Agency: The Experience of Self and Other in African Cultures,* 79–94. Michael Jackson and Ivan Karp, eds. Uppsala: Uppsala University.

Kennedy, Carolee
1978 *The Art and Material Culture of the Zulu-Speaking Peoples.* Pamphlet Series 1(3).

Los Angeles: UCLA Museum of Cultural History.

Klopper, Sandra
1991 "You need only one bull to cover fifty cows: Zulu Women and 'Traditional' Dress." *Southern African Studies* 6:147–177.

Klumpp, Donna Rey
1986 "An Historical Overview of Maasai Dress." In *Traditional Folk Textiles and Dress,* 31–34. Barbara Nordquist and Kendall Hunt, eds. Dubuque: Iowa: Kendall/Hunt Publishing Company.

Koloss, Hans-Joachim
1990 *Art of Central Africa: Masterpieces from the Berlin Museum für Volkerkunde.* New York: Metropolitan Museum of Art.

Kratz, Corrine
1988 "Okiek Ornaments of Transition and Transformation." *Kenya Past and Present* 20:21–26.
1994 *Affecting Performance: Meaning, Movement and Experience in Okiek Women's Initiation.* Washington, D. C.: Smithsonian Institution Press.

Krige, Eileen Jensen
1965 *The Social System of the Zulus.* 2nd ed. Piertermaritzburg: Shuter and Shooter.

Kriger, Colleen
1988 "Robes of the Sokoto Caliphate." *African Arts* 21(3):52–57, 78–79, notes 85–86.

Kristen, Christine
1980 "Sign-Painting in Ghana." *African Arts* 13(3):38–39.

Lamb, Venice
1975 *West African Weaving.* London: Gerald Duckworth and Company.

Lamb, Venice and Alastair Lamb
1981 *Au Cameroon: Weaving-Tissage.* Hertingfordburg: Roxford Books.
1984 *Sierra Leone Weaving.* Surrey: Unwin Brothers Ltd.

Lamp, Frederick
1978 "Frogs into Princes: The Temne Rabai Initiation." *African Arts* 11(2):38–49, notes 94–95.

Langmuir, E., S. Chojnacki, and P. Fetcko
1978 *Ethiopia: The Christian Art of an African Nation.* Salem, Massachusetts: Peabody Museum.

Lapsley, Samuel N.
1893 *Life and Letters of Samuel Norvell Lapsley, Missionary to the Congo Valley, West Africa, 1866–1892.* Richmond, Virginia: Whittet and Shepperson.

Last, Murray
1988 "The Sokoto Caliphate and Borno." In *General History of Africa, Vol 5. Africa in the Nineteenth Century until the 1880s,* 555–599. UNESCO. London: Heinemann.

Leach, Edmund
1958 "Magical Hair." *The Journal of the Royal Anthropologican Institute* 88 (part II):147–164.

Lerat, Jean-Marie
1992 *Ici Bon Coiffeur.* Paris: Éditions Syros-Alternatives.

Levinsohn, Rhoda
1984 *Art and Craft in Southern Africa.* Craighall, South Africa.: Delta Books.

Levtzion, Nehemia and J. F. Hopkins
1981 *Corpus of Early Arabic Sources for West African History.* London: Cambridge University Press.

Lewis, Herbert S.
1965 *A Galla Monarchy: Jimma Abba Jifar, Ethiopia 1830–1932.* Madison: University of Wisconsin Press.

Liu, Robert K.
1984 "The Bead in African Assembled Jewelry: Its Multiple Manifestations." In *Beauty by Design: the Aesthetic of African Adornment,* 40–45. Marie-Thérèse Brincard, ed. New York: The African-American Institute.

Locke, Margaret
1993 "Cultivating the Body: Anthropology and Epistemologies of Bodily Practice and Knowledge." *Annual Review of Anthropology* 22:133–55.

MacGaffey, Wyatt
1993 "The Eyes of Understanding: Kongo Minkisi." In *Astonishment and Power,* 21–88. Washington, D.C.: Smithsonian Institution Press.

Mack, John
1986 *Madagascar: Island of the Ancestors.* London: Trustees of the British Museum.

Mason, Michael Atwood
1994 "I Bow My Head to the Ground: The Creation of Daily Experience in a Cuban American Santeria Initiation." *Journal of American Folklore* 107(423):23–39.

Mauss, Marcel
1979 "Body Techniques." In *Sociology and Psychology,* 95–123. London: Routledge and Kegan Paul.

Morgan, David and Sue Scott
1993 "Bodies in a Social Landscape." In *Body Matters: Essays on the Sociology of the Body,* 1–21. Sue Scott and David Morgan, eds. London: The Falmer Press.

Mudindaambi, Lumbwe
1976 *Objets et Techniques de la Vie Quotidienne Mbala.* Vol 2. Bandundu, Zaire: Ceeba Publications

Mulyumba, Barnabe.
1968 "La croyance religieuse des Lega traditionnels." *Etudes congolaises* 11(3): 1–14; (11)4, 3–19.

Mulyumba wa Mamba Itongwa
1978 *Apercu sur la structure politique des Balega-Basile.* Brussels: Les cahiers du Cedaf.

Murdock, George P.
1959 *Africa: Its Peoples and Their Culture History.* New York: McGraw-Hill Book Company.

Murphy, Robert F.
1964 "Social Distance and the Veil." *American Anthropologist* 66(6, part 1):1257–1274.

Newman, Paul
1977 *Chadic classification and Reconstructions.* Malibu, California: Undena Publications.

Nicolas, Francis
1950 *Tamensna Les ioullemmeden de l'est ou Touareg "Kel Dinnik."* Paris: Imprimerie Nationale.

Nooter, Mary H.
1984 Luba Arts and Leadership. M. A. thesis, Columbia University.
1993 *Secrecy: African Art that Conceals and Reveals*. New York: The Museum for African Art.

Norden, Hermann
c. 1925 *Fresh Tracks in the Belgian Congo*. Boston: Small, Maynard & Company.

Northern, Tamara
1973 *Royal Art of Cameroon*. Hanover: Trustees of Dartmouth College.

Novelli, Bruno
1988 *Aspects of Karimojong Ethnosociology*. Verona: Museum Comboniaum.

Omari, Mikelle Smith
1984 *From the Inside to the Outside: The Art and Ritual of Bahian Condomblé*. Los Angeles: UCLA Museum of Cultural History.

Ortner, Sherry
1984 "Theory in Anthropology since the Sixties." *Comparative Studies in Society and History* 26:126–165.

Pazzaglia, Augusto
1982 *The Karimojong: Some Aspects*. Bologna: Museum Comboniaum.

Perani, Judith
1989 "Northern Nigerian Prestige Textiles: Production, Trade, Patronage and Use." In *Man Does Not Go Naked,* 64–81. Basel: Ethnologisches Seminar der Universität und Museum für Volkerkunde.

Perani, Judith and Norma Wolff
1992 "Embroidered Gown and Equestrian Ensembles of the Kano Aristocracy." *African Arts* 25(3): 70–81, notes 102–104.

Picton, John and John Mack
1979 *African Textiles*. London: The Trustees of the British Museum.

Pokornowski, Ila
1979 "Beads and Personal Adornment." In *The Fabrics of Culture: The Anthropology of Clothing and Adornment,* 103–118. Justine Cordwell and Ronald Schwartz, eds. New York: Mouton Publishers.

Polhemus, Ted
1975 "Social Bodies." In *The Body as a Medium of Expression,* 13–35. London: Institute of Contemporary Arts.

Rasmussen, Susan
1991a "Veiled Self, Transparent Meanings: Tuareg Headdress as Social Expression." *Ethnology* 30(2):101–117.
1991b "Lack of Prayer: Ritual Restrictions, Social Experience, and the Anthropology of Menstruation among the Tuareg." *American Ethnologist* 18(4):751–769.
1992 "Disputed Boundaries: Tuareg Discourse on Class and Ethnicity." *Ethnology* 31(4):351–365.
1994 "The 'Head Dance' contested Self, and Art as a balancing act in Tuareg spirit possession." *Africa* 64(1):74–98.

Ravenhill, Philip L.
1980 "Baule Statuary Art: Meaning and Modernization." *ISHI Working Papers in the Traditional Arts*, Nos. 5, 6. Philadelphia: Institute for the Study of Human Issues.

Roberts, Allen F.
1986a "Social and Historical Contexts of Tabwa Art." In *Tabwa, the Rising of a New Moon: A Century of Tabwa Art*. Evan M. Mauer and Allen F. Roberts, eds. Seattle: University of Washington Press.
1986b "Duality in Tabwa Art." *African Arts* 19 (4):54–73.
1988 "Through the Bamboo Thicket: The Social Process of Tabwa Ritual Performances." *The Drama Review* 32(2):123–138.
1990 "Tabwa Masks and Old Trick of the Human Race." *African Arts* 23(2):37–47, 101.

Ross, Doran H.
1979 *Fighting with Art: Appliqued Flags of the Fante Asafo*. Los Angeles: UCLA Museum of Cultural History.

Roy, Christopher
1979 Mossi Masks and Crests. Ph.D. dissertation, Indiana University.

Rubin, Barbara
1970 "Calabash Decoration in North East State, Nigeria." *African Arts* 4(1):20–25, note 80.

Schildkrout, Enid and Curtis Keim
1990 *African Reflections: Art from Northeastern Zaire*. Seattle: University of Washington Press.

Sechefo, Justinus
n.d. *The Old Clothing of the Basotho*. Mazenod: The Catholic Centre.

Sheppard, William
1917 *Presbyterian Pioneers in Congo*. Richmond, Virginia: Presbyterian Committee of Publication.

Sieber, Roy
1973 *African Textiles and Decorative Arts*. New York: Museum of Modern Art.

Smith, Robert
1976 *Kingdoms of the Yoruba*. New York: Harper and Row.

Sobania, Neal W. and Raymond A. Silverman
1992 *Art of Everyday Life in Ethiopia and Northern Kenya*. Holland, Michigan: Hope College.

Sontag, Susan
1977 *Illness as Metaphor*. New York: Farrar, Straus and Giroux.

Spencer, Paul
1965 *The Samburu: A Study of Gerontocracy in a Nomadic Tribe*. Berkeley and Los Angeles: University of California Press.

Spring, Christopher
1993 *African Arms and Armor*. Washington, D. C.: Smithsonian Institution Press.

Stone, Caroline
1987 "Embroidery from North Africa." *Aramco World* 38(6):12–19.

Sugier, Clémence
1968 "Les Coiffes féminines de Tunisie." Cahiers des Arts et Traditions populaires 2:61–78.

Sutton, J.
1979 "Towards a less orthodox history of

Hausaland." *Journal of African History* 20(2):179–202.

Tait, David
1961 *The Konkomba of northern Ghana.* London: Oxford University Press.

Thompson, Robert Farris
1970 "The Sign of the Divine King." *African Arts* 3(3):8–17, 74–80.
1971 *Black Gods and King: Yoruba Art at UCLA.* Los Angeles: UCLA Museum and Laboratories of Ethnic Arts and Technology..
1972 "The Sign of the Divine King: Yoruba Bead-Embroidered Crowns with Veil and Bird Decorations." In *African Art and Leadership,* 227–260. Douglas Fraser and Herbert M. Cole, eds. Madison: University of Wisconsin Press.
1993 *Face of the Gods Art and Altars of Africa and the African Americas.* New York: The Museum for African Art and Prestel, Munich.

Torday, Emil
1925 *On the trail of the Bushongo.* Philadelphia and London: J. B. Lippincott Company.

Torday, Emil, and T. A. Joyce
1910 *Notes éthnographiques sur les peuples communément appelés Bakuba, ainsi que* sur les peuplades apparentées: Les Bushongo. M.R.A.C.: Brussels.

Turner, Byran
1984 *The Body and Society: Explorations in Social Theory.* New York: Basil Blackwell.
1991 "Recent Developments in the Theory of the Body." In *The Body: Social Process and Cultural Theory,* 1–35. Mike Featherstone, Mike Hepworth, and Bryan Turner, eds. London: Sage Publications.

Turner, Terence
1980 "The Social Skin." In *Not Work Alone: A Cross-cultural View of Activities Superfluous to Survial,* 112–140. Jeremy Cherfas and Roger Lewin, eds. London: Temple Smith.

Turner, Victor
1970 *Forest of Symbols.* Ithaca: Cornell University Press.Tyrell, Barbara and Peter Jurgens
1983 *African Heritage.* Johannesburg: MacMillan.

Vansina, Jan
1955 "Initiation Rituals of the Bushoong." Africa 25:138–153.
1964 *Le royaume Kuba.* Ser. in 8, 49. M.R.A.C.: Tervuren.
1978 *The Children of Woot: A History of the Kuba Peoples.* Madison: University of Wisconsin Press.
1990 *Paths in the Rainforest.* Madison: University of Wisconsin Press.

Verner, Samuel P.
1903 *Pioneering in Central Africa.* Richmond, Virginia: Presbyterian Committee of Publication.

Vogel, Susan
1991 *Africa Explores: 20th Century African Art.* New York and Munich: The Center for African Art and Prestel-Verlag.

Voll, John Obert
1978 *Historical Dictionary of the Sudan* 17. Metuchen, New Jersey: Scarecrow Press.

Wass, Betty M.
1975 Yoruba Dress: A Systemic Case Study of Five Generations of a Lagos Family. Ph.D. dissertation, Michigan State University, East Lansing.

Webb, Virginia-Lee
1992 "Fact and Fiction: Nineteenth-Century Photographs of the Zulu." *African Arts* 25(1):50–59, 98–99.

Wilson, M. and Thompson
1969 *Oxford History of South Africa.* New York: Oxford University Press.

Yongolelo Tambwe ya Kasimba
1975 *Introduction a l'histoire des Lega. Problemes et methodes.* Brussels: Les cahiers du Cedaf.

Zahan, Dominque
1960 *Sociétés Initiation de Bambara, le Ntomo, le Komo.* The Hague: Mouton.

# UCLA FOWLER MUSEUM OF CULTURAL HISTORY

| | |
|---|---|
| **Christopher B. Donnan** | Director |
| **Doran H. Ross** | Deputy Director |
| **Donald H. McClelland** | Assistant Director |
| | |
| **Patricia B. Altman** | Curator Emeritus of Folk Art and Textiles |
| **Patricia Anawalt** | Director, Center for the Study of Regional Dress |
| **George Briggs** | Chief Security Supervisor |
| **Daniel R. Brauer** | Director of Publications |
| **Roger H. Colten** | Curator of Archaeology |
| **Clarissa M. Coyoca** | Accountant |
| **Kyrin Ealy** | Director of Development |
| **Cynthia D. Eckholm** | Associate Registrar |
| **Betsy R. Escandor** | Administrative Assistant |
| **Adana Gardner** | Administrative Assistant |
| **Roy W. Hamilton** | Curator of Southeast Asian and Oceanic Collections |
| **Jo A. Hill** | Conservator |
| **Sarah Jane Kennington** | Registrar |
| **Anthony A.G. Kluck** | Assistant Director of Publications |
| **Lori LaVelle** | Receptionist |
| **Victor Lozano, Jr.** | Exhibition Production |
| **David A. Mayo** | Exhibition Designer |
| **Owen F. Moore** | Collections Manager |
| **Denis J. Nervig** | Photographer |
| **Dina M. Ogle** | Accounting Assistant |
| **Betsy D. Quick** | Director of Education |
| **Christine Sellin** | Director of Public Relations |
| **Don Simmons** | Exhibition Production |
| **Barbara Sloan** | Assistant Director, Center for the Study of Regional Dress |
| **David Svenson** | Publications Processing Assistant |
| **Polly Svenson** | Museum Store Manager |
| **Fran Tabbush** | Associate Collections Manager |
| **Bobby Whitaker** | Director of Security |
| **Patrick White** | Exhibition Production |

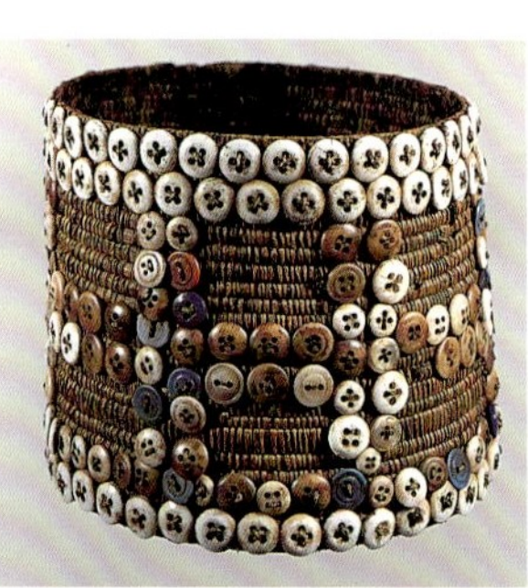

## PUBLICATION PRESENTATION

**Irina Averkieff**
Design and editing

**Daniel R. Brauer**
Publication Supervision

**Denis J. Nervig**
Photography

**Emily Meyer**
Research Assistant